Jones & Bartlett
Student Edition

Nursing Informatics

and the Foundation of Knowledge

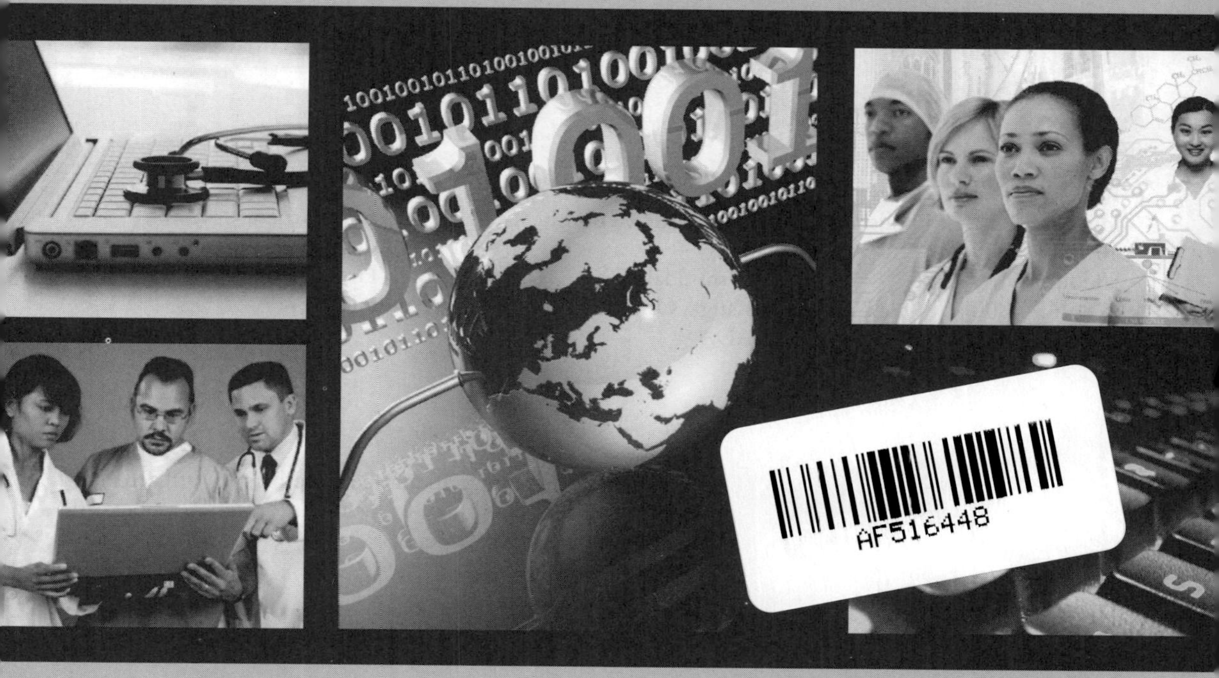

Dee McGonigle • Kathleen Mastrian

JONES AND BARTLETT
PUBLISHERS

BOSTON TORONTO LONDON SINGAPORE NEW DELHI

World Headquarters
Jones and Bartlett Publishers
40 Tall Pine Drive
Sudbury, MA 01776
978-443-5000
info@jbpub.com
www.jbpub.com

Jones and Bartlett Publishers
Canada
6339 Ormindale Way
Mississauga, Ontario L5V 1J2
CANADA

Jones and Bartlett
Publishers International
Barb House, Barb Mews
London W6 7PA
UK

First Indian Edition 2010

Jones and Bartlett India Pvt. Ltd.
4262/3, Ansari Road, Daryaganj
New Delhi – 110 002
Tel. 011–4361 3900
info@jbpubindia.net
www.jbpubindia.com

ISBN : 978-93-80108-48-3

Printed and bound in India by Sanat Printers, Kundli - 131 028, Sonepat, Haryana.

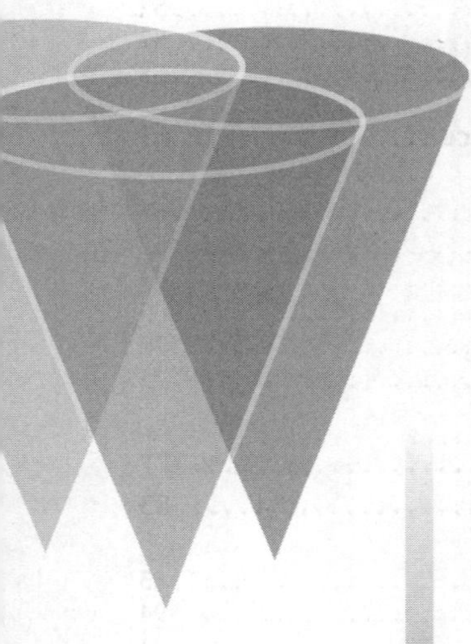

Contents

Preface

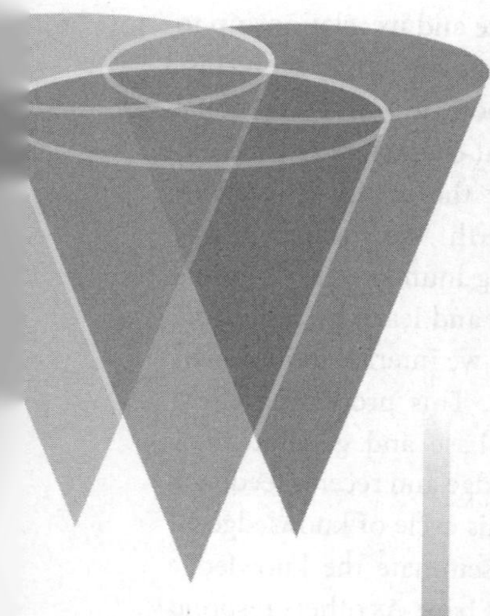

The idea for this book originated with the development of nursing informatics (NI) classes, the publication of articles related to technology-based education, and the creation of OJNI, the *Online Journal of Nursing Informatics,* of which Dee McGonigle is a founding editor. Like most nurse informaticists, we fell into the specialty; our love affair with technology and gadgets and our willingness to be the first to try new things helped to hook us into the informatics specialty. The rapid evolution of technology and its transformation of the ways of nursing prompted us to try to capture the essence of NI in a text.

We realized from the beginning that we could not possibly know all there is to know about informatics and how it supports nursing practice, education, administration, and research. We also knew that our faculty roles constrained the opportunities for exposure to changes in this rapidly evolving field. Therefore, we developed a tentative outline and a working model of the theoretical framework for the book and invited participation from informatics experts and specialists around the world. We were pleased with the enthusiastic responses we received from some of those invited contributors and a few volunteers who heard about the book and asked to participate in their particular area of expertise. Interestingly, one nonnurse suggested that we include a chapter in the education section on e-portfolios to showcase professional accomplishments, which we did! We believe that this book provides a comprehensive elucidation of this exciting field. You may notice that occasionally the contributing authors present similar information about a topic. This is especially true for Sections II and III of the book. We did not edit out those similarities because we believe that it is important to preserve the perspectives of our expert contributors, and similar presentations of materials will help to emphasize the importance of a particular topic.

The theoretical underpinning of the book is the Foundation of Knowledge model. The model is introduced in its entirety in Chapter 1, where we discuss nursing science and its relationship to NI. We believe that humans are organic information systems constantly acquiring, processing, and generating information or knowledge both in our professional and personal lives. It is our high degree of knowledge that characterizes us as extremely intelligent, organic machines. Individuals have the ability to manage knowledge. This ability is learned and honed from birth. We make our way through life interacting with our environment and being inundated with information and knowledge. We experience our environment and learn by acquiring, processing, generating, and disseminating knowledge. As we interact in our environment, we acquire knowledge that we must process. This processing effort causes us to redefine and restructure our knowledge base and generate new knowledge. We then share (disseminate) this new knowledge and receive feedback from others. The dissemination and feedback initiates this cycle of knowledge all over again since we acquire, process, generate, and disseminate the knowledge gained from sharing and reexploring our own knowledge base. As others respond to our knowledge dissemination and we acquire new knowledge, we engage in rethinking and reflecting on our knowledge, processing, generating, and then disseminating anew.

The purpose of this book is to provide a set of practical and powerful tools to help ensure that the reader will gain an understanding of NI and move from information through knowledge to wisdom. Defining demands of nurses and providing tools to help them survive and succeed in the Information Age remains a major challenge. Exposing nursing students and nurses to the principles and tools used in NI helps to prepare them to meet the challenge of practicing nursing in the Information Age while striving to improve patient care at all levels.

The text provides a comprehensive framework that embraces knowledge so that readers can develop their knowledge repositories and the wisdom necessary to act upon and apply that knowledge. The book is divided into five sections. Section I covers the building blocks of NI—nursing science, information science, computer science, cognitive science, and the human–technology interface. Section II provides readers with a look at various perspectives on NI and NI practice as described by experts in the field. Section III covers healthcare delivery applications and issues associated with the application of NI to nursing practice and nursing administration. Section IV presents subject matter on how informatics supports nursing education and nursing research. The future of NI and a summary of the relationship of informatics to the Foundation of Knowledge model are presented in Section V. The introductions to each section will explain the relationship between the content of that section and the Foundation of Knowledge model. The chapters within each section will provide practical application tips—

what you need to know in order to implement what you have learned—and the most important message that the author wants to leave with you.

This book places the material within the context of knowledge acquisition, processing, generation, and dissemination. It will serve both nursing students and professionals needing to understand, use, and evaluate NI knowledge. As nursing professors, our major responsibility is to prepare the practitioners and leaders in the field. Because NI permeates the entire scope of nursing—practice, administration, education, and research, nursing education curricula must include NI. Our primary objective was to develop the most comprehensive and user-friendly NI text on the market to prepare nurses for current and future practice challenges. In particular, this book provides a solid groundwork from which to integrate NI into practice, education, administration, and research.

Goals of this book are to:

1. impart core NI principles that should be familiar to every nurse and nursing student.
2. help the reader understand knowledge and how it is acquired, processed, generated, and disseminated.
3. explore the changing role of NI professionals.
4. demonstrate the value of the NI discipline as an attractive field of specialization.

These goals help nurses and nursing students understand and use fundamental NI principles so that they will efficiently and effectively function as current and future nursing professionals. The overall vision, framework, and pedagogy of this book offer benefits to the readers by highlighting established principles while drawing out new ones that continue to emerge as nursing and technology evolve.

Acknowledgments

We are deeply grateful to our contributors who provided this text with a richness and diversity of content that we could not have captured alone. We especially wish to acknowledge the superior work of Alicia Mastrian, graphic designer of the Foundation of Knowledge model which serves as the theoretical framework upon which the text is anchored. We could never have completed this project without the dedicated and patient efforts of the Jones and Bartlett staff, especially Emily Ekle and Carolyn Rogers. Both fielded our questions and concerns in a very professional and respectful manner.

Dee wishes to acknowledge the undying love, support, patience and continued encouragement of her best friend and husband, Craig, and her son, Craig, who has also made her so very proud. She would like to sincerely thank her mother Jennie, mother-in-law Ruth, aunt Rose, cousins Judi, John, Camille, Glenn, Mary Jane, and Sonny, and her dear friends for their support and encouragement, especially Renee, Nedra, Kate, and Hilde.

Finally, Kathy wishes to acknowledge the loving support of her family: husband Chip, children Ben and Alicia, sisters Carol and Sue, and parents Bob and Rosalie Garver. Kathy also wishes to acknowledge those friends who understand the importance of validation, especially Katie, Bobbie, Kathy, Anne, and Catherine.

Authors' Note

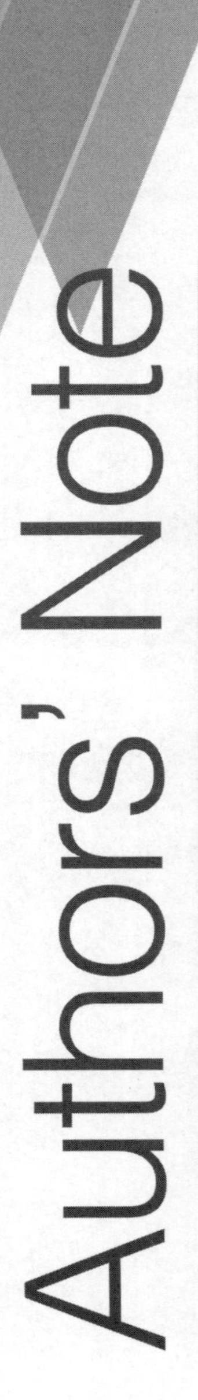

This text provides an overview of nursing informatics from the perspective of diverse experts in the field with a focus on nursing informatics and the foundation of knowledge. We want our readers and students to focus on the relationship of knowledge to informatics, a message all too often lost in the romance with technology. We hope you enjoy the text!

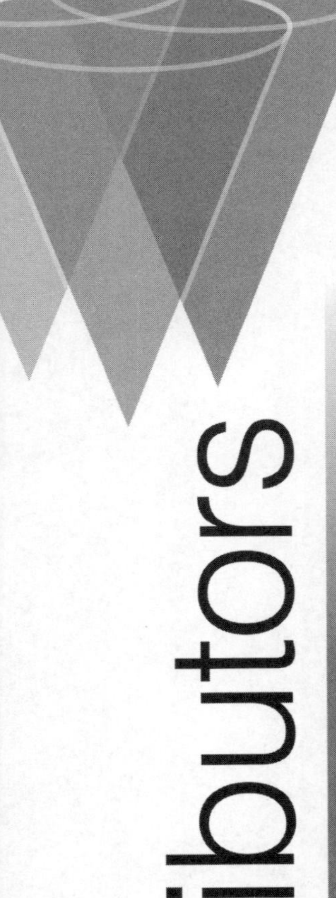

Contributors

Kathleen Albright, RN, BA
Honeywell HomMed

Ida Androwich, PhD, RN, BC, FAAN
Loyola University Chicago
School of Nursing
Maywood, IL

Emily Barey, RN, MSN
Director of Nursing Informatics
Epic Systems Corporation
Madison, WI

Lisa Reeves Bertin, BS, EMBA
Pennsylvania State University
Sharon, PA

Jennifer Bredemeyer, RN
Loyola University Chicago
School of Nursing
Skokie, IL

Sylvia M. DeSantis, MA
Pennsylvania State University
University Park, PA

Eric R. Doerfler, NP, PhD(c)
Pennsylvania State University
School of Nursing
Middletown, PA

Judith Effken, PhD, RN, FACMI
University of Arizona
College of Nursing
Tucson, AZ

William Scott Erdley, DNS, RN
University at Buffalo
State University of New York
School of Nursing
Buffalo, NY

Nedra Farcus, MSN, RN
Pennsylvania State University–Altoona
Altoona, PA

Nicholas Hardiker, RN, PhD
Senior Research Fellow
University of Salford
School of Nursing
Salford, England

Schuyler F. Hoss, BA
Northwest Healthcare Management
Vancouver, WA

Glenn Johnson, MLS
John A. Dutton e-Education Institute
Pennsylvania State University
University Park, PA

June Kaminski, RN, MSN
Kwantlen University College
Surrey, British Columbia, Canada

Julie Kenney, RNC, BSN
Loyola University Chicago
School of Nursing
Oak Lawn, IL

Audrey Kinsella, MA, MS
Information for Tomorrow
Telehealth Planning Services
Asheville, NC

Margaret Ross Kraft, PhD, RN
Loyola University Chicago
School of Nursing
Maywood, IL

Wendy L. Mahan, PhD, CRC, LPC
Pennsylvania State University
University Park, PA

Peter J. Murray, PhD, RN, FBCS
Founding Fellow
CHIRAD, UK
Nocton, England

Lynn M. Nagle, RN, PhD
Assistant Professor
University of Toronto
Toronto, Ontario, Canada

Ramona Nelson, PhD, BC-RN, FAAN, ANEF
Slippery Rock University
Slippery Rock, PA

Susan M. Paschke, MSN, RN–BC, CNA–BC
The Cleveland Clinic
Cleveland, OH

Sheldon Prial, RPH, BS Pharmacy
Sheldon Prial Consultance
Melbourne, FL

Jackie Ritzko
Pennsylvania State University
Hazelton, PA

Nancy Staggers, PhD, RN, FAAN
Associate Professor, Informatics
University of Utah
College of Nursing
Salt Lake City, UT

Patricia Sweeney, MS, CRNP, APRN, BC
Pennsylvania State University
Dunmore, PA

Denise D. Tyler, MSN/MBA, RN-BC
Clinical Specialist
Information Systems Services
Kaweah Delta Health Care District
Visalia, CA

Marianela Zytkowski, MS, BSN, RN-BC
The Cleveland Clinic
Cleveland, OH

The Building Blocks of Nursing Informatics

Nursing professionals are knowledge workers who are information dependent. As health care continues to evolve in an increasingly competitive information marketplace, professionals, the knowledge workers, must be well prepared to make significant contributions by harnessing appropriate, timely information. Nursing informatics (NI) is the product of the scientific synthesis of information in nursing because it uses concepts from computer science, cognitive science, information science, and nursing science. NI will continue to evolve as more and more professionals access, use, and develop the information, computer, and cognitive sciences necessary to advance nursing science for the dual betterment of our patients and our profession. Regardless of our future roles, it is clear that we need to understand computer, information, and cognitive sciences in order to be able to advance nursing science.

Nursing informatics implementation requires us to view nursing informatics from the perspective of our current healthcare delivery system and specific, individual organizational needs, while proactively anticipating and creating the future applications in both the healthcare system and our profession. We, as nursing professionals, should each be expected to discover opportunities to use nursing informatics, participate in the design of solutions, and be challenged to identify, develop, evaluate, modify, and enhance applications to improve patient care. This book is designed to provide you with the information and knowledge you need to meet this expectation.

Section I presents an overview of the building blocks of nursing informatics: nursing, information, computer, and cognitive sciences. Also included in this section is a chapter on improving the human–technology interface. This section will lay the foundation for the remainder of the book.

In Chapter 1, we describe nursing science and introduce the Foundation of Knowledge model as the conceptual framework for the book. In this chapter, we use a clinical case scenario to illustrate the concepts central to nursing science. We also derive a definition of nursing science from the American Nurses Association definition of nursing. Nursing science is the ethical application of knowledge acquired through education, research, and practice to provide services and interventions to patients in order to maintain, enhance, or restore their health, and to acquire, process, generate, and disseminate nursing knowledge to advance the nursing profession. Information is a central concept and health care's most valuable resource. Information science and systems, together with computers, are constantly changing the way healthcare organizations conduct their business. This will continue to evolve.

To prepare for these innovations, you need to understand fundamental information and computer concepts, covered in Chapters 2 and 3, respectively. Information science deals with the interchange (or flow) and scaffolding (or structure) of information and involves the application of information tools for solutions to patient care and business problems in healthcare. In order to be able to use and synthesize information effectively, we must be able to obtain, perceive, process, synthesize, comprehend, convey, and manage the information. Computer science deals with understanding the development, design, structure, and relationship of computer hardware and software. This science offers extremely valuable tools that, if used skillfully, can facilitate the acquisition and manipulation of data and information by nurses, who can then synthesize these into an ever-evolving knowledge and wisdom base. This can not only facilitate professional development and the ability to apply evidence-based practice decisions within nursing care, but if disseminated and shared, could advance the profession's knowledge base as well. The development of knowledge tools such as the automation of decision making and strides in artificial intelligence have altered the understanding of knowledge and its representation. The ability to structure knowledge electronically facilitates our ability to share our knowledge structures and enhance our collective knowledge.

Cognitive science, discussed in Chapter 4, deals with understanding how the mind functions. This science encompasses how people think, understand, remember, synthesize, and access stored information/knowledge. The nature of knowledge, how it is developed, used, modified, and shared provides the basis for our continued learning and intellectual growth.

Chapter 5, related to improving the human–technology interface, discusses the need to significantly improve quality and safety outcomes in this country. Through the use of information technology, we can radically improve the designs for human technology interfaces so that the technology better fits both human and task

FIGURE I-1
Foundation of Knowledge model. (Designed by Alicia Mastrian.)

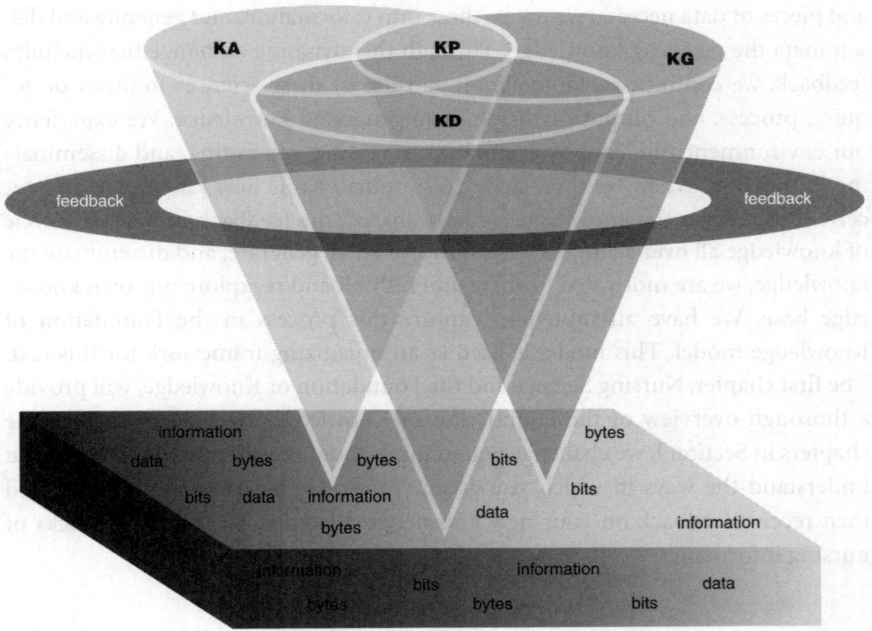

KA- Knowledge Acquisition
KD- Knowledge Dissemination
KG- Knowledge Generation
KP- Knowledge Processing

requirements. A number of useful tools are currently available for the analysis, design, and evaluation phases of development life cycles and should be used routinely by informatics professionals to ensure that technology better fits both task and user requirements. In this chapter, the author stresses that the focus on interface improvement using these tools has had a huge impact on patient safety in one area of health care—anesthesiology. With increased attention from informatics professionals and engineers, the same kinds of improvements should be possible in other areas. This human–technology interface is a crucial area if we are to implement the theories, architectures, and tools provided by the building block sciences.

The material within this book is placed within the context of the Foundation of Knowledge model (shown in Figure I-1 and periodically throughout the book, but more fully introduced and explained in Chapter 1). The Foundation of

Knowledge model is utilized throughout the text to illustrate how knowledge is used to meet healthcare delivery systems', organizations', patients', and nurses' needs. It is through our human–technology interfacing or interaction with these building blocks—the theories, architecture, and tools—that we acquire the bits and pieces of data necessary, process these into information, and generate and disseminate the resulting knowledge. Through this dynamic exchange that includes feedback, we continue our interaction and use of these sciences to input or acquire, process, and output or disseminate generated knowledge. We experience our environment and learn by acquiring, processing, generating, and disseminating knowledge. When we then share (disseminate) this new knowledge and receive feedback on the knowledge we have shared, the feedback initiates the cycle of knowledge all over again. As we acquire, process, generate, and disseminate the knowledge, we are motivated to share and rethink and reexplore our own knowledge base. We have attempted to capture this process in the Foundation of Knowledge model. This model is used as an organizing framework for this text. The first chapter, Nursing Science and the Foundation of Knowledge, will provide a thorough overview of the Foundation of Knowledge model. As you read the chapters in Section I, we challenge you to think about how the model can help you understand the ways in which you acquire, process, generate, disseminate, and then receive feedback on your new knowledge related to the building blocks of nursing informatics.

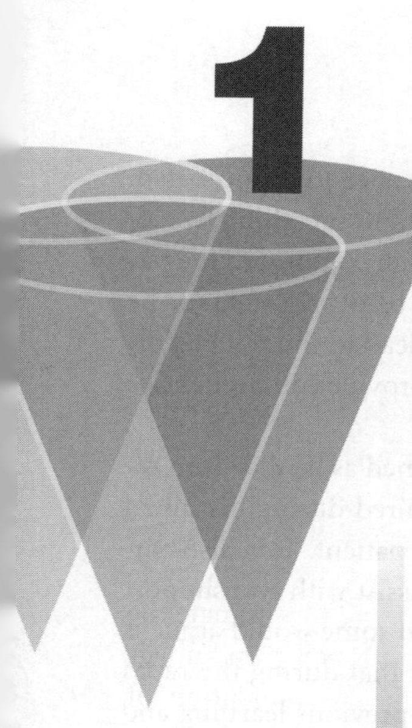

1 Nursing Science and the Foundation of Knowledge

Kathleen Mastrian and Dee McGonigle

Objectives

1. Define nursing science and its relationship to various nursing roles and nursing informatics.
2. Introduce the Foundation of Knowledge model as the organizing conceptual framework for the book.
3. Explain the relationship between knowledge acquisition, knowledge processing, knowledge generation, knowledge dissemination, and wisdom.

Key Terms

Borrowed theory
Building blocks
Clinical databases
Clinical practice guidelines
Conceptual framework
Data
Data mining
Evidence
Feedback
Foundation of Knowledge model
Information
Knowledge
Knowledge acquisition
Knowledge dissemination
Knowledge generation
Knowledge processing
Knowledge worker
Nursing informatics
Nursing science
Nursing theory
Relational database
Transparent

WISDOM

One of the most frequently quoted and widely accepted definitions of **nursing informatics** is that it is a combination of **nursing science**, information science, and computer science. In this chapter, we will focus on nursing science as one of the **building blocks** of nursing informatics, although in this text we extend the traditional definition of nursing informatics to include cognitive science as one of the building blocks. We will also introduce the **Foundation of Knowledge model** as the organizing **conceptual framework** of this text and tie the model to nursing science and the practice of nursing informatics. To lay the groundwork for this discussion, let's begin with a patient scenario.

Tom H. is a registered nurse who works in a very busy metropolitan hospital emergency room (ER). He has just admitted a 79-year-old male whose wife brought him to the hospital because he is having trouble breathing. Tom immediately clips a pulse oximeter to the patient's finger and performs a very quick assessment of the patient's other vital signs. He discovers a rapid pulse rate and a decreased oxygen saturation level in addition to the rapid and labored breathing. Tom determines that the patient is not in immediate danger and that he does not need to be intubated. Tom focuses his initial attention on easing the patient's labored breathing by elevating the head of the bed and initiating oxygen treatment; he then hooks the patient up to a heart monitor. Tom will continue to assess the breathing status as he performs a head-to-toe assessment of the patient that will lead to the nursing diagnoses and additional interventions that are necessary to provide comprehensive care to this patient.

Think about Tom's actions and how and why he intervened as he did. Tom relied on the immediate **data** and **information** that he acquired during his initial rapid assessment in order to deliver appropriate care to his patient. Tom also employed technology (pulse oximeter and heart monitor) to assist with and support the delivery of care. What is not immediately apparent, and some would argue is **transparent** (done without conscious thought), is the fact that during the rapid assessment, Tom was reaching into his knowledge base of previous learning and experiences to direct his care, so that he could act with wisdom. He used both **nursing theory** and **borrowed theory** to inform his practice. Tom certainly used nursing process theory, and he may have also used one of several other nursing theories such as Rogers's science of unitary human beings, Orem's theory of self-care deficit, or Roy's adaptation theory. In addition, Tom may also have applied his **knowledge** from some of the basic sciences like anatomy, physiology, psychology, and chemistry as he determined the patient's immediate needs. Information from Maslow's hierarchy of needs, Lazarus's transaction model of stress and coping and the health belief model may also have helped Tom practice professional nursing. He gathered data, then analyzed and interpreted that data to form a conclusion—the essence of science. In other words, Tom is illustrating the practice aspects of nursing science.

The American Nurses Association (2003) defines nursing in this way: "Nursing is the protection, promotion, and optimization of health and abilities, prevention of illness and injury, alleviation of suffering through the diagnosis and treatment of human response, and advocacy in the care of individuals, families, communities, and populations" (p. 6). Thus the focus of nursing is on the human responses to actual or potential health problems and advocacy for various clients. These human responses are varied and may change over time in a single case. Nurses must possess the technical skills to manage equipment and perform procedures; the interpersonal skills to interact appropriately with people; and the cognitive skills to observe, recognize, and collect data, analyze and interpret data, and reach a reasonable conclusion that forms the basis of a decision. At the heart of all of these skills lies the management of data and information. We are defining nursing science as the ethical application of knowledge acquired through education, research, and practice to provide services and interventions to patients in order to maintain, enhance, or restore their health and to acquire, process, generate, and disseminate nursing knowledge to advance the nursing profession.

Nursing is an information-intensive profession. The steps of utilizing information, applying knowledge to a problem, and acting with wisdom form the basis of nursing practice science. Let's examine the relationship between data and information and apply these ideas to our case scenario. Information is data that is processed using knowledge. In order for information to be valuable, it must be accessible, accurate, timely, complete, cost effective, flexible, reliable, relevant, simple, verifiable, and secure. Knowledge is the awareness and understanding of a set of information and ways that information can be made useful to support a specific task or arrive at a decision. In our case example, Tom utilized accessible, accurate, timely, relevant, and verifiable data and information. He compared that data and information to his knowledge base and previous experiences to determine which data and information were relevant to the current case. By applying previous knowledge to data, he converted data into information and information into new knowledge—understanding of what nursing interventions were appropriate in this case. Information, then, is data made functional through the application of knowledge.

We acquire data and information in bits and pieces and then transform the information into knowledge. The information-processing functions of the brain are frequently compared to those of a computer and vice versa. You will learn more about this comparison in Chapter 4, Introduction to Cognitive Science. Humans can be thought of as organic information systems constantly acquiring, processing, and generating information or knowledge both in our professional and personal lives. Individuals have an amazing ability to manage knowledge. This ability is learned and honed from birth. We make our way through life interacting with our environment and being inundated with data and information. We experience our environment and learn by acquiring, processing, generating, and disseminating knowledge. Tom acquired knowledge in his basic nursing education program and continues to build his foundation of knowledge by such activities as reading nursing research and theory articles, attending continuing education programs, consulting with expert colleagues, and utilizing **clinical databases** and **clinical practice guidelines**. As he interacts in the environment, he acquires knowledge that he must process. This processing effort causes him to redefine and restructure his knowledge base and generate new knowledge. He can then share (disseminate) this new knowledge with other colleagues, and he may receive **feedback** on the knowledge that he shares. The dissemination and feedback initiates the cycle of building the knowledge foundation all over again since he acquires, processes,

FIGURE 1-1
Foundation of Knowledge model. (Designed by Alicia Mastrian.)

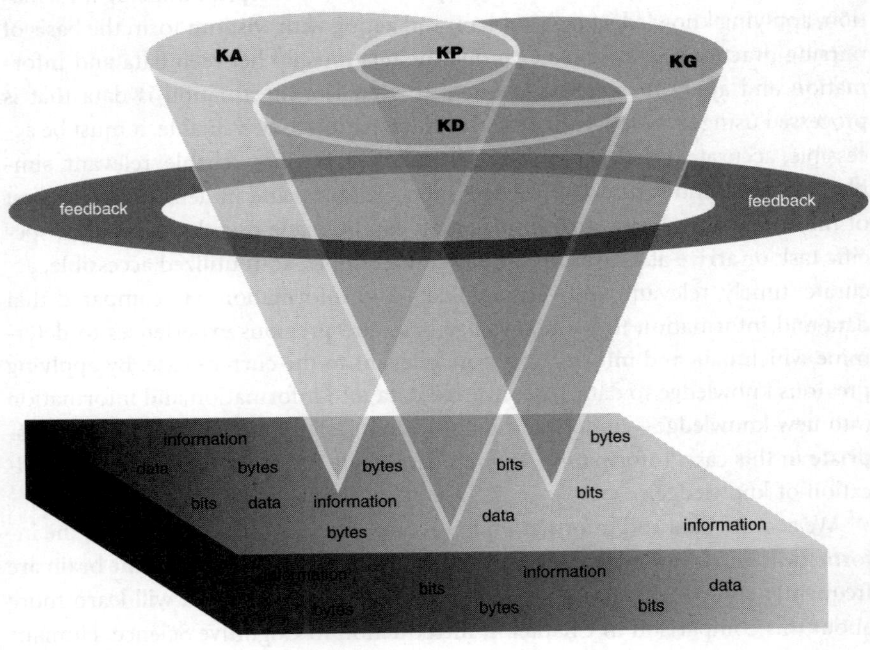

KA- Knowledge Acquisition
KD- Knowledge Dissemination
KG- Knowledge Generation
KP- Knowledge Processing

generates, and disseminates the new knowledge as a result of the interactions. As others respond to his **knowledge dissemination** and he acquires yet more knowledge, he is engaged to re-think about and reflect on and reexplore his **knowledge acquisition**, processing, generating, and then disseminating anew. We have attempted to capture this process in the Foundation of Knowledge model used as an organizing framework for this text.

At its base, the model has bits, bytes (computer terms for chunks of information), data, and information in a random representation. Growing out of the base are separate cones of light that expand as they reflect upward and represent knowledge acquisition, **knowledge generation**, and knowledge dissemination. At the intersection of the cones and forming a new cone is **knowledge processing**.

Encircling and cutting through the knowledge cones is feedback that acts on and may transform any or all aspects of knowledge represented by the cones. Now imagine the model as a dynamic figure with the cones of light and the feedback rotating and interacting rather than remaining static. In other words, knowledge acquisition, knowledge generation, knowledge dissemination, knowledge processing, and feedback are constantly evolving for us as nurse scientists. The transparent effect of the cones is deliberate and is intended to suggest that as knowledge grows and expands its use becomes more transparent—we use it without even being consciously aware of what aspect of knowledge we are using at any given moment during our practice.

If you are an experienced nurse, think back to when you were a novice. Did you feel like all you had in your head were bits of data and information that did not form any type of cohesive whole? As the model depicts, the processing of knowledge begins a bit later (imagine a time line applied vertically) with early experiences on the bottom and expertise growing as the processing of knowledge ensues. Early on in our education as nurses, we focus our conscious attention mainly on knowledge acquisition and depend on our instructors and others to process, generate, and disseminate knowledge. As we become more comfortable with the science of nursing, we begin to take over some of the other foundation of knowledge functions. However, in order to keep up with the explosion of information in nursing and health care, we must continue to rely on the knowledge generation of nursing theorists and researchers and the dissemination of their work. In this sense, we are committed to lifelong learning and the use of knowledge in the practice of nursing science.

This book uses the Foundation of Knowledge model, reflecting that knowledge is a powerful tool and for that reason, nurses focus on information as a key building block of knowledge. The application of the model will be described in each section of the book to help you understand and appreciate the foundation of knowledge in nursing science and how it applies to nursing informatics. All of the various nursing roles—practice, administration, education, research, informatics—involve the science of nursing. Nurses are **knowledge workers**, working with information and generating information and knowledge as a product. We are knowledge acquirers, providing convenient and efficient means of capturing and storing knowledge. We are knowledge users, individuals or groups who benefit from valuable, viable knowledge. Nurses are knowledge engineers, designing, developing, implementing, and maintaining knowledge. We are knowledge managers, capturing and processing collective expertise and distributing it where it can create the largest benefit. We are knowledge developers or generators, changing and evolving knowledge based on the tasks at hand and information available.

In our case scenario, at first glance, we might label Tom as a knowledge worker, a knowledge acquirer, and a knowledge user. However, if we stop here, we might be selling Tom short in his practice of nursing science. Yes, he *acquired* and used knowledge to help him achieve his work. He also *processed* the data and information he collected to develop a nursing diagnosis and a plan of care. We also need to recognize that the knowledge stores he used to develop and glean knowledge from valuable information is generative (having the ability to originate and produce or generate) in nature. For example, in our case scenario, Tom may have learned something new about his patient's culture from the patient or his wife that he will file away in the knowledge repository of his mind to be used in another similar situation. As he compares this new cultural information to what he already knows, he may gain insight into the effect of culture on a patient's response to illness. Thus Tom is a knowledge *generator*. If he shares this newly acquired knowledge with another practitioner, and as he records his observations and his conclusions, he is then *disseminating* knowledge. Tom is also using *feedback* from the various technologies he has employed to monitor his patient's status. He may also use feedback from lab reports or even other practitioners to help him rethink, revise, and apply the knowledge about this patient that he is generating.

Knowledge must also be viable. Knowledge viability refers to applications (most technology based) that offer easily accessible, accurate, and timely information obtained from a variety of resources and methods and presented in a manner so as to provide us with the necessary elements to generate new knowledge. In our case scenario, Tom may have felt the need to consult an electronic database or a clinical guidelines repository that he has downloaded on his PDA or that reside in the ER's networked computer system to assist him in the development of a comprehensive care plan for his patient. In this way, Tom is also using technology and **evidence** to support and inform his practice. It is also possible in this scenario that an alert may appear in the electronic health record or the clinical information system reminding Tom to ask about influenza and pneumonia vaccines, as many clinical information systems have such alerting functions. Clinical information technologies that support and inform nursing practice and nursing administration are an important part of nursing informatics and will be covered in detail in Section III of this text. Technologies that support and inform nursing education and nursing research will be covered in Section IV.

This book provides a framework that embraces knowledge so that the readers can develop the wisdom necessary to apply what they have learned. Wisdom is the application of knowledge to an appropriate situation. In the practice of nursing science, we expect action and/or actions directed by wisdom. Wisdom uses knowledge and experience to heighten common sense and insight to exercise sound judgment in practical matters. It is developed through knowledge, experience, insight, and reflection. Wisdom is sometimes thought of as the highest form of common sense resulting from accumulated knowledge or erudition (deep, thorough learning) or enlightenment (education that results in understanding and the dissemination of knowledge). Wisdom is the ability to apply valuable and viable knowledge, experience, understanding, and insight while being prudent and sensible. Knowledge and wisdom are not synonymous since knowledge abounds with others' thoughts and information while wisdom is focused on our own minds and the synthesis of our experience, insight, understanding, and knowledge. Some might call wisdom the foundation of the art of nursing.

As suggested earlier, some nursing roles might be viewed as more focused on certain aspects of the foundation of knowledge, rather than on other aspects. One might argue that nurse educators are primarily knowledge disseminators and nurse researchers are knowledge generators. While the more frequent output of their efforts can certainly be viewed in this way, it is important to realize that all nurses use all of the aspects of the Foundation of Knowledge model regardless of the area of practice. In order for nurse educators to be effective, they must be in the habit of constantly building and rebuilding their foundation of knowledge about nursing science. In addition, as they develop and implement curricular innovations, they must also evaluate the effectiveness of those changes. In some cases, they will utilize formal research techniques to do so and are therefore generating knowledge about the best and most effective teaching strategies. Similarly, nurse researchers must acquire and process new knowledge as they design and conduct their research studies. All nurses have the opportunity to be involved in the formal dissemination of knowledge via their participation in professional conferences either as presenters or attendees. In addition, some nurses will disseminate knowledge by formal publication of their ideas. In both cases, conference presentation and publication, nurses may receive feedback that stimulates rethinking about the knowledge they have generated and disseminated, thus prompting them to acquire and process anew.

All nurses, regardless of the practice arena, must use informatics and technology to inform and support that practice. In our case scenario, we discussed Tom's use of various monitoring devices that provide feedback on the physiological status of the patient. We also suggested that Tom might consult a clinical database or nursing practice guidelines residing on a PDA or a clinical agency network as he develops an appropriate plan of action for his nursing interventions. Perhaps the clinical information system (CIS) in the agency supports the collection of data about patients in a **relational database** that provides an opportunity for **data mining** by nursing administrators or nurse researchers. Thus, administrators and researchers can glean information about best practices and what improvements are necessary to deliver the best and most effective nursing care (Swan, Lang, & McGinley, 2004).

The future of nursing science and nursing informatics is intimately associated with the nursing education and nursing research arenas. Skiba (2007) suggests that we need techno-savvy and well-informed faculty who can demonstrate the appropriate use of technologies to enhance the delivery of nursing care. Along those lines, Greenfield (2007) conducted research among nursing students to determine the effectiveness of PDA technology applied to medication administration. Her study makes a good case for incorporating PDA technology into nursing curricula. Girard (2007) discussed cutting-edge operating room technologies such as nanosurgery using nanorobots, smart fabrics that aid in patient assessment during surgery, biopharmacy techniques for the safe and effective delivery of anesthesia, and virtual reality training. In the summary of her editorial, she makes an extremely provocative point about nursing education:

> Educators will need to expand their knowledge and teach for the future and not the past. They must take heed that the old tried-and true nursing education methods and curriculum that has lasted 100 years will have to change, and that change will be mandated for all areas of nursing … (p. 353)

Bassendowski (2007) specifically addresses the potential for the generation of knowledge in educational endeavors as faculty apply new technologies to teaching and the focus shifts away from individual to group instruction that promotes sharing and processing of knowledge.

Informatics and the use of technology in the practice of nursing are equally important in the nursing research arena. Participants in the development of the national nursing research agenda (NNRA) identified these two technology-related priorities (among other research priorities) for nursing research (NNRA, 2006, Chapter 2, p. 4):

- *Nursing Informatics: Enhancing Patient Care.* This area of research is designed to strengthen patient care. Priorities will be selected from research into the collection, organization, processing, and dissemination of information for clinical practice, including the design and development of databases, classification systems, computer models, and expert systems.

- *Technology Dependency Across the Life Span*: This research addresses technology used to support or replace lost function of body organs or systems when technology is an essential element in the treatment of chronic disease. Included are the study of individual and family responses, prevention of complications, bioethical issues, and demand for resources.

Goossen (2000) believes that the focus on nursing informatics research should be on the structuring and processing of patient information and how these inform nursing decision making in clinical practice. It is clear that the increasing use of technology to enhance nursing practice, nursing education, and nursing research will open new avenues for acquiring, processing, generating, and disseminating knowledge.

SUMMARY

In this chapter, we provided an overview of nursing science and how nursing science relates to typical nursing practice roles, nursing education, and nursing research. We also introduced the Foundation of Knowledge model as the organizing conceptual framework for this book. Finally, we introduced the relationship of nursing science to nursing informatics. In subsequent chapters, you will learn more about how nursing informatics supports nurses in their many and varied roles. **The most important thought we'd like to leave you with is** that nurses in the systematic application of nursing science are knowledge users, knowledge managers, knowledge developers, knowledge engineers, and knowledge workers.

THOUGHT-PROVOKING Questions

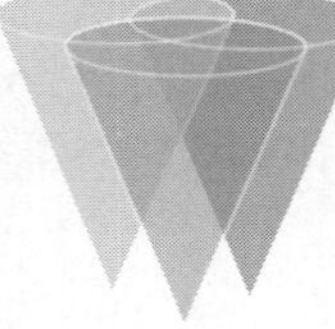

1. Imagine you are in a social situation and someone asks you, "What does a nurse do?" Think about how you will capture and convey the richness that is nursing science in your answer.
2. Choose a clinical scenario from your recent experience and analyze it using the Foundation of Knowledge model. How did you acquire knowledge? How did you process knowledge? How did you generate knowledge? How did you disseminate knowledge? How did you use feedback, and what was the effect of the feedback on the foundation of your knowledge?

References

American Nurses Association. (2003). *Nursing's social policy statement.* (2nd ed.). Silver Spring, MD: Author.

Bassendowski, S. (2007). NursingQuest: Supporting an analysis of nursing issues. *Journal of Nursing Education, 46*(2), 92–95. Retrieved January 27, 2008, from Education Module database [document ID: 1210832211].

Girard, N. (2007). Science fiction comes to the OR. Association of Operating Room Nurses. *AORN Journal, 86*(3), 351–353. Retrieved January 27, 2008, from Health Module database [document ID: 1333149261].

Goossen, W. (2000). Nursing informatics research. *Nurse Researcher, 8*(2), 42. Retrieved January 27, 2008, from ProQuest Nursing & Allied Health Source database [document ID: 67258628].

Greenfield, S. (2007). Medication error reduction and the use of PDA technology. *Journal of Nursing Education, 46*(3), 127–131. Retrieved January 27, 2008, from Education Module database [document ID: 1227347171].

Skiba, D. (2007). Faculty 2.0: Flipping the novice to expert continuum. *Nursing Education Perspectives, 28*(6), 342–344. Retrieved January 27, 2008, from ProQuest Nursing & Allied Health Source database [document ID: 1401240241].

Swan, B., Lang, N., & McGinley, A. (2004). Access to quality health care: Links between evidence, nursing language, and informatics. *Nursing Economics, 22*(6), 325–332. Retrieved January 27, 2008, from Health Module database [document ID: 768191851].

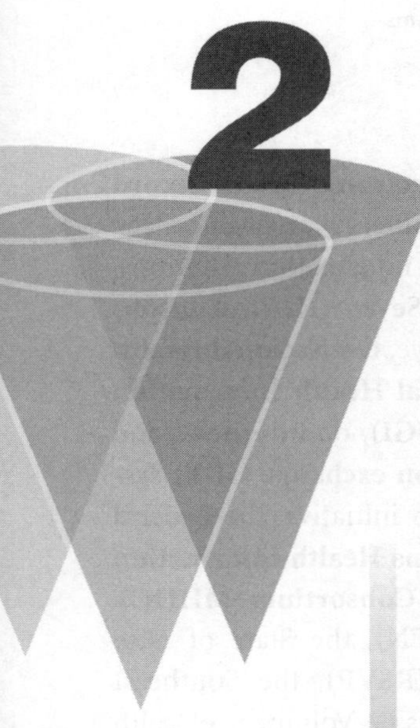

2 Introduction to Information, Information Science, and Information Systems

Dee McGonigle and Kathleen Mastrian

Objectives

1. Reflect on the progression from data to information to knowledge.
2. Describe the term *information.*
3. Assess how information is acquired.
4. Explore the characteristics of quality information.
5. Describe an information system.
6. Explore data acquisition or input and processing or retrieval, analysis, and synthesis of data.
7. Assess output or reports, documents, summaries alerts, and outcomes.
8. Describe information dissemination and feedback.
9. Define information science.
10. Assess how information is processed.
11. Explore how knowledge is generated in information science.

Key Terms

Acquisition
Alerts
Analysis
Chief information officers (CIO)
Chief technical officers (CTO)
Chief technology officers (CTO)
Cognitive science
Communication science
Computer-based information system (CBIS)
Computer science
Consolidated health informatics (CHI)
Data
Dissemination
Document
Electronic health record (EHR)
Federal Health Information Exchange (FHIE)
Feedback

INTRODUCTION

In this chapter, we will be exploring information, **information systems** (IS), and information science. The key word is information. As healthcare professionals, we are **knowledge workers**, and we deal with information on a daily basis. There are many concerns and issues that arise with healthcare information, such as ownership, access, disclosure, exchange, security, privacy, disposal,

Key Terms *Continued*
Health information exchange (HIE)
Health Level Seven (HL7)
Indiana Health Information Exchange (IHIE)
Information
Information science
Information system (IS)
Information technology (IT)
Infrastructure
Input
Interface
Internet2
Knowledge
Knowledge worker
Library science
Massachusetts Health Data Consortium (MHDC)
National Health Information Infrastructure (NHII)
National Health Information Network (NHIN)
New England Health EDI Network (NEHEN)
Next-Generation Internet (NGI)
Outcome
Output
Processing
Rapid Syndromic Validation Project (RSVP)
Report
Social sciences
Stakeholders
Summaries
Synthesis
Telecommunications

dissemination, etc. With the gauntlet of an **electronic health record (EHR)** being set, public and private sector **stakeholders** have been collaborating on a wide-ranging variety of healthcare information solutions. Some of these initiatives include **Health Level Seven (HL7)**, **Consolidated Health Informatics's (CHI's)** eGov initiative, the **National Health Information Infrastructure** (NHII), the **National Health Information Network (NHIN)**, **Next-Generation Internet** (NGI), or **Internet2**, and iHealth record. There are also **health information exchange (HIE)** systems such as Connecting for Health, the eHealth initiative, the **Federal Health Information Exchange** (FHIE), the **Indiana Health Information Exchange** (IHIE), the **Massachusetts Health Data Consortium** (MHDC), the **New England Health EDI Network** (NEHEN), the State of New Mexico **Rapid Syndromic Validation Project** (RSVP), the Southeast Michigan e-Prescribing Initiative, and the Tennessee Volunteer eHealth Initiative (Goldstein, Groen, Ponkshe, & Wine, 2007). It is quite evident from the brief listing above that there is need to remedy the healthcare information technology concerns, challenges, and issues that we face today. One of the main issues deals with how we manage healthcare information. It is important to understand how we obtain, manipulate, use, share, and dispose of information. This chapter will deal with the information piece of this complex puzzle.

INFORMATION

Suppose that someone tells you the number 99.5. What does that mean to you? It could be a radio station that you listen to or a score on a test. Now, if someone tells you that Ms. Howsunny's temperature is 99.5° Fahrenheit, what does that tell you? You know that 99.5 is a person's temperature. You processed **data** (99.5) to the information that 99.5° is a specific person's temperature. Data are raw facts. **Information** is processed data that has meaning. As healthcare professionals we are constantly **processing** data and information in order to provide the best care possible for our patients.

We will begin with data. There are many types of data that we must deal with such as alpha, numeric, audio, image, and video data. Alpha data refers to letters and numeric refers to numbers. Thus, alphanumeric data would include letters and numbers. This would include all text and the numeric **outputs** of digital monitors. Some of the alphanumeric data that we are concerned with is in the form of our patients' names, identification numbers, or medical record numbers. Audio data refers to sounds, noises, or tones. There are monitor **alerts** or alarms, taped or recorded messages, and other sounds. Image data would include graphics and pictures such as graphic monitor displays or recorded electrocardiograms, X-rays, MRIs, and CT scans, to name a few. Video data refers to animations, moving pictures, or moving graphics. You might review the ultrasound of your pregnant patient, examine a patient's echocardiogram, watch an animated video for professional development, or learn how to operate a new technology tool such as a pump or monitoring system.

The form does not matter. What matters is the integrity and quality of the data. Integrity refers to whole, complete, correct, and consistent data. Data integrity can be compromised through human error, viruses, worms, other bugs, hardware failures or crashes, transmission errors, and/or hackers entering the system. Information technologies can help to decrease these errors by putting safeguards in place such as backing up files on a routine basis, error detection for transmissions, and developing user **interfaces** that help people enter the data correctly. High quality data refers to data that are relevant and accurately represent their corresponding concepts. Data are dirty when there are errors in the database such as duplicate, incomplete, or outdated records. McGonigle found 50 cases of tongue cancer in one database she examined for data quality. When the records were tracked down and analyzed, and the dirty data were removed, there was only one case of tongue cancer. The same person had been entered erroneously 49 times. The major problem was with the patient's identification number and name. The numbers were changed or his name was misspelled repeatedly. If a researcher had just taken the number of cases in that defined population as 50, he would have concluded it was an epidemic, resulting in flawed information. Therefore, it is imperative that we have clean data if we want quality information. The data that we process into information must be of high quality and integrity to create meaning to inform our assessments and decision making.

Quality of information is necessary for it to be valuable. There are several characteristics of valuable, quality information such as accessibility, security, timeliness, accuracy, relevancy, completeness, flexibility, reliability, objectivity, utility, transparency, verifiability, and reproducibility. Accessibility is a must; the right user must be able to have the right information at the right time and in the right format to meet his/her needs. When we refer to the right user we mean an authorized user who has the right to obtain the data and information he/she is seeking. Security is a major challenge since we must block unauthorized users while providing open, easy access for the right user (see Chapter 12 in Section III). Timely information means that it is available when it is needed for the right purpose and at the right time. Knowing who won the lottery last week does not help you know if you won today. Accurate information means that there are no errors in the data and information. Relevant information is subjective in the fact that the user must have information that is relevant or applicable to her/his needs. If you are trying to decide whether or not your patient needs insulin and only the patient's CT scan information is available, this information would not be relevant for your current need. However, if you needed information about the CT scan, then the information would be relevant. Complete information contains all of the necessary essential data. If you need to contact the only relative listed for the patient and his or her contact information is listed but the approval for them to be a contact is missing, this information would be considered incomplete. Flexible information means that it can be used for a variety of purposes. Information concerning the inventory of supplies on a nursing unit can be used by the nurses who need to know if an item is available for use for a patient. The nurse manager would access this information to help him or her decide what supplies need to be ordered as well as determining what items are used often and to do an economic assessment of any waste. Reliable information comes from reliable or clean data and authoritative and credible sources. Objective information is as close to the truth as we can get. It is not subjective or biased but factual and impartial. If someone tells you something, you must determine if that person is reliable and if what she is telling you is objective or tainted by her perspective. Utility refers to the ability to provide the right information at the right time to the right person for the right purpose. Transparency allows users to apply their intellect to accomplish their tasks while the tools housing the information disappear. Verifiable information means that one can check to verify or prove that it is correct. Reproducibility refers to the ability to produce the information again. The value relates directly to how the information informs decision making.

The two ways that we acquire information are by either actively looking for it or having it conveyed to us by our environment. We use all of our senses (vision, hearing, touch, smell, and taste) to gather **input** from the world around us, and as technologies mature, we will have more and more input through more of our senses. Currently, we receive information from our computers (output), through our vision, hearing, or touch (input), and we respond (output), to the computer (input), and this is how we interface with technology. Many people access the Internet on a daily basis seeking information or imparting information. We are constantly becoming informed, discovering, or learning, becoming reinformed, rediscovering or relearning, and purging what we have acquired. The information we acquire is added to our knowledge base. **Knowledge** is the awareness and understanding of a set of information and ways that information can be made useful to support a specific task or arrive at a decision. This knowledge building is an ongoing process that we engage in while we are conscious and going about our normal daily activities.

INFORMATION SCIENCE

Information science has evolved over the last 50 or more years as a field of scientific inquiry and professional practice. **Information science** can be thought of as the science of information, studying the application and usage of information and knowledge in organizations and the interfacings or interaction between people, organizations, and information systems. It is an extensive, interdisciplinary science that integrates features from **cognitive science**, communication science, **computer science**, **library science**, and social sciences. Information science is primarily concerned with the input, processing, output, and feedback of data and information through technology integration with a focus on comprehending the perspective of the stakeholders involved and then applying information technology as needed. It is systemically based, dealing with the big picture rather than individual pieces of technology. Information science can be related to determinism. It is a response to technological determinism,

> the belief that technology develops by its own laws, that it realizes its own potential, limited only by the material resources available, and must therefore be regarded as an autonomous system controlling and ultimately permeating all other subsystems of society. (Web Dictionary of Cybernetics and Systems, 2007, ¶ 1)

This approach sets the tone for the study of information as it applies to itself, the people, the technology, and the varied sciences that are contextually related depending on the setting's or organization's needs; what is important is the interfacing of the stakeholders and their systems and how they generate, use, and locate information. According to Cornell University (2004), "Information Science brings together faculty, students and researchers who share an interest in combining computer science with the social sciences of how people and society interact with information" (¶ 1). Information science therefore is an interdisciplinary, people-oriented field that explores and enhances the interchange of information to transform society, communication science, computer science, cognitive science, library science, and social sciences. Our society is dominated by the need for information, and knowledge and information science focuses on systems as well as individual users fostering user-centered approaches that enhance society's information capabilities by effectively and efficiently linking people, information, and technology. This impacts the configuration and mix of organizations and influences the nature of work or how knowledge workers interact with and produce information and knowledge.

INFORMATION PROCESSING

According to O'Connor and Robertson (2005), "Shannon believed that information was no different than any other quantity and therefore could be manipulated by a machine" (¶ 13). Claude E. Shannon is considered the father of information theory (Horgan, 1990) and thought of information processing as the conversion of latent information into manifest information. Latent information is that which is not yet realized or apparent while manifest information is obvious or clearly apparent.

Information science enables the processing of information. This processing links people and technology. Humans are organic information systems, constantly acquiring, processing, and generating information or knowledge both in our professional and personal lives. It is our high degree of knowledge that characterizes us as extremely intelligent organic machines. The premise of this book revolves around this concept and is organized on the basis of the Foundation of Knowledge model: knowledge **acquisition**, knowledge processing, knowledge generation, and knowledge dissemination.

Information is data that is processed using knowledge. In order for information to be valuable, it must be accessible, accurate, timely, complete, cost effective, flexible, reliable, relevant, simple, verifiable, and secure. Knowledge is the awareness and understanding of a set of information and ways that information can be made useful to support a specific task or arrive at a decision. As an example, if you were going to design a building, part of the knowledge necessary for developing a new building is understanding how the building will be used, how large of a building is needed compared to the space available to build on, how many people will have or need access to this building, and so on. Therefore, the work of choosing or rejecting facts based on their significance or relevance to a particular task, such as designing a building, is also based on a type of knowledge used in the process of converting data into information. Information can then be considered data made functional through the application of knowledge. The knowledge used to develop and glean knowledge from valuable information is generative (having the ability to originate and produce or generate) in nature. Knowledge must be viable. Knowledge viability refers to applications that offer easily accessible, accurate, and timely information obtained from a variety of resources and methods and presented in a manner so as to provide us with the necessary elements to generate knowledge.

Information science and computational tools are extremely important in enabling the processing of data, information, and knowledge in health care. The hardware, software, networking, algorithms, and the human organic information system work together to create meaningful information and generate knowledge. The links between information processing and scientific discovery are paramount. However, without the ability to generate practical results that can be disseminated, the processing of data, information, and knowledge is for naught. It is the ability of the machines (inorganic information systems) to support and facilitate the functioning of people (human organic information systems) that refine, enhance, and evolve nursing practice by generating knowledge. This knowledge represents five rights: the *right information*, accessible by the *right people* in the *right settings*, applied the *right way* at the *right time*. It is also the struggle to integrate new knowledge and old knowledge to enhance wisdom. Wisdom is the ability to act; it assumes action and/or actions directed by one's own wisdom. Wisdom uses knowledge and experience to heighten common sense and insight to exercise sound judgment in practical matters. It is developed through knowledge, experience, insight, and reflection. Wisdom is sometimes thought of as the highest form of common sense resulting from accumulated knowledge or erudition (deep, thorough learning) or enlightenment (education that results in understanding and the dissemination of knowledge). It is the ability to apply valuable and viable knowledge, experience, understanding, and insight while being prudent and sensible. Knowledge and wisdom are not synonymous since knowledge abounds with others' thoughts and information while wisdom is focused on our own minds and the **synthesis** of our experience, insight, understanding, and knowledge. If clinicians are inundated with data without the ability to process it, the situation results in too much data and too little wisdom. That is why it is crucial that clinicians have viable information systems at their fingertips to facilitate the acquisition, sharing, and utilization of knowledge while maturing wisdom; it is a process of empowerment.

INFORMATION SCIENCE AND THE FOUNDATION OF KNOWLEDGE

Information science is a multidisciplinary science that involves aspects from computer science, cognitive science, social science, communication science, and library science to deal with obtaining, gathering, organizing, manipulating, managing, storing, retrieving, recapturing, disposing of, distributing, or broadcasting information. Information science studies everything that deals with information and can be defined as the study of information systems. This science originated as a subdiscipline of computer science, in an attempt to understand and rationalize the management of technology within organizations. It has matured into a major field of management that is increasingly being emphasized as an important area of research in management studies and has expanded to examine the human–computer interaction, interfacing, and interaction of people, information systems, and corporations. It is taught at all major universities and business schools around the world. Organizations have become intensely aware of the fact that information and knowledge are potent resources that must be cultivated and honed to meet their needs. Thus, information science or the study of information systems, the application and usage of knowledge, focuses on why and how technology can be put to best use to serve the information flow within the organization.

Information science impacts information interfacing, influencing how we interact with information and subsequently develop and use knowledge. The information we acquire is added to our knowledge base. Knowledge is the awareness and understanding of a set of information and ways that information can be made useful to support a specific task or arrive at a decision.

Healthcare organizations have been profoundly affected by and rely on the evolution of information science to enhance the recording and processing of routine and intimate information while facilitating human-to-human and human-to-systems communications, delivery of healthcare products, dissemination of information, and enhancing the organization's business transactions. The benefits and enhancements of information science technologies have also brought risks such as glitches and loss of information and hackers who can steal identities and information. This makes the importance of solid leadership, guidance, and vision vital for the maintenance of cost-effective business performance and cutting-edge, safe information technologies for the organization. This field studies all facets of information building and use. The emergence of information science and its impact on information has also influenced how we acquire and use knowledge.

One thing we would like to leave you with is that information science has had a tremendous impact on society and will expand its sphere of influence as it continues to evolve and innovate human activities at all levels, especially the nature of our work. What visionaries only dreamed of is now possible and part of our reality. The future has yet to unfold in this important arena.

INTRODUCTION TO INFORMATION SYSTEMS

Consider the following scenario. You have just been hired by a large healthcare facility. You enter the personnel office and are told that you will have to learn a new language in order to work on the unit where you have been assigned. This language is just used on this unit. If you had been assigned to a different unit, you would have to learn another language that is specific to that unit, and so on. Therefore, interdepartmental sharing and information exchange (known as interoperability) is severely hindered. This is how we used to operate in health care—in silos. We had a system for the lab, one for finance, one for clinical departments, and so on. Learning the importance of communication, tracking, and research, we now have integrated information systems that handle the needs of the entire organization.

Information and **information technology** have become major resources for organizations, and health care is no exception. Information technologies help to shape the healthcare organization, in conjunction with the personnel or people, money, materials, and equipment. Many healthcare facilities have hired **chief information officers (CIOs)** or **chief technical officers (CTOs)**, also known as **chief technology officers (CTOs).** The CIO is involved with the information technology **infrastructure** and this role is sometimes expanded to chief knowledge officer. The CTO is focused on organizationally based scientific and technical issues and is responsible for technological research and development as part of the organization's products and services. The CTO and CIO must be visionary leaders for the organization, since so much of the business of health care relies on solid infrastructures that generate potent and timely information and knowledge. The CTO and CIO are sometimes interchangeable positions. However, in some organizations, the CTO reports to the CIO. These positions will become paramount as companies continue to shift from being product oriented to knowledge oriented and as they begin emphasizing the production process itself rather than the product. In healthcare, information systems must be able to handle the volume of data and information necessary to generate the needed information and knowledge for best practices, the basis of our actions, since our goal is to provide the highest quality of patient care.

Information Systems

Information systems (ISs) can be manually based, but for the purposes of this text, the term refers to **computer-based information systems (CBISs)**. According to Jessup and Valacich (2008), computer-based information systems "are combinations of hardware, software and **telecommunications** networks that people build and use to collect, create, and distribute useful data, typically in organizational settings" (p. 10). Along those same lines, information systems are also defined as "A set of interrelated components that collect, manipulate, store and disseminate data and information and provide a feedback mechanism to meet an objective" (Stair & Reynolds, 2008, p. 4). ISs are designed for specific purposes within organizations. They are only as functional as the decision making, problem-solving skills, and programming potency built in and the quality of data and information inputted. The IS's capability to disseminate, provide feedback, and adjust the data and information based on these dynamic processes are what sets them apart. The IS should be a user-friendly entity that provides the right information at the right time and in the right place.

As defined previously, an IS acquires data or inputs; processes data that consists of the retrieval, **analysis**, and/or synthesis of data; disseminates or outputs in the form of **reports, documents, summaries**, alerts, and/or **outcomes**; and provides for responses or feedback. Input or data acquisition is the activity of collecting and acquiring raw data. Input devices are combinations of hardware, software, and telecommunications and include keyboards, light pens, touch screens, mice or other pointing devices, automatic scanners, and machines that can read magnetic ink characters or lettering. In receiving a pay-per-view movie, the viewer must input the chosen movie, verify the purchase, and have a payment method approved by the vendor. The IS must acquire this information before one can receive the movie.

Processing, the retrieval, analysis, and/or synthesis of data, refers to the alteration and transformation of the data into helpful or useful information and outputs. The processing of data can range from storing it for future use to comparing the data, making calculations, or applying formulas, to taking selective actions. Processing devices are combinations of hardware, software, and telecommunications and include processing chips where the central processing unit (CPU) and main memory are housed. According to Schupak (2005), there is a bunny chip that could save the pharmaceutical industry money while sparing "Millions of furry creatures, with a chip that mimics a living organism" (¶ 1). The HμREL Corporation has a chip to mimic the human body.

> A patented HμREL microfluidic circuit comprises an arrangement of separate but fluidically interconnected "organ" or "tissue" compartments. Each compartment contains a culture of living cells drawn from, or engineered to mimic the primary function(s) of, the respective organ or tissue of a living animal. Microfluidic channels between the compartments permit a culture medium that serves as a "blood surrogate" to re-circulate as in a living system. Drug candidates of interest are added to the culture medium and allowed to re-circulate through the device; they then distribute to and interact with the cells in the organ compartments much as they would in the human body. The effects of drug compounds and their metabolites on the cells within each respective organ compartment are detected by measuring or monitoring key physiological events. The cell types employed may be adherent or non-adherent, and derived from either standard cell culture lines or primary tissue. (HμREL Corporation, 2005, ¶ 1)

As these new technologies continue to evolve, we will see more and more robust ISs that can handle a variety of biological and clinical applications.

In the movie rental example, the IS must verify the data entered and then process the request by following the steps necessary to provide access to the movie that was ordered. This processing must be instantaneous in our world where everyone wants it now! After the data is processed, it is stored. In this case, the rental must also be processed so the vendor receives payment for the movie, whether electronically, via a credit card or checking account withdrawal, or by generating a bill for payment.

Output or **dissemination** produces helpful or useful information that can be in the form of reports, documents, summaries, alerts, or outcomes. Reports are designed to inform and are generally tailored to the context of a given situation and/or user or user group. Reports may include charts, figures, tables, graphics, pictures, hyperlinks, references, or other documentation necessary to meet the needs of the user. Documents represent information that can be printed, saved, e-mailed or shared, or displayed. Summaries are condensed versions of the original designed to highlight the major points. Alerts are warnings, feedback, or additional information necessary to assist the user in interacting with the system. Outcomes are the expected results of input and processing. Output devices are combinations of hardware, software, and telecommunications and include sound and speech synthesis outputs, printers, and monitors. Continuing with the movie rental example, the IS must be able to provide the consumer with the movie he ordered when he wants it and somehow notify him that he has indeed purchased the movie and is granted access. The IS must also be able to generate payment either electronically or by generating a bill, and storing the transactional record for future use.

Feedback or responses are reactions to the inputting, processing, and outputs. In ISs, feedback refers to information from the system that is used to make modifications in the input, processing actions, or outputs. In our movie rental example, what if the consumer accidentally entered the same movie order three times and only wanted to order the movie once? The IS would determine that more than one movie order is out of range for the same movie order at the same time and provide feedback. The feedback is used to verify and correct the input. If undetected, this error would result in an erroneous bill and decreased customer satisfaction while creating more work for the vendor who would have to deal with the customer to resolve this problem. Section III of this book provides detailed descriptions of clinical information systems that operate on these same principles to support healthcare delivery.

SUMMARY

Information systems deal with the development, use, and management of an organization's IT infrastructure. An IS acquires data or inputs; processes data that consists of the retrieval, analysis, and/or synthesis of data; disseminates or outputs in the form of reports, documents, summaries, alerts, and/or outcomes; and provides for responses or feedback. Quality decision-making and problem-solving skills are vital to the development of effective, valuable ISs. Organizations are recognizing that their most precious asset is their information, represented in their employees, experience, competence or know-how, and innovative or novel approaches, all of which are dependent on a robust information network that encompasses the information technology infrastructure.

One thing we would like to leave you with is the importance of continuing to develop and refine functional, robust, visionary ISs that meet the current information needs while being able to evolve to handle the future information and knowledge needs of our healthcare industry.

THOUGHT-PROVOKING Questions

1. How do you acquire information? Choose 2 hours out of your busy day and try to take note of all of the information that you receive from your environment. Keep a diary denoting where the information came from and how you knew it was information and not data.
2. Reflect on an information system that you are familiar with such as the automatic banking machine. How does this IS function? What are the advantages of using this system; i.e., why not use a bank teller instead? What are the disadvantages? Are there enhancements that you would add to this system?
3. In health care, think about a typical day of practice and describe the setting. How many times does the nurse interact with ISs? What are the ISs that we interact with, and how do we access them? Are they at the bedside, handheld or station based? How does their location and ease of access impact nursing care?
4. Briefly describe an organization and discuss how our need for information and knowledge impacts the configuration and mix of that organization with other organizations. Also discuss how the need for information and knowledge influences the nature of work or how knowledge workers interact with and produce information and knowledge in this organization.
5. If you could only meet four of the rights discussed in this chapter, which one would you omit and why? Also, provide your rationale for each right you chose to meet.

References

Cornell University. (2004). *Information science.* Retrieved October 21, 2007, from http://www.infosci.cornell.edu

Goldstein, D., Groen, P., Ponkshe, S., & Wine, M. (2007). *Medical informatics 20/20.* Sudbury, MA: Jones and Bartlett.

Horgan, J. (1990). *Claude E. Shannon: Unicyclist, juggler and father of information theory.* Retrieved March 11, 2008, from http://www.ecs.umass.edu/ece/hill/ece221.dir/shannon.html

HμREL Corporation. (2005). *Technology.* Retrieved October 22, 2007, from http://www.hurelcorp.com/technology.html

Jessup, L., & Valacich, J. (2008). *Information systems today* (3rd ed.). Upper Saddle River, NJ: Pearson Prentice Hall.

O'Connor, J., & Robertson, E. (2005). *Claude Elwood Shannon.* Retrieved October 29, 2007, from http://www.thocp.net/biographies/shannon_claude.htm

Schupak, A. (2005). *Technology: The bunny chip.* Retrieved October 23, 2007, from http://members.forbes.com/forbes/2005/0815/053.html

Stair, R., & Reynolds, G. (2008). *Principles of information systems* (8th ed.). Boston, MA: Thompson Course Technology.

Web Dictionary of Cybernetics and Systems. (2007). *Technological determinism.* Retrieved October 23, 2007, from http://pespmc1.vub.ac.be/asc/TECHNO_DETER.html

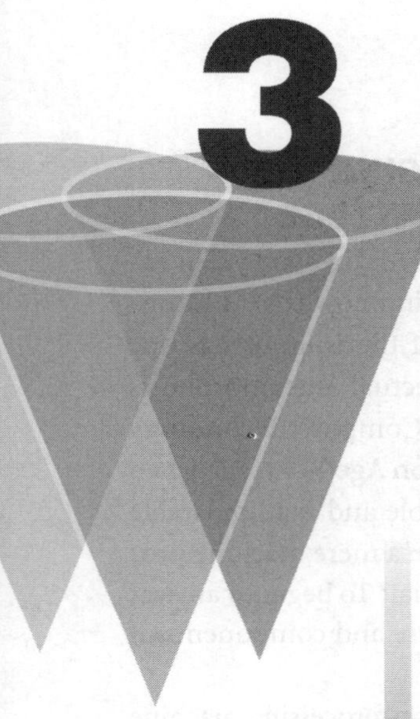

3 Computer Science and the Foundation of Knowedge Model

June Kaminski

Objectives

1. Describe the essential components of computer systems including hardware and software.
2. Appreciate the rapid evolution of computer systems and the benefit of keeping up to date with current trends and developments.
3. Analyze how computer systems function as tools for managing information and generating knowledge.
4. Define the concept of human–technology interfaces.
5. Articulate how computers can support collaboration and information exchange.

Key Terms

Acquisition
Applications
Arithmetic logic unit (ALU)
Binary system
Basic input/output system (BIOS)
Bit
Bus
Byte
Cache memory
Central processing unit (CPU)
Communication software
Compact disc read-only memory (CD-ROM)
Compact disc-recordable (CD-R)
Compact disc-rewritable (CD-RW)
Compatibility
Computer
Computer science
Conferencing software
Creativity software
Databases
Degradation

INTRODUCTION

In this chapter, the discipline of **computer science** is introduced through a focus on computers and the hardware and software that make up these evolving systems. Computer science offers extremely valuable tools that, if used skillfully, can facilitate the **acquisition** and manipulation of data and **information** by nurses, who can then synthesize these into an ever-evolving **knowledge** and wisdom base. This can not only facilitate **professional development** and the ability to apply evidence-based practice decisions within nursing care, but if disseminated and shared, could advance the profession's knowledge base as well. This chapter begins with a look at common computer hardware, followed by a brief overview of operating, productivity, creativity, and communication software. The chapter concludes with a glimpse at how computer systems help to shape knowledge and collaboration and support human–technology interface dynamics.

Key Terms *Continued*
Desktop
Digital video disc (DVD)
Digital video disc-recordable (DVD-R)
Digital video disk-rewritable (DVD-RW)
Dissemination
Dynamic random access memory (DRAM)
Electronically erasable programmable read-only memory (EEPROM)
E-mail
E-mail client
Erasable programmable read-only memory (EPROM)
Exabyte (EB)
Execute
Extensibility
FireWire
Firmware
Flash memory
Gigabyte (GB)
Gigahertz (GHz)
Graphical user interface (GUI)
Graphics card
Hard disk
Hardware
Information
Information Age
Input/output system (I/O)
Instant message (IM)
Integrated drive electronics (IDE)
Internet browser
Keyboard
Knowledge
Laptop
Mainframes
Main memory
Megabyte (MB)
Megahertz (MHz)
Memory

THE COMPUTER AS A TOOL FOR MANAGING INFORMATION AND GENERATING KNOWLEDGE

Throughout history, various milestones have signaled discoveries, inventions, or philosophical shifts that spurred a surge in knowledge and understanding within the human race. The advent of the computer is one such milestone, one that has sparked an intellectual metamorphosis whose boundaries have yet to be fully understood. Computer **technology** has ushered in what has been called the "**Information Age**"—an age when data, information, and knowledge are both accessible and manipulatable by more people than ever before in history. How can a mere machine provide such a revolutionary state of knowledge potential? To begin to answer this question, it is best to examine the basic structure and components of computer systems.

Essentially, a computer is an electronic information-processing machine that serves as a tool to manipulate data and information. These unique machines accept data inputted via a variety of devices, process data through logical and arithematic rendering, store the data in memory components, and output data and information to the user.

Since the advent of the first electronic computer in the mid-1940s, computers have evolved to become essential tools in every walk of life, including the profession of nursing. The complexity of today's computers has skyrocketed and will continue to do so. "For many applications, the highest-performance microprocessors of today outperform the **supercomputer** of less than 10 years ago" (Hennessy & Patterson, 2006, p. 2). Major computer manufacturers and researchers such as Intel have identified the need to design computers to mask this growing complexity. This is done by honing hardware and software capabilities until they work seamlessly together to ensure **user-friendly**, intuitive tools for users of all levels of expertise.

According to Intel Corporation's technology research team, the goal is "technology that just works" (Intel, 2008, ¶ 1). To conceal complexity, Intel research is looking at a number of solutions, by:

- Relating user mental models with complex systems and technology to improve the use and adaptation of systems across devices and contexts.
- Enabling devices to explore their environment to discover other devices and capabilities, and then form integrated teams that self-organize for higher functionality and performance.
- Better control of failure modes, graceful **degradation** and self-healing across ensembles of devices.

Key Terms *Continued*
Microprocessor
Modem
Monitor
Motherboard
Mouse
MPEG-1 Audio Layer-3 (MP3)
Nonsynchronous
Office suite
Open source software
Operating system (OS) software
Palm computers
Parallel port
Peripheral component interconnection (PCI)
Personal computer (PC)
Personal digital assistants (PDAs)
Plug and play
Port
Portability
Portable operating system interface for UNIX (POSIX)
Presentation
Processing
Productivity software
Professional development
Programmable read-only memory (PROM)
Publishing
QWERTY
Random-access memory (RAM)
Read-only memory (ROM)
Security
Serial port
Small computer system interface (SCSI)
Software
Sound card
Spreadsheet
Supercomputers
Synchronous

- Zero-knowledge applications and interoperation. (Intel Corporation, 2008, ¶ 2).

Computers are universal machines, since they are general-purpose, symbol-manipulating devices that can perform any task represented in specific programs. For instance, they can be used to draw an image, calculate statistics, write an essay, or record nursing care data. In a nutshell, computers can be used for data and information storage, retrieval, analysis, generation, and transformation.

Most computers are based on scientist John Von Neumann's model of a processor-memory-input-output architecture. The logic unit and control unit are parts of the processor, the **memory** is the storage region, and the input and output segments are provided by the various computer devices such as the keyboard, mouse, monitor, and so on. Recent developments show promise in modified or alternative configurations to the Von Neumann model, particularly the parallel computing model where multiple processors are set up to work together.

Components

Hardware

Computer **hardware** refers to the actual physical body of the computer and its components. There are several key components in the average computer that work together to shape a complex yet highly usable machine that serves as a tool for knowledge management, communication, and creativity.

Outer Protection: The Casing » The most noticeable component of any computer is the outer case. Desktop **personal computers (PCs)** have either a **desktop** case that lies flat, horizontally on a desk, often with the computer monitor positioned on top of it, or a tower case that stands vertically and usually sits beside the monitor or on a lower shelf or the floor. Most cases come equipped with a case fan, which is extremely critical for keeping the computer components cool when in use. **Laptop**

Key Terms *Continued*
Synchronous dynamic random-access memory (SDRAM)
Technology
Terabyte (TB)
Throughput
Touch screen
Universal serial bus (USB)
User friendly
User interface
Video adapter card
Virtual memory
Wisdom
Word processing
World Wide Web (WWW)
Yottabyte (YB)
Zettabyte (ZB)

computers combine the casing in a flat rectangular casing that is attached to the hinged liquid crystal display (LCD) monitor. **Palm computers** and **personal digital assistants (PDAs)** also have a protective outer plastic and metal case with an embedded LCD screen.

Central Processing Unit » Sometimes conceptualized as the "brain" of the computer, the **central processing unit (CPU)** is the computer component that actually **executes**, calculates, and processes the binary computer code (comprised of various configurations of zeros and ones) instigated by the operating system and other applications on the computer. It serves as the command center that directs the actions of all other computer components and manages both incoming and outgoing data that is processed across components. Common CPUs include the Pentium, K6, PowerPC and Sparc models.

The CPU contains specific mechanical units, including registers, **arithmetic logic units (ALUs)**, a floating point unit (FPU), control circuitry, and cache memory. Together, these inner components form the computer's central processor. Registers consist of data-storing circuits that are processed by the adjacent ALUs or the FPU. **Cache memory** is extremely quick memory that holds whatever data and code is being used at any one time. The CPU uses the cache to store in-process data so that it is quickly retrieved as needed. Also, the CPU is protected by a heat sink, a copper or aluminum metal block that cools the processor (often with the help of a fan) to prevent overheating.

The speed and power of a CPU used to be measured in **megahertz** and was written as a value in MHz, e.g., 400 MHz (meaning the microprocessor ran at 400 MHz, executing 400 million cycles per second). Now it is more common to see the speed measured in gigahertz (1 **gigahertz** or GHz is equal to 1,000 megahertz), thus a CPU that operates at 4 GHz is a thousand times faster than one set at 4 MHz. The more cycles a processor can engage in per second, the faster computer programs can run.

In recent years, processor manufacturers such as Intel have moved to multicore **microprocessors**, which are chips that combine two or more processors (Hennessy & Patterson, 2006). In fact, multiple microprocessors have replaced many formerly popular computer types.

> Minicomputers, which were traditionally made from off-the-shelf logic or from gate arrays, have been replaced by servers made using microprocessors. **Mainframes** [bold added] have been almost replaced with multiprocessors consisting of small numbers of off-the-shelf microprocessors. Even high-end supercomputers are being built with collections of microprocessors. (Hennessy & Patterson, 2006, p. 3)

Motherboard » The **motherboard** has been called the central nervous system of the computer and is a key foundational component since all other components are connected to it in some way (either via local sockets, attached directly to it, or connected via cables). The essential structures of the motherboard include the major chip set, super input/output (I/O) chip, basic input/output system (BIOS), read-only memory (ROM), **bus** communications pathways, and a variety of sockets that allow components to plug into it. The chip set (often a pair of chips), determines the computer's CPU type and memory. It also houses the north bridge and south bridge controllers that allow the buses to transfer data from one to another.

Power Supply » The power supply is a critical component of any computer, since it provides the essential electrical energy needed to allow a computer to operate. The power supply unit converts the 240-volt alternating current (AC) main power provided via the power cable from the wall socket the computer is plugged into, into low-voltage direct current (DC) power. Computers are dependent on a reliable, steady supply of DC power to function properly. The more devices and programs used on a computer, the higher the power supply should be to avoid damage and malfunctioning. Power supplies normally range from 160 to 700 watts, with an average of 300 to 400 watts. Most contemporary power supply units come equipped with at least one fan to cool the unit under heavy use. The power supply is controlled by pressing the on and off switch, as well as the reset switch (which restarts the system) of a computer.

Hard Disk » The **hard disk** is so named because of the rigid hard disks that reside in it, which are mounted to a spindle that is spun by a motor when in use. Drive heads (most computers have two heads) produce a magnetic field through their transducers that magnetize the disk surface as a voltage is applied to the disk. The hard disk acts as a permanent data storage area that holds the data, information, documents, and programs saved on the computer, even when the computer is shut off. Disk drives are not infallible, though, thus making the backup of important data imperative.

The computer writes binary data to the hard disk by magnetizing small areas of its surface. Each drive head is connected to an actuator that moves along the disk to hover over any point on the disk surface as it spins. The parts of the hard disk are encased in a sealed unit. The hard drive is managed by a disk controller, which is a circuit board that controls the motor and actuator arm assembly and produces the voltage waveform that contacts the heads to write and read data and handles communications with the motherboard. The hard drive is usually located within the computer's hard outer casing. Some people also attach a second hard drive externally to increase available memory or to back up data.

Main Memory or Random Access Memory » **Random access memory (RAM)** is considered to be volatile memory since it is a temporary storage system that allows the processor to access program codes and data while working on a task. RAM is lost once the system is rebooted, shut off, or loses power.

The memory is actually situated on small chip boards that sport rows of pins along the bottom edge and are plugged into the motherboard of the computer. These memory chips contain complex arrays of tiny memory circuits that can be either set by the CPU during write operations (puts them into storage) or read by the CPU during data retrieval. The circuits store the data in binary form as either a low (on) voltage stage, expressed as a zero, or a high (off) voltage stage, expressed as a one. All of the work being done on a computer resides in this RAM until it is saved onto the hard disk or other storage device. Computers generally come with 2 gigabytes of RAM or more, and may offer more RAM via graphics cards and other expansion cards.

A select portion of the RAM is called the **main memory**, which serves the hard disk and facilitates the interactions between the hard disk and central processor. Main memory is provided by **dynamic random access memory (DRAM)** and is attached to the processor using specific addresses and data buses.

Synchronous dynamic random access memory (SDRAM) is "much faster than conventional (**nonsynchronous**) [bold added] memory because it can synchronize itself with a microprocessor's bus" (Null & Lobur, 2006, p. 8).

Read-Only Memory » **Read-only memory (ROM)** is essential permanent or semipermanent nonvolatile memory that stores saved data and is critical in the working of the computer's operating system and other activities. ROM is primarily stored in the motherboard but may also be available through the graphics card, other expansion cards, and peripherals. In recent years, rewritable ROM chips have become available. This may include other forms of ROM such as **programmable read-only memory (PROM)**, **erasable programmable read-only memory (EPROM)**, **electronically erasable programmable read-only memory (EEPROM)**, and a **flash memory** (a variation of EEPROM).

Basic Input/Output System » The **basic input/output system (BIOS)** is a specific type of ROM used by the computer when it first boots up, to establish basic communication between the processor, motherboard, and other components. It is often called boot **firmware**, which controls the computer from the time it is switched on until the primary operating system (such as Windows XP or Vista, Mac OS X, or Linux) takes over. The firmware initializes the hardware and then boots (loads and executes) the primary operating system.

Virtual Memory » **Virtual memory** is a special type of memory that is stored on the hard disk to provide temporary data storage so data can be swapped in and out of the RAM as needed. This is particularly handy when working with large data-intensive programs such as games, multimedia, and so on.

Integrated Drive Electronics Controller » The **integrated drive electronics (IDE)** controller is the primary interface for the hard drive, compact disc (CD-ROM) or digital video disc (DVD) drive, and the floppy disk drive.

Peripheral Component Interconnection Bus » The **peripheral component interconnection (PCI)** bus is important for connecting additional plug-in components to the computer, since it utilizes a series of slots on the motherboard that allow PCI card plug-ins.

Small Computer System Interface » The **small computer system interface (SCSI)** provides the means to attach additional devices such as scanners, extra hard drives, and so on to the computer.

Digital Video Disc/Compact Disc Drive » The **compact disc read-only memory (CD-ROM)** drive reads and records data to portable compact discs (CDs), using a laser diode and a mirror positioned by a motor to emit an infrared light beam that reflects onto a track on the CD. The light reflected on the disc is directed by a system of lenses to a photo detector that converts the light pulses into an electrical signal that is then decoded by the drive electronics to the motherboard. Both **compact disc-recordable (CD-R)** and **compact disc-recordable and rewritable (CD-RW)** drives are common. The same principle applies to **digital video discs (DVDs)**, which come in **DVD-R** and **DVD-RW** formats. A DVD drive can do everything a CD drive can do, plus it can play DVDs, and if it is a recordable unit, it can record onto blank DVDs.

Floppy Drive » The floppy disk drive is becoming less commonly used on many contemporary computers, since its permanent storage space is very limited (usually no more than 2 megabytes [MB]). Users can insert plastic-coated 3.5″ disks into the floppy drive to save data as backup or for document portability. The drive itself is usually made of polyester film coated with a magnetic material and enclosed in a rigid plastic case that is housed in the computer case and attached to the inner computer components.

Flash Drive » A flash drive is a portable memory device that uses electrically erasable programmable read-only memory (EEPROM) to provide fast, permanent memory.

Modem » The **modem** is a component that can either be situated externally or internally and enables Internet connectivity via a telephone line or cable connection through network adapters situated within the computer apparatus.

Connection Ports » All computers have connection **ports** made to fit only one type of plug-in device. The ports include a monitor cable port, keyboard/mouse ports, a network cable port, microphone/speaker/auxiliary input ports and printer ports (SCSI or parallel). "Ports allow movement of data to and from devices external to the computer" (Null & Lobur, 2006, p. 11).

Specific Ports »

Parallel port—connects to a printer

Serial port—connects to an external modem

Universal serial bus (USB) port—connects to a myriad of plug-in devices, such as portable flash drives, digital cameras, MP3 players, graphics tablets, light pens, and so on using a **plug and play** connection (the ability to add devices automatically).

FireWire (IEEE 1394)—is often used to connect digital-video devices to the computer.

Graphics Card » Most computers come equipped with a graphics accelerator card slotted in the microprocessor of a computer to process image data and output it to the monitor. These in situ **graphics cards** provide satisfactory graphics quality for two-dimensional (2D) art and general text and numerical data. However, if a user intends to create or view three-dimensional (3D) images or is an active game user, an enhancement graphics card is often sought.

Video Adapter Cards » Video adapter cards provide video memory, a video processor, and a digital-to-analog converter that works with the CPU to output higher quality video images to the monitor.

Sound Card » The **sound card** converts digital data into an analog signal that is then outputted to the computer's speakers or headphones. The reverse is also accomplished by inputting a signal from a microphone or other audio recording equipment, which then converts the analog signal to a digital one.

Bit » A **bit** is the smallest possible chunk of data memory used in computer processing, exhibited as either a one or a zero, making up the **binary system** of the computer.

Byte » A **byte** is a chunk of memory that consists of eight bits and is considered to be the best way to indicate computer memory or storage capacity. In modern computers, bytes are reflected as **megabytes (MB)** or **gigabytes (GB)**. See Box 3-1 for more about storage capacities.

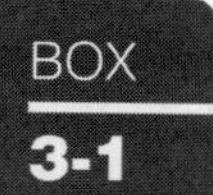

Storage Capacities

Dee McGonigle and Kathleen Mastrian

Yottabyte into learning about storage and memory capacities since they are evolving. We have seen great leaps in data storage. It all begins with the bit, the basic unit of data storage, composed of zeros and ones or **b**inary dig**its** (bit). A byte is generally considered to be equal to 8 bits or 23. The files on your computer are stored as binary files. The software that you are using translates these binary files into words, numbers, pictures, images, and/or video. Using this binary code in the binary numbering system, measurement is counted by factors of two such as 1, 2, 4, 8, 16, 32, 64, 128, etc. To add confusion, the multiples of the binary system in computer usage are prefixed based on the metric system. Therefore, a kilobyte (KB) is actually two to the 10th power (2^{10}) or 1,024 bytes, but is typically considered to be 1,000 bytes. This is why you see 1,024 or multiples of that number instead of an even one thousand mentioned at times in relation to kilobytes.

In the early 1980s, kilobytes were the norm as far as computer capacity and 128 KB machines were launched for personal use. The next couple of decades have advanced our computing power and storage capacity. As our capabilities soared so did our ability to save and store what we had used and created. Megabytes (MB) emerged and we thought we had it all. MBs are actually 1,048,576 bytes but are considered to be one million bytes. The next leap was one that some people could not even imagine. Gigabytes (GB) emerged; they are actually 1,073,741,824 bytes but are considered to be one billion bytes. Some experts are very concerned that we are losing valuable bytes when we round these measurements while the hard drive manufacturers are using the decimal system so their capacity is expressed as an even billion bytes per GB.

Our next advancements are moving into terabytes (TB), petabytes (PB), exabytes (EB), zettabytes (ZB) and yottabytes (YB).

Term	Storage Capacity
TB	1,000 GB
PB	1,000,000 GB
EB	1,000 PB
ZB	1,000 EB
YB	1,000 ZB

To put all of this in perspective, Williams (n.d., ¶ 5) wrote about the data powers of 10:

2 kilobytes: A typewritten page

2 megabytes: A high resolution photograph

10 megabytes: A minute of high-fidelity sound **OR** a digital chest X-ray

50 megabytes: A digital mammogram

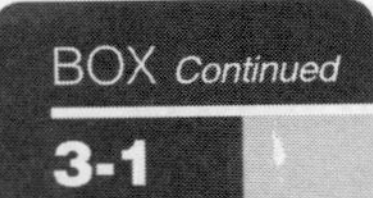

1 gigabyte: A symphony in high-fidelity sound **OR** a movie at TV quality
1 terabyte: All the X-ray films in a large technological hospital
2 petabytes: All U.S. academic research libraries
5 exabytes: All words ever spoken by human beings
We have not even addressed ZB and YB, stay tuned. . .

Reference

Williams, R. (n.d.). *Data powers of ten.* Retrieved on March 17, 2008, from http://www.cch.kcl.ac.uk/legacy/teaching/avmmet/data-powers-of-ten.html

Software

Software is the application programs developed to facilitate various user functions such as writing, artwork, organizing meetings, surfing the Internet, communicating with others, and so on. For this overview, software has been divided into four main categories: **operating system software, productivity software, creativity software**, and **communication software.**

User friendliness is a critical condition for effective software adoption. "End user performance is likely to be facilitated by user friendliness of software packages" (Mahmood, 2003, p. 71). The easier and more intuitive a software package seems to be to a user influences the user's perception of how clear the package is to understand and to use. The rapid evolution of hardware mentioned earlier has been equally matched by the phenomenal development in software over the past 3 or 4 decades.

Commercial Software » Several large commercial software companies such as Microsoft, Adobe, and Corel dominate the market shares in software sales and have done so since the advent of the personal computer. Licensed software has evolved over time, hence most programs have a long version history. Many software packages such as **office suites** are expensive to purchase, hence there is a definitive divide as far as access and affordability goes across societal spheres, especially when viewed from a global perspective.

Open Source Software » The open source movement began several years ago, but just recently has become a powerful phenomena that is changing the software production and consumer market. In addition to commercially available software, there are a growing number of **open source software** programs being developed in all four of the categories being addressed in this chapter. Open source is a very unique movement begun by developers who wished to offer their creations to others for the good of the community and encouraged others to do the same.

Users who modify or contribute to the evolution of the software are obligated to share their new code as well, but essentially the software is free to all. Open Office and KOffice are both examples of open source productivity software.

Operating System Software » The **operating system (OS) software** is the most important software on any computer. It is the very first program to load on computer start-up, and it is fundamental for the operation of all other software and the computer hardware. Examples of commonly used operating systems include the Microsoft Windows family, Linux, Mac OS X, and Unix. The operating system manages both the hardware and software and provides a reliable, consistent interface for the software **applications** to work with the computer's hardware. An operating system must be both powerful and flexible to adapt to the myriad of types of software available, made by a variety of development companies. New versions of the major operating systems are equipped to deal with multiple users and handle multitasking with ease. For instance, a user can work on a **word processing** document, listen for an **e-mail**–received signal, have an **Internet browser** window open to look for references on the Internet as needed, listen to music in the CD drive, and download a file all at the same time.

Operating system tasks can be summarized into six basic processes:

1. Memory management
2. Device management
3. Processor management
4. Storage management
5. Application interface
6. **User interface** (usually a **graphical user interface**, also known as **GUI**)

Designers of operating systems should take into consideration user goals and system goals. Operating systems should be convenient to use, easy to learn, reliable, safe, and fast. They should be easy to design, implement, and maintain, as well as flexible, reliable, error free, and efficient.

Silbershatz, Baer Galvin, and Gagne (2004) described how the Windows operating system has been designed with the following goals from Microsoft (MS):

- **Portability**—The OS can be moved from one hardware architecture to another with few changes needed.
- **Security**—The OS incorporates hardware protection for virtual memory and software protection mechanisms for OS resources.
- **POSIX** compliance—Applications designed to follow the portable operating system interface for UNIX (POSIX) (IEEE 1003.1) standard can be compiled to run on Windows without changing the source code.
- Multiprocessor support—The OS is designed for symmetrical multiprocessing.

- **Extensibility**—This is provided by using a layered architecture with a protected executive layer for basic system services, several server subsystems that operate in user mode, and a modular structure that allows additional environmental subsystems to be added without affecting the executive layer.
- International support—The Windows OS supports different locales via the national language support (NLS) application programming interface (API).
- **Compatibility** with MS-DOS and MS-Windows applications.

Productivity Software » Productivity software such as office suites are the most common software used both in the workplace and on personal computers. Several software companies produce these multiple program software suites, which usually combine word processing, **spreadsheet**, **database**, **presentation**, Web development, and e-mail programs all bundled together.

The intent of office suites is generally to provide all of the basic programs that an office or knowledge worker would need to do his or her work. The bundled

TABLE 3-1
Office Suite Software Features and Examples

Program	Application	Examples
Word processing	Composition, editing, formatting and producing text documents	Microsoft Word, Open Office Writer, KOffice KWord, Corel WordPerfect, Apple Pages
Spreadsheets	Grid-based documents in ledger format, organizes numbers and text and calculates statistical formulas	Microsoft Excel, Open Office Calc, KOffice Kspread, Corel Quattro Pro, Apple Numbers
Presentations	Slide show software, usually used for business or classroom presentations using text, images, graphs, and media	Microsoft PowerPoint, Open Office Impress, KOffice Kpresenter, Corel Presentations, Apple Keynote
Databases	Database creation for text and numbers	Microsoft Access (in elite packages), Open Office Base
E-mail	Integrated e-mail program to send and receive electronic mail	Microsoft Outlook, Corel WordPerfect Mail
Drawing	Graphics and diagram drawing	Open Office Draw, Corel Presentation Graphics, KChart
Math formulas	Inserts math equations in word processing and presentation work	Open Office Math, KOffice KFormula
Desktop publishing	Page layouts and publication-ready documents	Microsoft Publisher (in elite packages), Apple Pages

TABLE 3-2
Creative Software Features and Examples

Program	Application	Examples
Raster graphics programs	Draw, paint, render, manipulate and edit images, fonts, and photographs to create pixel-based (dot points) digital art and graphics.	Adobe Photoshop and Fireworks, Ulead Photo Impact, Corel Draw, Paint, and Paint Shop Pro, GIMP (open source), KOffice's Krita (open source)
Vector graphics programs	Mathematically rendered, geometric modeling is applied through shapes, curves, lines, points, and manipulated for shape, color, size. Ideal for printing and 3D modeling.	Adobe Flash, Freehand, and Illustrator, Corel Draw and Designer, Open Office Draw (open source), Mirosoft Visio, Xara Xtreme, KOffice Karbon14 (open source)
Desktop publishing programs	Page layout and publishing preparation for printed and Web documents, such as magazines, journals, books, newsletters, and brochures.	Adobe InDesign, Corel PageMaker, Microsoft Publisher, Scribus (open source), QuarkXPress, Apple Pages
Web design programs	Create, edit, and update Web pages using specific coding languages such as XML, CSS, HTML, and Java.	Adobe Dreamweaver, Coffee Cup, Microsoft FrontPage, Nvu (open source), W3C's Amaya (open source)
Multimedia programs	Combines text, audio, images, animation, and video into interactive content for electronic presentation.	Microsoft Movie Maker, Apple Quicktime and FinalCut Studio, Ulead VideoStudio, CamStudio (open source), Real Studio, Adobe Flash

Note: Many of the graphics programs can also be used for desktop publishing.

programs within the suite are organized to be compatible with one another, are designed to look similar to one another for ease of use, and provide a powerful array of tools for data manipulation, information gathering and knowledge generation. Some office suites add other programs such as database creation software, mathematical editors, drawing programs, and desktop **publishing** programs. Table 3-1 provides a summary of common programs included in five of the most popular office suites: Microsoft Office, Open Office, KOffice, Corel WordPerfect Suite, and Apple iWorks (for Mac computers). Of these five, Open Office (for Windows, Linux, Solaris, Mac OS X, FreeBSD, and HP-UX operating systems) and KOffice (for Linux environments) are open source software.

Creative Software » Creative software includes programs that allow users to draw, paint, render, record music and sound, and incorporate digital video and other multimedia in professional aesthetic ways to share and convey information and knowledge. See examples in Table 3-2.

Communication Software » Networking and communication software (see examples in Table 3-3) enable users to dialogue, share, and network with other users via

TABLE 3-3
Communication Software Features and Examples

Program	Application	Examples
E-mail client	Allows users to read, edit, forward, and send e-mail messages to other users via an Internet connection. The software can reside on the computer or accessed via the World Wide Web.	**Resident programs:** Microsoft Outlook and Outlook Express, Eudora, Pegasus, Mozilla Thunderbird, Lotus Notes **Web-based programs:** Gmail, Yahoo Mail, Hotmail
Internet browsers	Enables users to access, browse, download, upload, and interact with text, audio, video, and other Web-based documents.	Mozilla Firefox, Microsoft Internet Explorer, Apple Safari, Opera, Microbrowser (for mobile access)
Instant messaging (IM)	Real-time text messaging between users, who can attach images, videos, and other documents via personal computers, cell phones, and handheld devices.	MSN Instant Messenger, Microsoft Live Messenger, Yahoo Messenger, Apple iChat
Conferencing	Enables users to communicate in a virtual meeting room setting to share work, have discussions, and plan, using an intranet or Internet environment. Can exhibit files, video, and screenshots of content.	Adobe Acrobat Connect, Microsoft Live Meeting or Meeting Space, GotoMeeting, Meeting Bridge, Free Conference, RainDance, WebEx

the exchange of e-mail or **instant messages (IMs)**, by accessing the **World Wide Web (WWW)**, or by engaging in virtual meetings using **conferencing software.**

Acquisition of Data and Information (Input Components)

Input devices include the **keyboard**, mouse, joysticks (usually used for playing computer games), game controllers or pads, Web cameras, styli (often used with tablets or PDAs), image scanners for copying digital images of documents or pictures, or other plug and play input devices such as digital cameras, digital video recorders (or camcorders), MPEG-1 Audio Layer-3 (MP3) players, electronic musical instruments, or physiological monitors. These devices are the origin or medium used to input text, visual, audio, or multimedia data into the computer system for viewing, listening, manipulating, creating, or editing. The two primary input devices on a computer are the keyboard and mouse. Figure 3-1 shows a diagram of a complete computer system, including input, throughput/processing, and output components.

Keyboard

Computer keyboards are very similar to typewriter keyboards and usually serve as the prime input device that enables the user to type words, numbers, and com-

FIGURE 3-1
Components of a computer system.

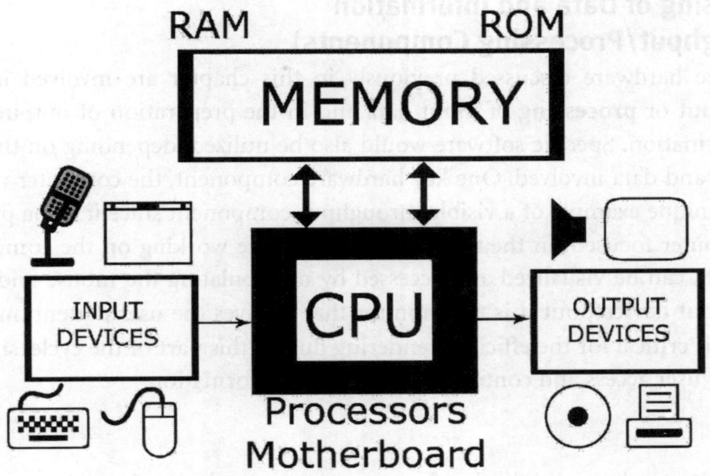

mands into the computer's programs. Standard computer keyboards have 101 keys and are organized to facilitate Latin-based languages using a **QWERTY** layout (so named because these letters are on the first six keys in the first row of letters).

Select keys are used as command keys, particularly the control (CTRL), alternate (Alt), Delete (Del), and Shift keys, which can all be used to activate useful commands. Also, the escape (Esc) key allows the user to instantly exit a process or program. The function keys are labeled F1 through F12. These are used in different ways by different programs. For example, on some computers, the F2 key could toggle or change the wireless Internet connection on and off. A program might instruct the user to press the F8 key in order to toggle the display between the CRT (computer monitor) and LCD (projector) for purposes of displaying the contents of the monitor screen or presenting to a group or class. The Print Screen (PrtSc) key sends a graphical picture or screen shot of a computer screen to the clipboard. This copied screen shot can then be pasted in any graphics program that can work with bitmap (bmp) files.

Mouse

The **mouse** is the second most common input device; it is manipulated by the user's hand to point, click, and move objects around on the computer screen. A mouse can come in a number of different configurations, including a standard mechanical trackball serial mouse, a bus mouse, a PS/2 mouse, a USB-connected mouse, an optical lens mouse, a cordless mouse, and an optomechanical mouse.

Processing of Data and Information (Throughput/Processing Components)

All of the hardware discussed previously in this chapter are involved in the **throughput** or **processing** of input data and in the preparation of output data and information. Specific software would also be utilized, depending on the application and data involved. One key hardware component, the computer monitor, is a unique example of a visible throughput component since it is the part of the computer focused on the most by users who are working on the computer. Input data can be visualized and accessed by manipulating the mouse and keyboard input devices, but it is the monitor that receives the user's attention. The monitor is critical for the efficient rendering during this part of the cycle, since it facilitates user access and control of the data and information.

Monitor

The **monitor** is the visual display that serves as the landscape for all interactions between user and machine. It typically resembles a television screen and comes in various sizes (usually ranging from 15 to 21 inches) and configurations. Monitors have either a cathode ray tube (CRT), as is the case with the conventional monitors with a large section behind the screen, or they feature thinner, flat-screen liquid crystal displays (LCD). Some computer monitors also have a **touch screen**, which can serve as an input device when the user touches key areas of the screen.

Monitors vary in refresh rate (usually measured in MHz) and in dot pitch. Both of these characteristics are important for user comfort. The faster the refresh rate, the more frequently the monitor refreshes the screen contents, resulting in a cleaner and clearer image on the screen. For instance, a monitor with a 100 MHz refresh rate will refresh the screen contents 100 times per second. Also, the higher the dot pitch factor, the smaller the dots that make up the screen image, meaning it provides a more detailed display on the monitor, which also facilitates clarity and ease of viewing.

If equipped with a touch screen, a monitor can also serve as an input device when activated by a stylus or finger pressure. Some might also consider the monitor to be an output device as well, since access to input and stored documents is often performed via the screen (for instance, reading a document that is stored on the computer or viewable from the Internet).

Dissemination (Output Components)

Output devices carry data in a usable form called **dissemination** through exit devices in or attached to a computer. Common forms of output forms include printed documents, audio or video files, physiological summaries, scan results, or saved files on portable disk drives such as a floppy disk, CD, DVD, or flash disks. Output devices literally put data and information at a user's fingertips, which can be used to develop knowledge and even **wisdom**. The most commonly used output devices include printers, speakers, and portable disk drives.

Printers

Printers are external components that can be attached to a computer using a printer cord that is secured into the computer's printer port. Printers enable users to print a paper copy of documents that are housed on the computer.

The most common printer types are the ink-jet printer and the laser printer. Ink-jet printers are more economical to use, with quite good quality, and apply ink to paper using a jet spray mechanism. Laser printers produce publisher-ready quality printing if combined with good quality paper, but it costs more to print. Both types of printers can print in black and white or in color.

Speakers

Most computers have some sort of speaker setup; they are often small speakers embedded in the monitor or tower case, or in the case of the laptop, close to the keyboard. Often, external speakers are added to a computer system by the user, using speaker connectors for enhanced sound and a more enjoyable listening experience.

WHAT IS THE RELATIONSHIP OF COMPUTER SCIENCE TO KNOWLEDGE?

Scholars and researchers are just beginning to understand the effect that computer systems, architecture, applications, and processes have on the potential for knowledge acquisition and development. Users who have access to contemporary computers equipped with full Internet access have resources at their fingertips that were only dreamed of before the 21st century. Entire library collections are accessible, with many documents available in full printable form. Users are able to contribute to the development of knowledge as well through the use of productivity, creativity, and communication software. Utilizing the World Wide Web interface, users are also able to disseminate knowledge on a grand scale with other users. The deluge of information available via computers must be mastered and organized by the user in order for knowledge to emerge. Discernment and the ability to critique and filter this information must also be present in order to facilitate the further development of wisdom.

The development of an understanding of computer science principles as they apply to technology used in nursing can facilitate optimal usage of the technology for knowledge development in the profession. The maxim that "knowledge is power" and that the skillful use of computers is at the heart of this power is a presumption (Richards, 2001). "The computer literate nurse will have knowledge, and as a result, power and influence. Society has accepted computers as standard elements, and as such, computers will continue to shape nurses' psychological, social, economic, and political existence in innumerable ways. Nursing, in order to interface with other spheres of society, must be computer literate. In short, society has accepted computer technology as a means to enhance life; so must nursing" (Richards, 2001, p. 9). Once nurses become comfortable with various technologies, they can shape them, refine them, and apply them in new and different ways—just as they have always adapted to earlier equipment and technologies.

HOW DOES THE COMPUTER SUPPORT COLLABORATION AND INFORMATION EXCHANGE?

Computers can be linked to other computers through networking software and hardware to promote communication, information exchange, work sharing, and collaboration. Networks can be local and/or organizationally based, joined together into a local area network (LAN), or on a wider area scope (such as a city or district) using a metropolitan area network (MAN) or from an even greater distance (e.g., a whole country or continent, or the Internet itself) using a wide area network (WAN) configuration (Sarkar, 2006). Network interface cards (NIC) are used to connect a computer and its modem to a network.

Networks within health care can manifest in several different configurations, including client-focused networks such as in telenursing, e-health, and client support networks; work-related networks including virtual work and virtual social networks; and learning and research networks as in communities of practice. These trends are still in their infancy in most nursing work environments (and personal lives) but they are predicted to be a strong trend in the future.

> As the Net generation grows in influence, the trend will be toward networks, not hierarchies, toward open collaboration rather than authority; toward consensus rather than arbitrary edict. The communication support provided by networks and information systems will also alter patterns of social interaction within a health care organization. This technology provides a medium for greater accessibility to shared information and support for rich

> interpersonal exchange and collaboration across departmental boundaries. (Richards, 2001, p. 10).

Virtual social networks are another form of professional network that have expanded phenomenally since the advent of the Internet and other computer software and hardware.

> Electronic media do more than just expand access to vast bodies of information. They also serve as a convenient vehicle for building virtual social networks for creating shared knowledge through collaborative learning and problem solving. Cross pollination of ideas through worldwide connectivity can boost creativity synergistically in the co-construction of knowledge. (Bandura, 2002, p. 4)

Basically, nursing-related virtual social networks provide a cyberspace for nurses to make contacts, share information and ideas, and build a sense of community.

Social communication software programs are used to provide a dynamic virtual environment, and often virtual social networks provide communicative capabilities through posting tools like blogs, forums, and wikis; e-mail for sharing ideas on a smaller scale; collaborative areas for interaction, creating and building digital artifacts or planning projects; navigation tools for moving through the virtual network landscape; and profiles to provide a space for each member to disclose personal information with others. Nurses who have to engage in shift work often find that virtual social networks can provide a sense of around-the-clock connection with other professionals. Since time is often a factor in any social interchange, virtual communication often offers an alternative for practicing nurses who can access information and interchange at any time of day. With active participation, the interchanges and shared information/ideas of the network can culminate into valuable social and cultural capital, available to all members. Often, nursing virtual social networks are created for the purpose of exchanging ideas on practice issues and best practices; becoming more knowledgable about new trends, research, and innovations in health care; or participating in advocacy, activist, and educational initiatives.

Through the use of portable disk devices such as floppy disks, compact discs (CDs) and DVDs, people can share information, documents, and communications by exchanging files. Since the advent of the Internet in the mid-1980s, the World Wide Web has evolved to become a viable and user-friendly way for people to collaborate and exchange information, projects, and other knowledge-based files such as Web sites, e-mail, social networking applications, and Web conferencing logs. See Box 3-2 for more about the new Web 2.0 tools.

BOX 3-2

Web 2.0 Tools

Dee McGonigle, Kathleen Mastrian, and Wendy Mahan

Web 2.0, the new World Wide Web tools, enable users to collaborate, network socially and disseminate knowledge with other users on a scale that was once not even comprehensible. These programs promote data/information exchange, feedback, and knowledge development and dissemination.

In order to facilitate a selective review of the Web 2.0 tools available, we have categorized them into three areas: tools for creating and sharing information, tools for collaborating, and tools for communicating. Examples of creating and sharing information tools include blogs, podcasts, Flickr, YouTube, Hellodeo, jing, Screencast-o-matic, Facebook, MySpace, and MakeBeliefsComix. Examples of tools for collaborating with others include Google Docs, Zoho, wikis, Del.icio.us, and Gliffy. Finally, some tools for communicating with others include Adobe Connect, Vyew, Skype, Twitter, and IM.

Through the use of the creating and sharing information tools we have seen an explosion of social networking on the Web. YouTube has promoted the "broadcast yourself" proliferation. You can launch a video onto YouTube that will be shared with others over the Web. Similarly, Flickr allows you to upload and tag personal photos to share either privately or publicly. Facebook and MySpace both promote socializing on the Web. Facebook is a social utility and MySpace is a place for friends according to each of their Web sites. Other tools let you create and share recorded messages, diagrams, screen captures, and even custom comic strips.

Collaborating over the Web has become easier. It is a way of life for many. Google Docs and Zoho allow you to create online and share and collaborate in real time. Wikis are server-based software programs that enable you to generate and edit web page content using any browser. Del.icio.us is a social bookmarking manager that uses tags to identify or describe the bookmarks that can be shared with others.

Communicating with others includes audio and video conferencing in real time. Adobe Connect is a comprehensive Web communications solution. It is a fee-based service that does provide a free trial. Make sure that you read all of the documentation on their site before downloading, installing and using this software. Vyew is free, always-on collaboration plus live Web conferencing. Skype allows you to make calls in audio only or with video as well. You can download Skype for free but depending on the type of calls you make, fees or charges could be assessed. Make sure you read through all of the information before downloading, installing, and using this software. Twitter allows you to answer the question, what are you doing, in 140 characters or less. Although you can use Twitter to keep the friends in your network updated on your daily activities, it can also be used for other purposes like asking questions or expressing thoughts. In addition, Twitter can be accessed by cell phones, so one can stay in touch on the go.

BOX *Continued*

3-2

Along with all of the advantages and intellectual harvesting capabilities from the use of these tools come security issues. Wagner (2007) warns you to "bear in mind before you jump in that you're giving information to a third-party company to store" (¶ 5). He also states that "you should talk to your company's legal and compliance offices to be sure you're obeying the law and regulations with regard to managing company's information" (¶ 5). One suggestion that he offers is that if you do not want to involve a third party, "Wikis provide a good alternative for organizations looking to maintain control of their own software. Organizations can install wiki software on their own, internal servers" (¶ 6).

This new wave of Web-based tools has presented us with the ability to interact, exchange, collaborate, communicate and share in ways we have only begun to envision. As the tools and their innovative uses continue to increase, we will need to stay vigilant to handle the associated security challenges. These Web 2.0 tools are providing us with a new cyber playground that is only limited by our own imaginations and intelligence. We encourage you to explore these tools. Refer to this book's companion Web site http://nursing.jbpub.com/informatics for more information.

Reference

Wagner, M. (2007). *Nine easy web-based collaborative tools.* Retrieved on March 17, 2008, from http://www.forbes.com/2007/02/26/google-microsoft-bluetie-ent-tech-cx_mw_0226smallbizresource.html

WHAT IS THE HUMAN–TECHNOLOGY INTERFACE?

In the context of using a computer system, the human–technology interface is facilitated by the input and output devices discussed earlier in this chapter. Specifically, the keyboard, mouse, monitor, laser pen, joystick, stylus or game pads and controls, and other USB or plug and play devices such as MP3 players, digital cameras, digital camcorders, musical instruments, and handheld computers such as PDAs are all viable devices for interfacing with a computer.

Also, the GUI afforded by the operating system of a computer provides the on-screen environment for direct interaction between the user and the computer. The typical GUI provided by Windows or Mac's OS X provide a user-friendly desktop interface that is made up of the input and output devices as well as icons that represent files, programs, actions, and processes. These interface icons can be activated by clicking the mouse buttons to perform various actions such as provide information, execute functions, open and manipulate folders (directories), select options, and so forth.

Although these aspects of a computer system may be taken for granted, they are critical in facilitating a sense of comfort and competency in users of the system. This is particularly critical in nursing, when computers are used in the context of nursing care. One question that arises is do nurses control these information technology tools, or do the tools shape the activities, decisions, and attention of the nurses as users of technology? Both possibilities could be answered in the affirmative to some extent, but the former—the nurse or user being in control is the safest situation as far as nursing care goes. If the nurse user needs to focus on the software or hardware due to difficult programs, confusing GUI schema, or sheer complexity in the programming, the provision of client care is going to suffer. It is critical that software and hardware used in the nursing milieu is expertly designed to actually facilitate nursing care in a user-friendly, intuitive way. This is one reason that informatics experts called nurse informaticians are being placed in positions of authority in order to facilitate the adoption of computer systems within nursing care environments. It is essential that the activities of the staff nurses are reflected well within the software that is utilized in the care setting. If nurses are knowledgable about computers and related technologies, they will be able to provide meaningful data and information about how computer systems will best work within their particular care areas. The human–technology interface is covered in detail in Chapter 5.

SUMMARY

The field of computer science is one of the fastest growing disciplines on the planet. Astonishing innovations in computer hardware, software, and architecture have occurred over the past few decades, and there are no indications that this trend will stop anytime soon. Computers have improved in speed, accuracy, and efficiency, yet also cost less and have reduced physical size, and are predicted to continue to follow these trends in the future. Current computer hardware and software offer vital and valuable tools for both nurses and clients to engage in on-screen and online activities that provide rich access to data and information. The productivity, creative, and communicative software tools can also support nurses who work with computers to further foster knowledge acquisition and development. Wide access to vast stores of information and knowledge shared by others also facilitates the emergence of wisdom in users that can be applied to nursing in meaningful and creative ways. It is imperative that nurses become discerning yet skilled users of computer technology in order to apply the principles of nursing informatics to practice and to contribute to the profession's ever-growing body of knowledge.

Working Wisdom

Since the beginning of the profession, nurses have applied their ingenuity, resourcefulness, and professional awareness of what works to adapt technology and objects to support nursing care, usually with the intent to promote efficiency but also client comfort and healing. This resourcefulness could also be applied effectively to the adaptation of information technology within the care environment, to ensure that the technology truly does serve clients and nurses as well as the rest of the interdisciplinary team.

Consider how you can develop competency in using the various computer hardware and software to not only promote efficient nursing care and develop yourself professionally, but to also further the development of the profession's body of knowledge.

Application Scenario

Dan P. is a first-year student in graduate studies in nursing. In the past, he has learned to use his family's personal computer to surf the World Wide Web, exchange e-mail with friends, and play some computer games. However, now he is realizing that the computer will be a vital tool for his academic success and has saved up enough money to purchase a laptop computer of his own. He has decided on a Pentium CPU system with 150 GB of ROM and 1 GB of RAM. Now he wishes to choose appropriate software for his system. He is on a limited budget, but wants to make the most of his investment.

1. Which of the four categories of software discussed in this chapter (operating system, productivity, creativity, or communication) would benefit Dan the most in his studies?
2. How could Dan afford to install software from all four groups on his new laptop?

THOUGHT-PROVOKING Questions

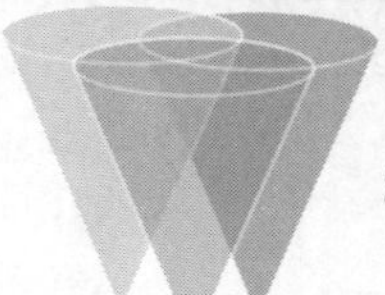

1. How can knowledge of computer hardware and software help nurses to participate in information technology adoption decisions in the practice area?
2. How can new computer software help nurses engage in professional development, collaboration, and knowledge dissemination activities at their own pace?

References

Bandura, A. (2002). Growing primacy of human agency in adaptation and change in the electronic era. *European Psychologist, 7*(1), 2–16.

Hennessy, J., & Patterson, D. (2006). *Computer architecture: A quantitative approach* (4th ed.). San Francisco: Morgan Kaufmann.

Intel Corporation. (2008). *Concealing complexity.* Retrieved on March 16, 2008, from http://techresearch.intel.com/articles/Exploratory/1430.htm

Mahmood, M. (2003). *Advanced topics in end user computing.* Hershey, PA: Idea Group Inc.

Null, L., & Lobur, J. (2006). *The essentials of computer organization and architecture* (2nd ed.). Boston, MA: Jones and Bartlett.

Richards, J. A. (2001, January/February). Nursing in a digital age. *Nursing Economic$, 19*(1), 6–12.

Sarkar, N. (2006). *Tools for teaching computer networking and hardware concepts.* Hershey, PA: Idea Group Inc.

Silbershatz, A., Baer Galvin, P., & Gagne, G. (2004). *Operating system concepts* (7th ed.). Hoboken, NJ: John Wiley & Sons.

Wagner, M. (2007). *Nine easy web-based collaborative tools.* Retrieved on March 17, 2008, from http://www.forbes.com/2007/02/26/google-microsoft-bluetie-ent-tech-cx_mw_0226smallbizresource.html

Williams, R. (n.d.). *Data powers of ten.* Retrieved on March 17, 2008, from http://www.cch.kcl.ac.uk/legacy/teaching/avmmet/data-powers-of-ten.html

Internet and Software Resources

BBC. (n.d.). *BBC absolute beginner's guide to using your computer. A WebWise guide.* Available at: http://www.bbc.co.uk/webwise/abbeg/abbeg.shtml

BBC. (2008). *BBC's computer tutor: The BBC's guide to using a computer.* Available at: http://www.bbc.co.uk/computertutor/computertutorone/index.shtml

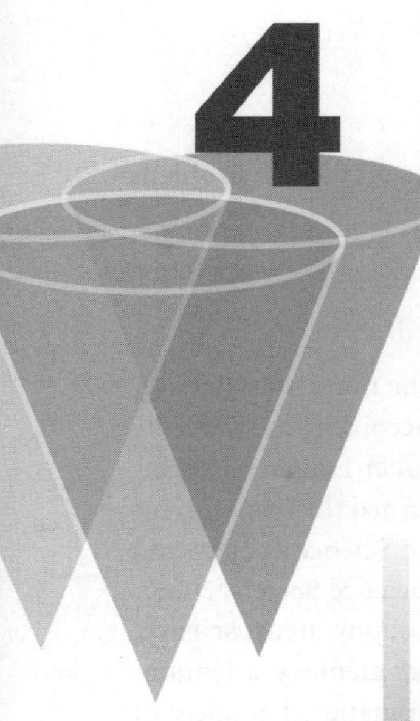

4 Introduction to Cognitive Science

Dee McGonigle and Kathleen Mastrian

Objectives

1. Describe cognitive science.
2. Assess how our minds process and generate information and knowledge.
3. Explore cognitive informatics.
4. Examine artificial intelligence (AI) and its relationship to cognitive science and computer science.

Key Terms

Artificial intelligence (AI)
Brain
Cognitive informatics
Cognitive science
Computer science
Decision making
Empiricism
Epistemology
Intelligence
Intuition
Knowledge
Logic
Memory
Mind
Neuroscience
Perception
Problem solving
Psychology
Rationalism
Reasoning
Wisdom

INTRODUCTION

Cognitive science is the third part of the three basic building blocks used to understand informatics. We began Section I by examining information science and then computer science and how each relates to and helps us understand the concept of informatics. We will conclude this exploration of the building blocks of informatics with an exploration of cognitive science, cognitive informatics, and **artificial intelligence**.

Throughout the centuries, cognitive science has intrigued philosophers and educators alike. Beginning in Greece, the ancient philosophers sought to comprehend how the **mind** worked, as well as the nature of knowledge. This age-old quest for unraveling the processes inherent in the working **brain** has been under study by the greatest minds. However, it was only 50 or so years ago that computer operations and actions were linked to cognitive science, theories of the mind, intellect, or brain. This led to the expansion of cognitive science to examine the complete array of cognitive processes from lower-level perceptions to high-level critical thinking, logical analysis, and **reasoning**. The focus of our text will be on its impact on nursing informatics (NI). This section will provide you with an introduction and overview of cognitive science, nature of knowledge, wisdom, and artificial intelligence (AI) as they apply to the

Foundation of Knowledge model and NI. The applications to NI include **problem solving,** decision support systems, usability issues, user-centered interfaces and systems, and the development and use of terminologies.

COGNITIVE SCIENCE

Cognitive science is the interdisciplinary field that studies the mind, **intelligence**, and behavior from an information processing perspective. According to *Wikipedia* (2007), "The term cognitive science was coined by Christopher Longuet-Higgins in his 1973 commentary on the Lighthill report, which concerned the then-current state of artificial intelligence research" (¶ 1). The Cognitive Science Society and the *Cognitive Science Journal* date back to 1980 (Cognitive Science Society, 2005). Their interdisciplinary base arises from **psychology**, philosophy, **neuroscience**, **computer science**, linguistics, biology, and physics and covers **memory**, attention, perception, reasoning, language, mental ability, and computational models of cognitive processes as well as the nature of the mind, knowledge representation, language, problem solving, **decision making**, and the social factors influencing the design and use of technology. Simply defined, cognitive science is the study of the mind and how information is processed in the mind. As described in the *Stanford Encyclopedia of Philosophy*, "The central hypothesis of cognitive science is that thinking can best be understood in terms of representational structures in the mind and computational processes that operate on those structures" (2007, ¶ 10). The mind is frequently compared to a computer and experts in computer science strive to understand how the mind processes data and information while experts in cognitive science attempt to model human thinking using artificial networks provided by computers. Some refer to the latter as **artificial intelligence.** How does the mind process all of the inputs received? What and how are things stored or placed into memory, accessed, augmented, changed, reconfigured, and restored? Cognitive science provides the scaffolding for the analysis and modeling of complicated, multifaceted human performance and therefore has a tremendous effect on the issues impacting informatics. The end user is the focus since we are concerned with enhancing the performance in the workplace; in nursing, the end user could be the actual clinician in the clinical setting, and cognitive science can enhance the integration and implementation of the technologies being designed to facilitate this knowledge worker with the ultimate goal of improving patient care. Technologies change rapidly, and this evolution must be harnessed for the clinician at the bedside. In order to do this at all levels of nursing practice, we must understand the nature of knowledge, the information and knowledge needed, and how the nurse processes this information/knowledge in his/her situational context.

SOURCES OF KNOWLEDGE

As philosophers have questioned what **knowledge** is, they have also strived to determine how it arises since the origins of knowledge can help us understand its nature. How do we come to know what we know about ourselves, others, and our world? There are many viewpoints on this issue, both scientific and nonscientific.

Holt (2006) stated that "There are two competing traditions concerning the ultimate source of our knowledge: empiricism and rationalism" (¶ 3). **Empiricism** is based on our knowledge being derived from our experiences or senses while **rationalism** contends that "some of our knowledge is derived from reason alone and that reason plays an important role in the acquisition of all of our knowledge" (Holt, ¶ 5). Empiricists do not recognize innate knowledge while rationalists believe that reason is more essential in the acquisition of knowledge than the senses.

According to others, there are three sources of knowledge: instinct, reason, and intuition. Instinct is when one reacts without reason, such as when a car is heading toward him and he jumps out of the way instinctively. Instinct is found in both humans and animals while reason and intuition are found only in humans. Reason "Collects facts, generalizes, reasons out from cause to effect, from effect to cause, from premises to conclusions, from propositions to proofs" (Sivananda, 2004, ¶ 4). **Intuition** is a way of acquiring knowledge that cannot be obtained by inference, deduction, observation, reason, analysis, or experience. Intuition was termed by Aristotle as "A leap of understanding, a grasping of a larger concept unreachable by other intellectual means, yet fundamentally an intellectual process" (Shallcross & Sisk, 1999, ¶ 4).

Some believe that knowledge is acquired through perception and logic. **Perception** is the process of acquiring knowledge about our environment or situation by obtaining, interpreting, selecting, and organizing sensory information from seeing, hearing, touching, tasting, and smelling. **Logic** is "[a] science that deals with the principles and criteria of validity of inference and demonstration: the science of the formal principles of reasoning" (Merriam-Webster, 2007, ¶ 1). Acquiring knowledge through logic requires reasoned action to make valid inferences.

The sources of knowledge provide a variety of inputs, throughputs, and outputs through which we process knowledge. No matter how we believe one acquires knowledge, it is important to be able to explain or describe our beliefs, communicate our thoughts, enhance shared understanding, and discover the nature of knowledge.

NATURE OF KNOWLEDGE

Epistemology is the study of the nature and origin of knowledge—what it means to know. Everyone has a conception of what it means to know based on their own perceptions, education, and experiences; knowledge is a part of life that continues to grow with us. Thus, a definition of knowledge is somewhat difficult to agree on since it reflects the viewpoints, beliefs, and understandings of the person or group defining it. Some people believe that it is a sequential process resembling a pyramid with data on the bottom, rising to information, then knowledge, and finally wisdom. Others believe that knowledge arises from our interactions and experience with our environment, and still others think that it is religiously or culturally bound. It is thought to be an internal process derived through our thinking/cognition and/or an external process from our senses, observations, studies, and interactions. Descartes' important premise "called 'the way of ideas' represents the attempt in epistemology to provide a foundation for our knowledge of the external world (as well as our knowledge of the past and of other minds) in the mental experiences of the individual" (*Encyclopedia Britannica*, 2007, ¶ 4). For the purpose of this text, we have defined knowledge as the awareness and understanding of a set of information and ways that information can be made useful to support a specific task or arrive at a decision; it abounds with others' thoughts and information or is information that is synthesized so that relationships are identified and formalized.

HOW IS KNOWLEDGE/WISDOM USED IN DECISION MAKING?

The whole point in collecting and building data, information, and knowledge is to be able to make informed, judicious, prudent, and intelligent decisions. When one considers the nature of knowledge and its applications, one must also examine the concept of wisdom. We have defined **wisdom** as knowledge applied in a practical way or translated into actions; to use knowledge and experience to heighten common sense and insight to exercise sound judgment in practical matters; sometimes thought of as the highest form of common sense resulting from accumulated knowledge or erudition (deep, thorough learning) or enlightenment (education that results in understanding and the dissemination of knowledge); it is the ability to apply valuable and viable knowledge, experience, understanding and insight while being prudent and sensible; is focused on our own minds; the synthesis of our experience, insight, understanding, and knowledge; the appropriate use of knowledge to solve human problems. It is knowing when and how to apply knowledge. The decision-making process evolves around knowledge and wisdom. It is through our efforts to understand the nature of knowledge and its evolution to wisdom that we can conceive of, build, and implement informatics tools that enhance and mimic our mind's processes to facilitate decision making and job performance.

COGNITIVE INFORMATICS

Wang (2003) describes **cognitive informatics** (CI) as an emerging transdisciplinary field of study that attempts to bridge the gap of understanding how information is processed in the mind and in the computer. Computing and informatics theories can be applied to help understand the information processing of the brain, and cognitive and neurological sciences can likewise be applied to build better and more efficient computer processing systems. Wang suggests that the common issue among the human knowledge sciences is developing an understanding of natural intelligence and human problem solving. Pacific Northwest National Laboratory (PNNL), operated for the U.S. Department of Energy (2007) suggests the disciplines of neuroscience, linguistics, artificial intelligence, and psychology make up this field. It defines CI as "the multidisciplinary study of cognition and information sciences, which investigates human information processing mechanisms and processes and their engineering applications in computing" (¶ 1). CI attempts to help bridge this gap by systematically exploring the mechanisms of the brain and mind and exploring specifically how information is acquired, represented, remembered, retrieved, generated, and communicated. This dawning of understanding can then be applied and modeled in artificial intelligence situations resulting in more efficient computing applications. Wang explains further:

> Cognitive informatics attempts to solve problems in two connected areas in a bidirectional and multidisciplinary approach. In one direction, CI uses informatics and computing techniques to investigate cognitive science problems, such as memory, learning and reasoning; in the other direction, CI uses cognitive theories to investigate the problems in informatics, computing, and software engineering. (p. 120)

WHAT IS ARTIFICIAL INTELLIGENCE?

Artificial intelligence (AI) is the field that deals with the conception, development, and implementation of informatics tools based on intelligent technologies. This field attempts to capture the complex processes of human thought and intelligence. Herbert Simon believes that the field of AI could have two functions: "One is to use the power of computers to augment human thinking, just as we use motors to augment human or horse power. The other is to use a computer's artificial intelligence to understand how humans think. In a humanoid way" (Association for the Advancement of Artificial Intelligence [AAAI], 2007a, ¶ 1). According to the AAAI (2007b), AI is the "scientific understanding of the mechanisms underlying thought and intelligent behavior and their embodiment in machines" (¶ 2).

John McCarthy, one of the men credited with founding the field of AI in the 1950s, stated that AI "is the science and engineering of making intelligent machines, especially intelligent computer programs. It is related to the similar task of using computers to understand human intelligence, but AI does not have to confine itself to methods that are biologically observable" (AAAI, 2007b, ¶ 4). Lamont (2007) interviewed Ray Kurzweil, a visionary who defined AI as "the ability to perform a task that is normally performed by natural intelligence, particularly human natural intelligence. We have in fact artificial intelligence that can perform many tasks that used to require—and could only be done by—human intelligence" (¶ 6). The intelligence factor is extremely important in AI and has been defined by McCarthy as "the computational part of the ability to achieve goals in the world. Varying kinds and degrees of intelligence occur in people, many animals and some machines" (AAAI, 2007b, ¶ 4).

The challenge of this field rests in capturing, mimicking, and creating the complex processes of the mind in our informatics tools, including software, hardware, and other machine technologies with the goal of the tool to be able to initiate and generate its own mechanical thought processing. As we have discussed, the brain's processing is highly intricate and complicated. This complexity is reflected in Cohn's (2006) comment that "Artificial intelligence is 50 years old this summer, and while computers can beat the world's best chess players, we still can't get them to think like a 4-year-old" (¶ 1). AI uses cognitive science and computer science to replicate and generate human intelligence. This field will continue to evolve and produce artificially intelligent tools to enhance our personal and professional lives.

SUMMARY

Cognitive science is the interdisciplinary field that studies the mind, intelligence, and behavior from an information processing perspective. Cognitive informatics (CI) is a field of study that attempts to bridge the gap of understanding how information is processed in the mind and in the computer. Computing and informatics theories can be applied to help understand the information processing of the brain, and cognitive and neurological sciences can likewise be applied to build better and more efficient computer processing systems. Artificial intelligence (AI) is the field that deals with the conception, development, and implementation of informatics tools based on intelligent technologies. This field attempts to capture the complex processes of human thought and intelligence. AI uses cognitive science and computer science to replicate and generate human intelligence. The sources of knowledge, nature of knowledge, and rapidly changing technologies must be able to be harnessed by the clinicians to enhance their bedside care. Therefore, we must understand the nature of knowledge, the information and knowledge needed, and how the nurse processes this information/knowledge in his/her situational context. The whole point in collecting and building data, information, and knowledge is to be able to build wisdom, the ability to apply valuable and viable knowledge, experience, understanding and insight while being prudent and sensible; it is focused on our own minds, the synthesis of our experience, insight, understanding, and knowledge. Nurses must use their wisdom and make informed, judicious, prudent, and intelligent decisions while enacting care. Cognitive science, cognitive informatics, and artificial intelligence will continue to evolve to help us build knowledge and wisdom.

THOUGHT-PROVOKING Questions

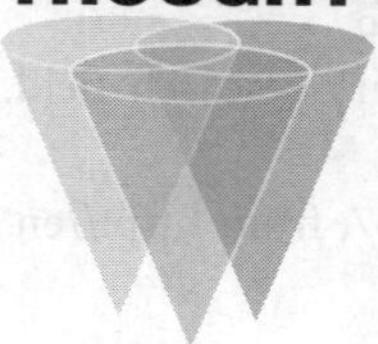

1. How would you describe cognitive informatics (CI)? Reflect on a plan of care that you have developed for a patient. How could cognitive informatics be used to create tools to help with this important work?
2. Think of a clinical setting you are familiar with and envision artificial intelligence tools. Are there any current tools in use? What tools would enhance practice in this setting and why?

References

Association for the Advancement of Artificial Intelligence (AAAI). (2007a). *AI overview.* Retrieved October 27, 2007, from http://www.aaai.org/AITopics/ html/overview.html

Association for the Advancement of Artificial Intelligence (AAAI). (2007b). *Cognitive science.* Retrieved on March 17, 2008, from http://www.aaai.org/aitopics/pmwiki/pmwiki.php/AITopics/CognitiveScience

Cognitive Science Society. (2005). *CSJ archive.* Retrieved October 28, 2007, from http://www.cogsci.rpi.edu/CSJarchive/1980v04/index.html

Cohn, D. (2006). *AI reaches the golden years.* Retrieved October 25, 2007, from http://www.wired.com/news/technology/0,71389-0.html

Encyclopedia Britannica. (2007). Epistemology. Retrieved January 2, 2008, from http://www.britannica.com/eb/article-247960/epistemology

Holt, T. (2006). *Sources of knowledge.* Retrieved January 2, 2008, from http://www.theoryofknowledge.info/sourcesofknowledge.html

Lamont, I. (2007). *The grill: Ray Kurzweil talks about 'augmented reality' and the singularity.* Retrieved October 28, 2007, from http://www.computerworld.com/action/article.do?command=viewArticleBasic&articleId=306176

Merriam-Webster Online Dictionary. (2007). Logic. Retrieved January 2, 2008, from http://www.m-w.com/cgi-bin/netdict?logic

Pacific Northwest National Laboratory (PNNL) (U.S. Department of Energy). (2007). *Cognitive informatics.* Retrieved January 8, 2008, from http://www. pnl.gov/cogInformatics

Shallcross, D. J., & Sisk, D. A. (1999). What is intuition? In T. Arnold (Ed.), *Hyponoesis glossary: Intuition.* Retrieved on March 17, 2008, from http://www. hyponoesis.org/html/glossary/intu_n.html

Sivananda, S. (2004). *Four sources of knowledge.* Retrieved January 2, 2008, from http://www.dlshq.org/messages/knowledge.htm

Stanford Encyclopedia of Philosophy. (2007). *Cognitive science.* Retrieved March 17, 2008 from http://plato.stanford.edu/entries/cognitive-science

Wang, Y. (2003). Cognitive informatics: A new transdisciplinary research field. *Brain and Mind, 4*(2), 115–127.

Wikipedia. (2007). *Cognitive science.* Retrieved October 28, 2007, from http://en. wikipedia.org/wiki/Cognitive_science

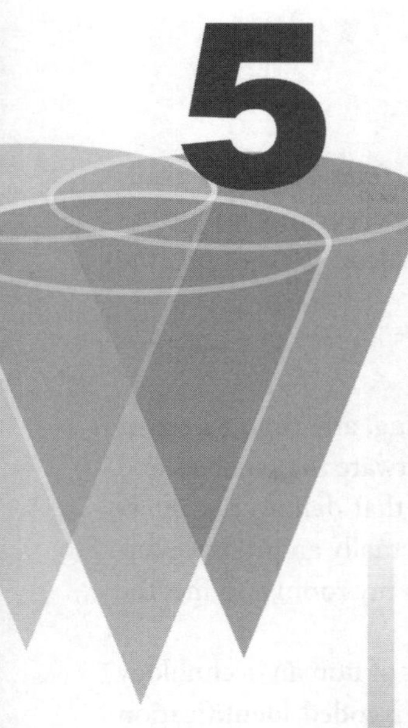

Improving the Human–Technology Interface

Judith A. Effken

Objectives

1. Describe human–technology interface.
2. Explore human–technology interface problems.
3. Reflect on the future of the human–technology interface.

Key Terms

Cognitive task analysis (CTA)
Cognitive walkthrough
Cognitive work analysis (CWA)
Ergonomics
Field study
Gulf of evaluation
Gulf of execution
Heuristic evaluation
Human–computer interaction (HCI)
Human factors
Human–technology interaction
Human–technology interface
Situational awareness
Task analysis
Usability
Workaround

INTRODUCTION

Several years ago I stayed in a new hotel on the edge of London. When I entered my room, I encountered three wall-mounted light switches in a row—but with no indication of which lights they operated. In fact, the mapping of switches to lights was so peculiar that I was more often than not surprised by the light that came on when I pressed a particular switch. You might conclude that I have a serious problem—but I would attribute my difficulty to poor design.

In his classic book, *The Psychology of Everyday Things*, Norman (1988) argued that life would be a lot simpler if people who built the things we encounter (like light switches) paid more attention to how we would use them. At least one everyday thing meets Norman's criteria for good design: the scythe. Even people who have never encountered one will pick up a scythe in the manner needed to use it because the design makes only one way feasible. The scythe's design fits perfectly with its intended use and a human user. Wouldn't it be great if all our technology were so well fit to our use? In fact, this is not such a far-fetched idea. Scientists and engineers are making excellent strides in understanding human–technology interface problems and proposing solutions.

By the end of this section, you should be able to: (1) define what we mean the "human–technology interface," (2) describe problems with human–technology interfaces currently available in health care, and (3) describe models, strategies, and exemplars for improving interfaces during the analysis, design, and evaluation phases of the development life cycle.

THE HUMAN–TECHNOLOGY INTERFACE

What is the **human–technology interface**? Broadly speaking, any time a human uses technology, there is some type of hardware and/or software that enables and supports the interaction. It is this hardware and software that defines the interface. So the array of light switches I described earlier was actually an interface (although not a great one) between the lighting technology in my room and me, the human user.

In today's healthcare settings, we encounter a wide variety of human–technology interfaces. Those of us who work in hospitals may use bar-coded identification cards to log our arrival time into a human resources management system. Using the same cards, we might log into our patients' electronic medical record, access their drugs from a drug administration system, and even administer their drugs using bar-coding technology. Other examples of human–technology interfaces we might encounter include a defibrillator, a patient-controlled analgesia (PCA) pump, any number of physiologic monitoring systems, electronic thermometers, and, of course, telephones and pagers.

The human interfaces for each of these technologies are different—and can even differ among different brands or versions of the same device. For example, to enter data into an electronic health record we might use a keyboard, a light pen, a touch screen, or our voices. Our healthcare technologies may present information to us via computer screen, printer, or a personal data assistant (PDA). Patient data might be displayed in the form of text, pictures (e.g., the results of a brain scan), or even sound (an echocardiogram); and the information may be arrayed or presented differently, based on our roles and preferences. Some human–technology interfaces mimic face-to-face human encounters. For example, faculty increasingly use videoconferencing technology to communicate with students. Similarly, telehealth allows nurses to use telecommunication and videoconferencing software to communicate more effectively and more frequently with patients at home by using the technology to monitor patients' vital signs, supervise their wound care, or demonstrate a procedure. Telehealth technology has fostered other virtual interfaces, such as in systemwide intensive care units (eICUs) in which intensivists and specially trained nurses monitor critically ill patients in intensive care units, some of which may be in rural locations. Sometimes telehealth interfaces allow patients to interact with a virtual clinician (actually a computer program) that will ask questions, provide social support, and tailor education to identify patient needs based on the answers to screening questions. These human–technology interfaces have been remarkably successful; sometimes patients prefer them to real clinicians!

Human–technology interfaces may present information using text, numbers, pictures, icons, or sound. Auditory, visual—or even tactile—alarms may alert us to important information. We interact with (or control) the technology using keyboards, digital pens, voice activation, or even touch.

A small, but growing number of clinical and educational interfaces rely heavily on tactile input. For example, many students learn to access an intravenous site using virtual technology. Other, more sophisticated virtual reality applications help physicians learn to do endoscopies or practice complex surgical procedures in a safe environment. Still others allow drug researchers to design new medications by combining virtual molecules (here, the tactile response is quite different for molecules that can be joined from those that cannot). In each of these training environments, accurately depicting tactile sensations is critical. For example, feeling the kind and amount of pressure required to penetrate the desired tissues, but not others, is essential to a realistic and effective learning experience.

The growing use of large databases for research has led to the design of novel human–technology interfaces that help researchers visualize and understand patterns in the data that generate new knowledge or lead to new questions. Many of these interfaces now incorporate multidimensional visualizations, in addition to scatter plots, histograms, or cluster representations. Some designers, like Quinn (the founder of the Design Rhythmics Sonification Research Laboratory at the University of New Hampshire) and Meeker (2000), use variations in sound to help researchers hear the patterns in large data sets. In Quinn's (2000) "climate symphony," different musical instruments, tones, pitches, and phrases are mapped onto variables such as the amounts and relative concentrations of minerals to help researchers detect patterns in ice core data covering over 110,000 years. Climate patterns take centuries to emerge and can be difficult to detect. The music allows the entire 110,000 years to be condensed into just a few minutes, making detection of patterns and changes much easier.

The human–technology interface is ubiquitous in health care and takes many forms. Next we will look at the quality of these interfaces, but it isn't always a pretty picture.

THE HUMAN–TECHNOLOGY INTERFACE PROBLEM

In *The Human Factor,* Vicente (2004) cited the many safety problems in health care identified by the Institute of Medicine's (1999) report and how the technology (defined broadly) we use often doesn't fit well with human characteristics. As a case in point, Vicente described his own studies of nurses' PCA pump errors. Nurses made the errors, in large part, because of the complexity of the user interface, which required up to 27 steps to program the device. Vicente and his colleagues developed a PCA in which programming required no more than 12 steps. Nurses who used it in laboratory experiments made fewer errors, programmed drug delivery faster, and reported lower cognitive workloads compared to the commercial device. Further evidence that our human–technology interfaces do not work as well as they might is evident in the following:

- Doyle (2005) reported that when a bar-coding medication system interfered with their workflow, nurses devised **workarounds**, such as removing the armband from the patient and attaching it to the bed because the barcode reader failed to interpret bar codes when the bracelet curved tightly around a small arm.
- Koppel et al. (2005) reported that a widely used computer-based provider order entry (CPOE) system meant to decrease medication errors actually facilitated 22 types of errors because the information needed to order medications was fragmented across as many as 20 screens, available medication dosages differed from those the physicians expected, and allergy alerts were triggered only *after* an order was written.
- Han et al. (2005) reported increased mortality among children admitted to Children's Hospital in Pittsburgh after CPOE implementation. Three reasons were cited for this unexpected outcome: (1) CPOE changed the workflow in the emergency room. Before CPOE, orders were written for critical time-sensitive treatment based on radio communication with the incoming transport team before the child arrived. After CPOE implementation, orders could not be written until the patient arrived and was registered in the system (a policy that was later changed). (2) Entering an order required as many as ten clicks and took as long as 2 minutes; moreover, computer screens sometimes froze or response time was slow. (3) When the team changed its workflow to accommodate CPOE, face-to-face contact among team members diminished. Despite the problems with study methods identified by some of the informatics community, there certainly were serious human–technology interface problems.
- In 2005, a *Washington Post* article reported that Cedars-Sinai Medical Center in Los Angeles had shut down a $34 million system after 3 months due to the medical staff's rebellion. Reasons for the rebellion included the additional time it took to complete the structured information forms, failure of the system to recognize misspellings (as nurses had previously done), and intrusive and in-

terruptive automated alerts (Connolly, 2005). Even though physicians actually responded appropriately to the alerts, modifying or cancelling 35% of the orders that triggered them, designers had not found the right balance of helpful-to-interruptive alerts. The system simply did not fit the clinicians' workflow.

Such unintended consequences (Ash, Berg, & Coiera, 2004) or unpredictable outcomes (Aarts, Doorewaard, & Berg, 2004) of healthcare information systems may be attributed, in part, to a flawed implementation process; but there were clearly **human–technology interaction** issues as well. That is, the technology was not well matched to the users and the context of care. In the pediatric case, a system developed for medical–surgical units was implemented in a critical care unit.

Human–technology interface problems are the major cause of up to 87% of all patient monitoring incidents (Walsh & Beatty, 2002). It is not always that the technology itself is faulty. In fact the technology may perform flawlessly, but the interface design may lead the human user to make errors (Vicente, 2004).

IMPROVING THE HUMAN–TECHNOLOGY INTERFACE

We can learn a lot from the related fields of cognitive engineering, **human factors**, and **ergonomics** about how to make our interfaces more compatible with their human users and the context of care. Each of these areas of study is multidisciplinary and integrates knowledge from multiple disciplines (e.g., computer science, engineering, cognitive engineering, psychology, and sociology). Over the years, the following three axioms have evolved for developing **effective human–computer interactions** (HCIs) (Staggers, 2003):

1. Users must be an early and continuous focus during interface design.
2. The design process should be iterative, allowing for evaluation and correction of identified problems.
3. Formal evaluation should take place using rigorous experimental and/or qualitative methods.

We will discuss each of these in turn.

Axiom 1: Users Must Be an Early and Continuous Focus During Interface Design

Rubin (1994) uses the term *user-centered design* to describe the process of designing products (human–technology interfaces, for example) so that users can carry out the tasks needed to achieve their goals with "minimal effort and maximal efficiency" (p. 10). Thus, in user-centered design, the end user is emphasized.

Vicente (2004) argued that technology should fit human requirements at five levels of analysis (physical, psychological, team, organizational, and political). Physical characteristics of the technology (e.g., size, shape, or location) should conform to the user's size, grasp, and available space). Information should be presented in ways that are consistent with known human psychological capabilities (e.g., the number of items that can be remembered is seven plus or minus two). In addition, systems should conform to the communication, workflow, and authority structures of work teams, as well as to organizational factors such as culture and staffing levels, and even to political factors (e.g., budget constraints, laws, or regulations).

A number of analysis tools and techniques have been developed to help designers better understand the task and user environment for which they are designing. These include the following:

- **Task analysis** examines how a task must be accomplished. Generally, analysts describe the task in terms of inputs needed for the task, outputs (what is achieved by the task), and any constraints on actors' choices on carrying out the task. Analysts then lay out the sequence of temporally ordered actions that must be carried out to complete the task in flow charts (Vicente, 1999). Task analysis is very useful in defining what human workers must do and what functions might be distributed between the worker and technology.
- **Cognitive task analysis (CTA)** usually starts by identifying, through interviews or questionnaires, the particular task and its typicality and frequency. Analysts then may review the written materials that describe the job or are used for training and determine, through structured interviews or observing experts perform the task, what knowledge is involved and how that knowledge might be represented.
- **Cognitive work analysis (CWA)** was developed specifically for the analysis of complex, high technology work domains such as nuclear power plants, intensive care units, or emergency departments where workers need considerable flexibility in responding to external demands (Burns & Hajdukiewicz, 2004; Vicente, 1999). A complete CWA includes five types of analysis: work domain, control tasks, strategies, social-organizational, and worker competencies. The *work domain analysis* describes the functions of the system and what information users need to accomplish task goals. The *control task analysis* investigates the control structures through which the user interacts with or controls the system. The analysis also identifies which variables—and relations among variables—discovered in the work domain analysis are relevant for particular situations so that context-sensitive interfaces can present the right information

(e.g., prompts or alerts) at the right time. The *strategies analysis* looks at how work is actually done by users to facilitate the design of appropriate human–computer dialogues. The *social-organizational analysis* identifies the responsibilities of various users (e.g., doctors, nurses, clerks, or therapists) so that the system can support collaboration, communication, and a viable organizational structure. Finally, the *worker competencies analysis* identifies design constraints related to the users themselves (Effken, 2002). Specialized tools are available for the first three types of analysis (Vicente, 1999). Analysts typically borrow tools (e.g., ethnography) from the social sciences for the two remaining types. Hajdukiewicz, Vicente, Doyle, Milgram, and Burns (2001) used CWA to model an operating room environment. Effken (2002) and Effken, Loeb, Johnson, Johnson, and Reyna (2001) used CWA to analyze the information needs for an oxygenation management display for an ICU. Other examples of the application of CWA in health care are described by Burns and Hajdukiewicz (2004) in their chapter on medical systems (pp. 201–238).

Axiom 2: The Design Process Should Be Iterative, Allowing for Evaluation and Correction of Identified Problems

Today there are available both principles and techniques for developing human–technology interfaces that people will be able to use with minimal stress and maximal efficiency. An excellent place to start is with Norman's (1988, pp. 188–189) principles (in the following list, Norman's own text is italicized):

1. *Use both knowledge in the world and knowledge in the head.* In other words, pay attention not only to the environment or to the user, but to both—and to how they relate. By using both, the problem actually may be simplified.
2. *Simplify the structure of tasks.* For example, reduce the number of steps and/or even computer screens needed to accomplish the goal.
3. *Make things visible: bridge the Gulfs of Execution and Evaluation.* Users need to be able to see how to use the technology to accomplish a goal (for example, what buttons does one press and in which order to program this PCA?); if they do, then designers have bridged the **gulf of execution**. They also need to be able to see the effects of their actions on the technology (e.g., if a nurse practitioner prescribes a drug to treat a certain condition, the actual patient response may not be perfectly clear). This bridges the **gulf of evaluation**.
4. *Get the mappings right.* Here, the term *mapping* is used to describe how environmental facts (such as the order of light switches or variables in a physiologic monitoring display) are accurately depicted by the information presentation.

5. *Exploit the power of constraints, both natural and artificial.* Because of where our eyes are located in our heads, we have to turn our heads to see what is happening behind us; however, that is not true of all animals. As the location of our eyes constrains what we can see, so also physical elements, social factors, and even organizational policy constrains how we accomplish tasks. By taking these constraints into account when designing technology, it can be made easier for humans to use.
6. *Design for error.* Mistakes happen. Technology should eliminate predictable errors and be sufficiently flexible to allow humans to identify and recover from unpredictable errors.
7. *When all else fails, standardize.* To get a feel for this principle, think how difficult it is to change from a Macintosh to a Windows environment or from the Windows operating system to Vista.

Kirlik and Maruyama (2004) described a real-world human–technology interface that follows Norman's principles. The authors observed how a busy expert short-order cook strategy managed to grill many hamburgers at the same time, but each to the customer's desired level of doneness. The cook put those burgers that were to be well-done on the back and far right portion of the grill, those to be medium-well done in the center of the grill, and those to be rare at the front of the grill, but farther to the left. The cook moved all burgers to the left as grilling proceeded and turned them over during their travel across the grill. Everything the cook needed to know was available in this simple interface. As a human–technology interface, the grill layout was elegant. The interface used knowledge housed both in the environment and in the expert cook's head; and things were clearly visible—both in the position of the burgers and the way they were moved. The process was clearly and effectively standardized, and constraints were built in. What might it take to create such an intuitive human–technology interface in health care?

Several useful books have been written about effective interface design (e.g., Burns & Hajdukiewicz, 2004; Cooper, 1995; Mandel, 1997). In addition, there is a growing body of research exploring new ways to present clinical data that might facilitate clinicians' problem identification and accurate treatment. Often designers use graphical objects to show how variables relate. The first to do so were likely Cole and Stewart (1993), who used changes in the lengths of the sides and area of a four-sided object to show the relationship of respiratory rate to tidal volume. Other researchers have demonstrated that histograms and polygon displays are better than numeric displays for detecting changes in patients' physiologic variables (Gurushanthaiah, Weinger, & Englund, 1995). When Horn, Popow, and Unterasinger (2001) presented physiologic data via a single circular object with 12 sectors (where each sector represented a different variable), nurses reported that it was easy to recognize abnormal conditions, but difficult to comprehend the patient's overall status. This kind of graphical object approach has been most widely utilized in anesthesiology, where a number of researchers have shown improved clinician **situational awareness** or problem detection time by mapping physiologic variables onto display objects that have meaningful shapes, for example, using a bellows-like object to represent ventilation (e.g., Agutter et al., 2003; Blike, Surgenor, Whallen, & Jensen, 2000; Michels, Gravenstein, & Westenskow, 1997; Zhang et al., 2002).

Effken (2006) compared a prototype display that represented physiological data in a structured pictorial format with two bar graph displays. The first bar graph display and the prototype both presented data in the order that experts were observed to use them. The second bar graph display presented the data in the way that nurses collected them. In an experiment in which resident physicians and novice nurses used simulated drugs to treat observed oxygenation management problems using each display, residents' performance was improved with the displays ordered as experts used them, but nurses' performance was not improved. Nurses performed better when the variables were ordered as they were used to collecting them, demonstrating the importance of understanding user roles and the tasks they need to accomplish.

But data need not only be represented visually. Gaver (1993) proposed that because ordinary sounds map onto familiar events, they could be used as icons to facilitate easier technology navigation and use and also to provide continuous background information about how a system is functioning. In health care, auditory displays have been used to provide clinicians with information about patients' vital signs (e.g., in pulse oximetry), for example, by changing in volume or tone when there is a significant change (Sanderson, 2006).

Admittedly, auditory displays are probably more useful for quieter areas of the hospital, such as the operating room. Perhaps that is why researchers have most frequently applied the approach in anesthesiology. For example, Loeb and Fitch (2002) reported that anesthesiologists detected critical events more quickly when auditory information about heart rate, blood pressure, and respiratory parameters was added to a visual display. Auditory tones also have been combined as "earcons" to represent relationships among data elements, for example, the relationship of systolic to diastolic blood pressure (Watson & Gill, 2004).

Axiom 3: Formal Evaluation Should Take Place Using Rigorous Experimental and/or Qualitative Methods

Perhaps one of the highest accolades that any interface can achieve is that it is transparent. An interface becomes transparent when it is so easy to use that users no longer think about it, but only about the task at hand. For example, a transparent

FIGURE 5-1
Nurse–patient interaction framework in which the technology supports the interaction.

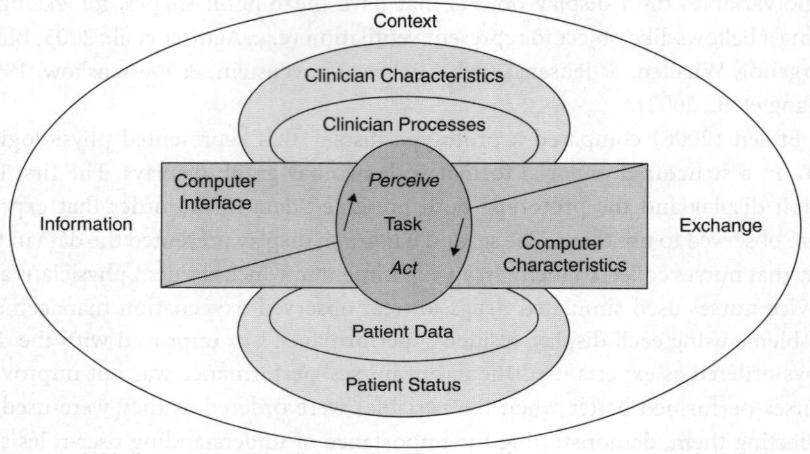

SOURCE: Adapted from Staggers, N. & Parks, P. L. (1993). Description and initial applications of the Staggers & Parks nurse–computer interaction framework. *Computers in Nursing, 11,* 282–290.

clinical interface would enable clinicians to focus on patient decisions rather than on how to access or combine patient data from multiple sources. In Figure 5-1, instead of the nurse interacting with the computer, the nurse and patient interact through the technology interface. The more transparent the interface, the easier the interaction should be.

Usability is a term that denotes the ease with which people can use an interface to achieve a particular goal. Usability of a new human–technology interface needs to be evaluated early and often throughout its development. Typical usability indicators include ease of use, ease of learning, satisfaction with using, efficiency of use, error tolerance, and fit of the system to the task (Staggers, 2003). Some of the more commonly used approaches to usability evaluation are:

- *Surveys of Potential or Actual Users.* Chernecky, Macklin, and Waller (2006) assessed cancer patients' preferences for Web site design. Participants were asked their preferences for a number of design characteristics such as display color, menu buttons, text, photo size, icon metaphor, and layout by selecting, on a computer screen, their preferences for each item from two or three options.

- *Focus Group.* Typically used at the very start of the design process, focus groups can help the designer better understand users' responses to potential interface designs as well as to content that might be included in the interface.
- *Cognitive Walkthrough.* In a **cognitive walkthrough**, evaluators assess a paper mock-up, working prototype, or completed interface by observing the steps users are likely to take to use the interface to accomplish typical tasks. The analysis helps designers determine how understandable and easy to learn the interface is likely to be for these users and the typical tasks (Wharton, Rieman, Lewis, & Polson, 1994).
- *Heuristic Evaluation.* A **heuristic evaluation** has become the most popular of what are called "discount usability evaluation" methods. The objective of a heuristic evaluation is to detect problems early in the design process when they can be most easily and economically corrected. The methods are termed *discount* because they typically are easy to do, involve fewer than 10 experts (often expert in relevant fields such as human computer technology [HCT] or cognitive engineering), and are therefore much less expensive than other methods. They are called *heuristic* because evaluators assess the degree to which the design complies with recognized usability rules of thumb or principles (the heuristics), such as those proposed by Nielsen (1994) and available on his Web site (http://www.useit.com/papers/heuristic/heuristic_list.html). For example, McDaniel and colleagues (2002) conducted a usability test of an interactive computer-based program to encourage smoking cessation by low-income women. As part of the initial evaluation, healthcare professionals familiar with intended users reviewed the design and layout of the program. The usability test revealed several problems with the decision rules used to tailor content to users that were corrected prior to implementation.
- *Formal Usability Test.* Formal usability tests typically use either experimental or observational studies of actual users using the interface to accomplish real-world tasks. A number of researchers use these methods. For example, Staggers, Kobus, and Brown (2007) conducted a usability study of a prototype electronic medication administration record. Participants were asked to add, modify, or discontinue medications using the system. The time they needed to complete the task, their accuracy in the task, and their satisfaction with the prototype were assessed (the latter through a questionnaire). Although satisfaction was high, the evaluation also revealed design flaws that could be corrected before implementation.
- *Field Study.* In a **field study**, end users evaluate a prototype in the actual work setting just prior to its general release. For example, Thompson, Lozano, and Christakis (2007) evaluated the use of touch screen computer kiosks containing

child health-promoting information in several low-income, urban community settings using an online questionnaire that could be completed after the kiosk was used. Most users found the kiosk easy to use and the information it provided easy to understand. Researchers also gained a better understanding of the characteristics of the likely users (e.g., 26% had never used the Internet and 48% had less than a high school education), as well as the information most often accessed (television/media use and smoke exposure).

Dykes and her colleagues (2006) used a field test to investigate the feasibility of using digital pen and paper technology to record vital signs as a way to bridge an organization from a paper to an electronic health record. In general, satisfaction with the tool increased with use; and the devices conformed well to nurses' workflow. However, 8% of the vital sign entries were recorded inaccurately because of inaccurate handwriting recognition, entries outside the recording box, or inaccurate data entry (data entered were not valid values). The number of modifications needed in the tool and the time that would be required to make them ruled out using the digital pen and paper as a bridging technology.

FUTURE OF THE HUMAN–TECHNOLOGY INTERFACE

Increased attention to improving the human–technology interface through human factors approaches has already led to significant improvement in one area of health care—anesthesiology. Anesthesia machines that used to have hoses that would fit into any delivery port now have hoses that can only be plugged into the proper port. Anesthesiologists have also been actively working with engineers to improve the computer interface through which they monitor their patients' status and are among the leaders in investigating the use of audio techniques as an alternative way to help anesthesiologists stay situationally aware. As a result, anesthesia-related deaths dropped from 2 in 20,000 to 1 in 200,000 in under 10 years (Vicente, 2004). We can hope that continued emphasis on the human factor (Vicente, 2004) and user-centered design (Rubin, 1994) by informatics professionals and HCI experts will be equally successful in other parts of the healthcare system. The increased amount of informatics research in this area is encouraging, but there is a long way to go.

SUMMARY

There are at least three messages that I hope you will take away from this discussion: First, if we are to significantly improve quality and safety outcomes in this country through the use of information technology, the designs for human–technology interfaces must be radically improved so that the technology better fits human and task requirements. Second, a number of useful tools are currently available for the analysis, design, and evaluation phases of development life cycles and should be used routinely by informatics professionals to ensure that technology better fits both task and user requirements. Finally, focusing on interface improvement using these tools has had a huge impact on patient safety in one area of health care—anesthesiology. With increased attention from informatics professionals and engineers, the same kind of improvement should be possible in other areas.

THOUGHT-PROVOKING Questions

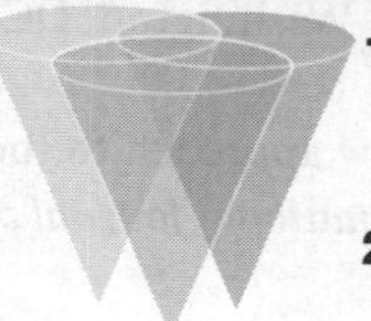

1. You are a member of a team that has been asked to evaluate a prototype PDA-based application for calculating drug dosages. Based on what you know about usability testing, what kind of test (or tests) might you do and why?
2. Is there a human–technology interface that you have encountered that you think needs improving? If you were to design a replacement, what of the analysis techniques that you read about would you choose? Why?

References

Aarts, J., Doorewaard, H., & Berg, M. (2004). Understanding implementation: The case of a computerized physician order entry system in a large Dutch university medical center. *Journal of the American Medical Association, 11*, 207–216.

Agutter, J., Drews, F., Syroid, N., Westneskow, D., Albert, R., Strayer, D., et al. (2003). Evaluation of graphic cardiovascular display in a high-fidelity simulator. *Anesthesia and Analgesia, 97,* 1403–1413.

Ash, J. S., Berg, M., & Coiera, E. (2004). Some unintended consequences of information technology in health care: The nature of patient care information system-related errors. *Journal of the American Medical Informatics Association, 11,* 104–112.

Blike, G. T., Surgenor, S. D., Whallen, K., & Jensen, J. (2000). Specific elements of a new hemodynamics display improves the performance of anesthesiologists. *Journal of Clinical Monitoring & Computing, 16,* 485–491.

Burns, C. M., & Hajdukiewicz, J. R. (2004). *Ecological interface design.* Boca Raton, FL: CRC Press.

Chernecky, C., Macklin, D., & Waller, J. (2006). Internet design preferences of patients with cancer. *Oncology Nursing Forum, 33,* 787–792.

Cole, W. G., & Stewart, J. G. (1993). Metaphor graphics to support integrated decision making with respiratory data. *International Journal of Clinical Monitoring and Computing, 10,* 91–100.

Connolly, C. (2005, March 21). Cedars-Sinai doctors cling to pen and paper. *Washington Post*, p. A01.

Cooper, A. (1995). *About face: Essentials of window interface design.* New York: Hungry Minds, Inc.

Doyle, M. (2005). *Impact of the Bar Code Medication Administration (BCMA) system on medication administration errors.* Unpublished doctoral dissertation, University of Arizona, Tucson.

Dykes, P. C., Benoit, A., Chang, F., Gallagher, J., Li, Q., et al. (2006). The feasibility of digital pen and paper technology for vital sign data capture in acute care settings. In *AMIA 2006 Symposium Proceedings* (pp. 229–233). Washington, DC: American Medical Informatics Association.

Effken, J. A. (2002). Different lenses, improved outcomes: A new approach to the analysis and design of healthcare information systems. *International Journal of Medical Informatics, 65*, 59–74.

Effken, J. A. (2006). Improving clinical decision making through ecological interfaces. *Ecological Psychology, 18*(4), 283–318.

Effken, J., Loeb, R., Johnson, K., Johnson, S., & Reyna, V. (2001). Using cognitive work analysis to design clinical displays. In V. L. Patel, R. Rogers, & R. Haux (Eds.). *Proceedings of MedInfo-2001* (pp. 27–31). London: IOS Press.

Gaver, W. W. (1993). What in the world do we hear? An ecological approach to auditory event perception. *Ecological Psychology, 5*, 1–30.

Gurushanthaiah, K. I., Weinger, M. B., & Englund, C. E. (1995). Visual display format affects the ability of anesthesiologists to detect acute physiologic changes: A laboratory study employing a clinical display simulator. *Anesthesiology, 83*, 1184–1193.

Hajdukiewicz, J. R., Vicente, K. J., Doyle, D. J., Milgram, P., & Burns, C. M. (2001). Modeling a medical environment: An ontology for integrated medical informatics design. *International Journal of Medical Informatics, 62*, 79–99.

Han, Y. Y., Carcillo, J. A., Venkataraman, S. T., Clark, R. S. B., Watson, R. S., Nguyen, T. C., et al. (2005). Unexpected increased mortality after implementation of a commercially sold computerized physician order entry system. *Pediatrics, 116*, 1506–1512.

Horn, W., Popow, C., & Unterasinger, L. (2001). Support for fast comprehension of ICU data: Visualization using metaphor graphics. *Methods in Informatics Medicine, 40*, 421–424.

Institute of Medicine. (1999). *To err is human: Building a safer health system.* Washington, DC: Institute of Medicine.

Kirlik, A., & Maruyama, S. (2004). Human–technology interaction and music perception and performance: Toward the robust design of sociotechnical systems. *Proceedings of the IEEE, 92*(4), 616–631.

Koppel, R., Metlay, J. P., Cohen, A., Abaluck, B., Localio, A. R., Kimmel, S. E., et al. (2005). Role of computerized physician order entry systems in facilitating medication errors. *Journal of the American Medical Association, 293*(10), 1197–1203.

Loeb, R. G., & Fitch, W. T. (2002). A laboratory evaluation of an auditory display designed to enhance intraoperative monitoring. *Anesthesia and Analgesia, 94*, 362–368.

Mandel, T. (1997). *The elements of user interface design.* New York: John Wiley & Sons.

McDaniel, A., Hutchinson, S., Casper, G. R., Ford, R. T., Stratton, R., & Rembush, M. (2002). Usability testing and outcomes of an interactive computer program to promote smoking cessation in low income women. In *Proceedings AMIA 2002* (pp. 509–513). Washington, DC: American Medical Informatics Association.

Michels, P., Gravenstein, D., & Westenskow, D. R. (1997). An integrated graphic data display improves detection and identification of critical events during anesthesia. *Journal of Clinical Monitoring & Computing, 13*, 249–259.

Nielsen, J. (1994). Heuristic evaluation. In J. Nielsen & R. L. Mack (Eds.), *Usability inspection methods* (pp. 25–62). New York: John Wiley & Sons.

Norman, D. A. (1988). *The psychology of everyday things.* New York: Basic Books.

Quinn, M. (2000). *The climate symphony: Rhythmic techniques applied to the sonification of ice core data.* Retrieved September 21, 2007, from http://www.bcca.org/ief/dquin00c.htm

Quinn, M., & Meeker, L. (2000). *Research set to music: The climate symphony and other sonifications of ice core, radar, DNA, seismic and solar wind data.* Retrieved March 17, 2008, from http://www.drsrl.com/climate_paper.html

Rubin, J. (1994). *Handbook of usability testing: How to plan, design, and conduct effective tests.* New York: Wiley & Sons.

Sanderson, P. (2006). The multimodal world of medical monitoring displays. *Applied Ergonomics, 37*, 501–512.

Staggers, N. (2003). Human factors: Imperative concepts for information systems in critical care. *AACN Clinical Issues, 14*(3), 310–319.

Staggers, N. & Parks, P. L. (1993). Description and initial applications of the Staggers & Parks nurse–computer interaction framework. *Computers in Nursing, 11*, 282–290.

Staggers, N., Kobus, D., & Brown, C. (2007). Nurses' evaluations of a novel design for an electronic medication administration record. *CIN: Computers, Informatics, Nursing, 25*(2), 67–75.

Thompson, D. A., Lozano, P., & Christakis, D. A. (2007). Parent use of touchscreen computer kiosks for child health promotion in community settings. *Pediatrics, 119*(3), 427–434.

Vicente, K. (2004). *The human factor.* New York: Routledge.

Vicente, K. J. (1999). *Cognitive work analysis: Toward safe, productive, and healthy computer-based work.* Mahwah, NJ: Lawrence Erlbaum Associates.

Walsh, T., & Beatty, P. C. W. (2002). Human factor error and patient monitoring. *Physiological Measurement, 23,* R111–R132.

Watson, G., & Gill, T. (2004). Earcon for intermittent information in monitoring environments. In *Proceedings of the 2004 Conference of the Computer-Human Interaction Special Interest Group of the Human Factors and Ergonomics Society of Australia (OzCHI2004)*, Wollonggong, New South Wales, 22–24 November.

Wharton, C., Rieman, J., Lewis, C., & Polson, P. (1994). The cognitive walk-through: A practitioner's guide. In J. Nielsen & R. L. Mack (Eds.), *Usability inspection methods* (pp. 105–139). New York: John Wiley & Sons, Inc.

Zhang, Y., Drews, F. A., Westenskow, D. R., Foresti, S., Agutter, J., et al. (2002). Effects of integrated graphical displays on situation awareness in anaesthesiology. *Cognition, Technology & Work, 4,* 82–90.

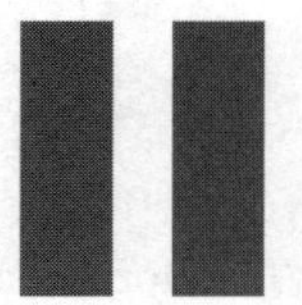

section

Perspectives on Nursing Informatics

Nursing informatics (NI) is the synthesis of nursing science, information science, computer science, and cognitive science to manage and enhance the healthcare data, information, knowledge, and wisdom for the dual betterment of patient care and the nursing profession. In Section I you learned about the four sciences of NI, also referred to as the four building blocks. Nursing knowledge workers must be able to understand the evolving specialty, nursing informatics, in order to begin to harness and use the tools available for managing the vast amount of healthcare data and information. It is essential that nursing informatics capabilities be appreciated, promoted, expanded, and advanced to facilitate the work of the nurse, improve patient care, and enhance the nursing profession.

Section II presents the perspectives of nursing experts on nursing informatics. Chapter 6 is an overview of nursing informatics, and in Chapter 7, you will learn about the development of standardized terminologies in nursing informatics. Chapter 8 is where nursing informatics roles, competencies, and skills are explored, and Section II concludes with Chapter 9 reviewing the information and knowledge needs of nurses in the 21st century. While some of the information presented by our expert contributing authors may seem duplicated in the chapters, we believe that it is important to expose you to the various perspectives about NI as they are provided by our contributors.

In the overview of nursing informatics (NI), interrelationships among major NI concepts are discussed. As data are transformed into information and information into knowledge, increasing complexity and interrelationships ensue. The boundaries between concepts can be blurred, and feedback loops from one concept level to another occur. Structured languages and human–computer interaction

(HCI) concepts, which are critical elements for NI, are noted. Taxonomies and other current structured languages for nursing are listed. HCI concepts are briefly defined and discussed because they are critical to the success of informatics solutions. Last and importantly, the construct of decision making is added to the traditional nursing metaparadigms: nurse, person, health, and environment. Decision making is not only at the crux of nursing practice in all settings and roles; it is a fundamental concern of NI. Nursing's work is centered in the concepts of NI: data, information, knowledge, and wisdom. Information technology per se is not the focus; it is the information that the technology conveys that is central. Nursing informatics is no longer the domain of experts in the field. More interestingly, one does not need technology to be performing informatics. The centerpiece of informatics is the manipulation of data, information, and knowledge, especially related to the decision making in any aspect of nursing or in any setting. In a way, we are all already informatics nurses.

In Chapter 7, Developing Standardized Terminologies in Nursing Informatics, different approaches to terminology development are discussed. Standardized nursing terminologies (and the structures and systems that support their implementation and use) are merely a means to an end; they do not obviate the need to think and work creatively, to do right by the people in our care, and to continue to advance nursing.

Chapter 8, Nursing Informatics Roles, Competencies, and Skills, discusses NI as a relatively new nursing specialty that combines the building block sciences covered in Section I. Combining these sciences results in nurses being able to effectively and safely care for their patients as the information that they need is readily available. Nurses have been actively involved in NI since computers were introduced into health care. With the advent of electronic health records (EHRs), it became apparent that nursing needed to develop its own language. NI was instrumental in assisting in the nursing language development. The healthcare industry employs the largest number of knowledge workers. This is resulting in the realization that healthcare administrators must begin to change the way that they look at their employees. The nurses and physicians are bright, highly skilled, and dedicated to giving the best patient care. Administrators who tap into this wealth of knowledge will find that the patients' care will become safer and more efficient. NI is a specialty that is governed by the standards that have been established by the American Nurses Association (ANA) and is a very diverse field that results in many nurse informaticist specialists (NISs) becoming focused on one segment of NI. Although NI is a recognized specialty area of practice, all nurses will be expected to have some knowledge of the field. Nursing informatics competencies have been developed to ensure that all entry level nurses will be ready to enter a field that is becoming more technologically advanced. The competencies may also be used to determine the educational needs of currently practicing nurses. Nurse informatics specialists no longer have to enter the field as a result of on-the-job exposure, but can now obtain an advanced degree in NI at many well-established universities throughout the country. NI has grown tremendously as a specialty since its inception and is predicted to continue growing.

Chapter 9, Information and Knowledge Needs of Nurses in the 21st Century, states that the core concepts and competencies of informatics are particularly well suited to a model of interprofessional education. Ideally, when emulating clinical settings, informatics knowledge should be integrated with the processes of interprofessional teams and decision making. As simulation laboratories are becoming increasingly common fixtures in the delivery of health-related professional education, they provide a perfect opportunity to incorporate the EHR applications. The learning laboratory for nursing education will then more closely approximate the information technology-enabled clinical settings that are emerging. A presumption is often made that future graduates will be more computer literate than nurses currently in practice. Although this may be true, computer literacy or comfort does not equate to an understanding of the facilitative and transformative role of information technology. It is essential that the future curricula of basic nursing programs embed the concepts of the role of information technology in supporting clinical care delivery. A majority of nurses have yet to embrace the notion of informatics and understand its meaning and relevance to their work. There is an emerging global focus on information technology to support clinical care and on the potential benefits for clinicians and patients. Anticipate that in the future, we will have the computing power to aggregate and transform additional multidimensional data and information sources (e.g., historical, multisensory, experiential, genetic) into a clinical information system (CIS) to engage with individuals, families, and groups in ways not yet imagined. Every nurse's practice will make contributions to new nursing knowledge in these dynamically interactive CIS environments. Afforded with the right tools to support the management of data, complex information processing and ready access to knowledge, the core concepts and competencies associated with informatics will be embedded in the practice of every nurse, whether administrator, researcher, educator, or practitioner. Information technology is not a panacea, but it will provide the profession with unprecedented capacity to more rapidly generate and disseminate new knowledge.

As you are aware, the material within this book is placed within the context of the Foundation of Knowledge model (Figure II-1) to meet healthcare delivery systems', organizations', patients', and nurses' needs. Through our involvement in nursing informatics and learning about this evolving specialty, we will be able to

FIGURE II-1
Foundation of Knowledge model. (Designed by Alicia Mastrian.)

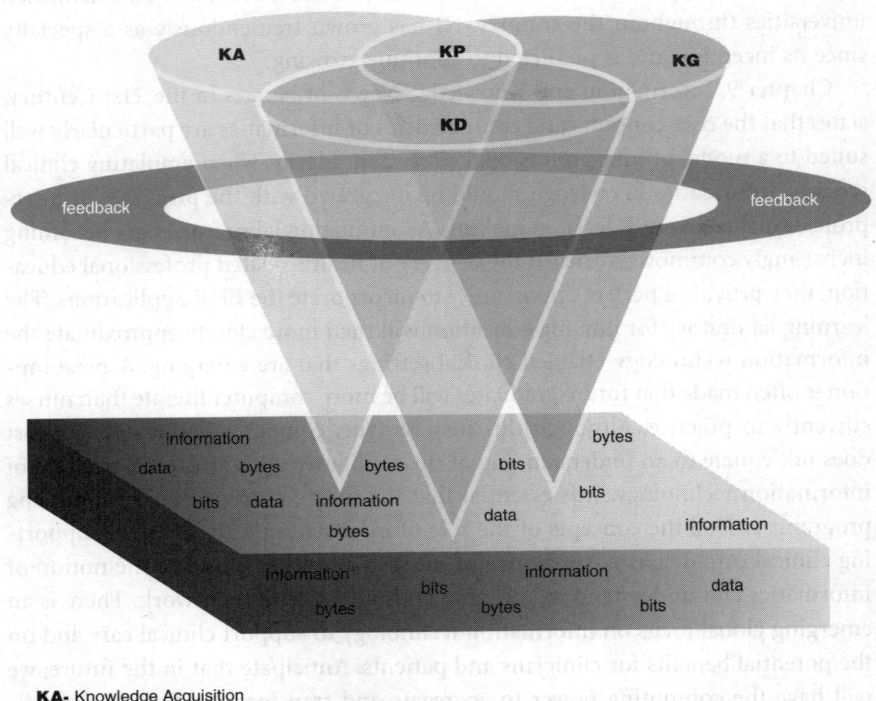

use the current theories, architecture, and tools, while beginning to challenge what is known. This questioning and search for what could be will provide the basis for the future landscape of nursing. We have attempted to capture this process in the Foundation of Knowledge model used as an organizing framework for this text. In this section, you will learn about nursing informatics. If you are beginning your education, you will consciously focus on input and knowledge acquisition, trying to glean as much information and knowledge as possible. As you become more comfortable in your clinical setting and with nursing science, you will begin to take over some of the other knowledge functions. Experienced nurses, also known as seasoned nurses, question what is known and search for ways to enhance their knowledge and the knowledge of others. What is not available must be created. It is through these leaders, researchers, or clinicians that new knowledge is generated and disseminated and nursing science advanced. Sometimes, however, in order to keep up with the explosion of information in nursing and health care, we must continue to rely on the knowledge generation and dissemination of others. In this sense, we are committed to lifelong learning and the use of knowledge in the practice of nursing science. How you interact within your environment and apply what you learn will depend on your placement in the Foundation of Knowledge model. Where do you currently function?

As you read through this section, we challenge you to ask yourself, how can I:

- apply the knowledge I gain from my practice setting to benefit my patients and enhance my practice?
- help my colleagues and patients understand and use the current technology that is available?
- use my wisdom to help create the theories, tools, and knowledge of the future?

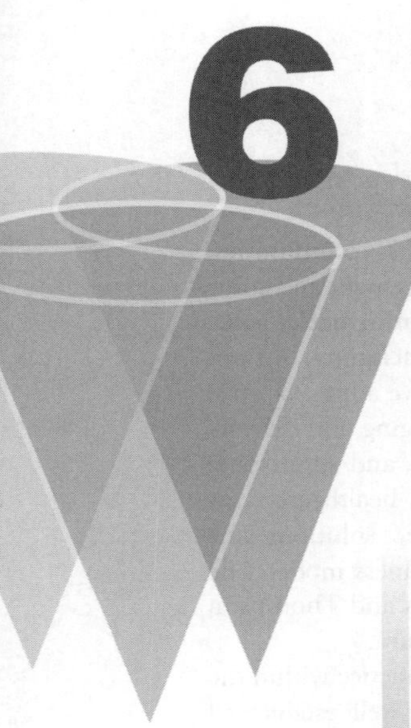

6 Overview of Nursing Informatics

Nancy Staggers and Ramona Nelson

Objectives

1. Define nursing informatics (NI) and key terminology
2. Explore NI metastructures, concepts, and tools
3. Reflect on the sciences underpinning NI
4. Describe phenomena of nursing

Key Terms

Decision support system
Ergonomics
Expert system
Human–computer interaction
Informatics nurse
Informatics nurse specialist
Informatics solution
Information
Knowledge
Nanotechnology
Nursing informatics (NI)
Usability
Wisdom

INTRODUCTION

The foundations of nursing informatics exactly underpin the topic of **knowledge** generation in nursing. As will be seen, **nursing informatics (NI)** centers on the concepts of data, **information**, knowledge, and **wisdom**. More to the point, nurses in all settings and areas of practice are considered knowledge workers. These salient concepts are described in this chapter in more detail.

The following pages were crafted by a panel of NI experts as they revised the metastructures portion of the American Nurses Association's *Scope and Standards for Nursing Informatics Practice* during 2005–2007.[1,2]

> Nursing informatics (NI) is a specialty that integrates nursing science, computer science, and information science to manage and communicate data, information, knowledge and wisdom in nursing practice. NI supports consumers, patients, nurses, and other providers in their decision-making in all roles and settings. This

[1]Acknowledgment: The authors would like to thank Paulette Fraser, MS, RN, BC, for her work as coleader of the metastructures section of the American Nurses Association's 2007 revision of the *Scope and Standards for Nursing Informatics Practice.*

[2]The following passage is reprinted with permission of the American Nurses Association. Boldface type has been applied to key terms, and figure and table numbers have been changed to correspond to this chapter.

support is accomplished through the use of information structures, information processes, and information technology.

The goal of NI is to improve the health of populations, communities, families, and individuals by optimizing information management and communication. These activities include the design and use of **informatics solutions** and/or technology to support all areas of nursing, including, but not limited to, the direct provision of care, establishing effective administrative systems, designing useful decision support systems, managing and delivering educational experiences, enhancing life-long learning, and supporting nursing research. The term individuals refer to patients, healthcare consumers and any other recipient of nursing care or informatics solutions. The term patient refers to consumers in both a wellness and illness model. The definition and goal of NI is based upon work by Staggers and Thompson (2002) and evolved in 2007 to include the concept of wisdom.

NI is one example of a discipline-specific informatics practice within the broader category of health informatics. NI has become well established within nursing since its recognition as a specialty for registered nurses by the American Nurses Association (ANA) in 1992. It focuses on the representation of nursing data, information, knowledge (Graves & Corcoran, 1989) and wisdom (Nelson & Joos, 1989) as well as the management and communication of nursing information within the broader context of health informatics. Nursing informatics (1) provides a nursing perspective, (2) illuminates nursing values and beliefs, (3) denotes a practice base for nurses in NI, (4) produces unique knowledge, (5) distinguishes groups of practitioners, (6) focuses on the phenomena of interest for nursing, and (7) provides needed nursing language and word context (Brennan, 2003) to health informatics.

METASTRUCTURES, CONCEPTS, AND TOOLS OF NURSING INFORMATICS

To understand NI, its metastructures, sciences, concepts and tools are first explained. Metastructures are overarching concepts used in theory and science. Also of interest are the sciences underpinning NI, concepts and tools from information science and computer science, human–computer interaction and ergonomics concepts, and the phenomena of nursing.

Metastructures: Data, Information, and Knowledge

In the mid 1980's Blum (1986) introduced the concepts of data, information and knowledge as a framework for understanding clinical information systems and their impact on health care. He did this by classifying the then current clinical information systems by the three types of objects that these systems processed. These were data, information and knowledge. He noted that the classification was artificial with no clear boundaries; however, increasing complexity between the concepts existed. In 1989, Graves and Corcoran

FIGURE 6-1
Conceptual framework for the study of nursing knowledge.

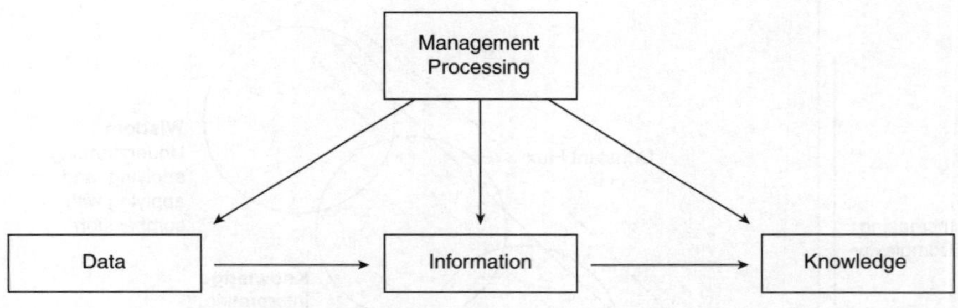

built on this work when they published their seminal work that described the study of nursing informatics using the concepts of data, information and knowledge. The article contributed two broad principles to NI that will be acknowledged here. The first contribution was a definition of NI that has been widely accepted in the field.

The second contribution of Graves and Corcoran (1989) was an information model that identified data, information, and knowledge as key components of NI practice. The Graves model is presented in Figure 6-1.

Graves and Corcoran (1989) drew from Blum (1986) to define the three concepts as follows:

- Data are discrete entities that are described objectively without interpretation,
- Information is data that are interpreted, organized, or structured, and
- Knowledge is information that is synthesized so that relationships are identified and formalized.

Data, which are processed to information and then knowledge, may be obtained from individuals, families, communities, and populations. Data, information, and knowledge are of concern to nurses in all areas of practice. For example, data derived from direct care of an individual may then be compiled across persons and aggregated for decision-making by nurses, nurse administrators, or other health professionals. Further aggregation may address communities and populations. Nurse-educators may create case studies using these data, and nurse-researchers may access aggregated data for systematic study.

As an example, an instance of vital signs for an individual—heart rate, respiration, temperature, and blood pressure—can be considered (a set of) data. A serial set of vital signs taken over time, placed into a context, and used for longitudinal comparisons is considered information. That is, a dropping blood pressure, increasing heart rate, respiratory rate, and fever in

FIGURE 6-2
The relationship of data, information, knowledge, and wisdom.

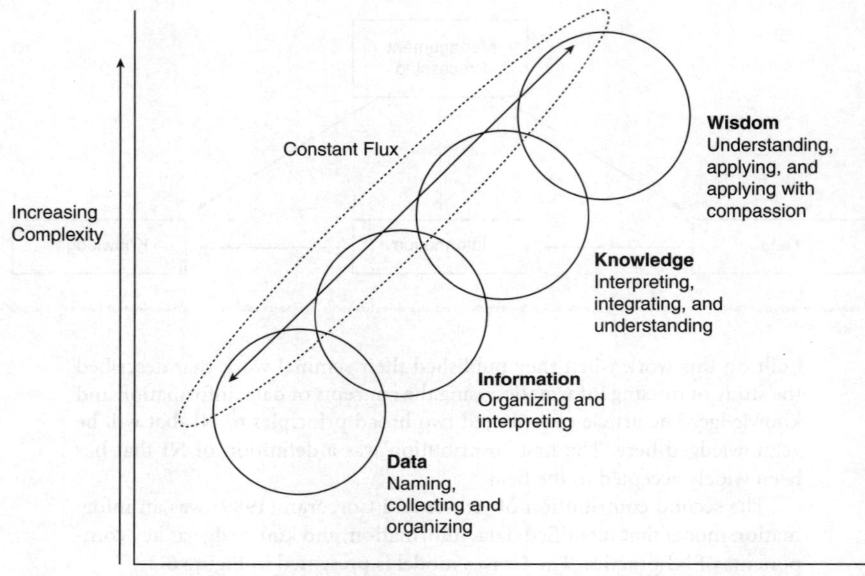

SOURCE: Reprinted with modification from Englebardt, S. & Nelson, R. (2002). *Health care informatics: An interdisciplinary approach* (Figure 1-4, page 13). St. Louis, MO: Elsevier, Reprinted with permission from Elsevier.

an elderly, catheterized person are recognized as being abnormal for this person. The recognition that the person may be septic and, therefore may need certain nursing interventions reflects information synthesis (knowledge) based on nursing knowledge and experience.

Figure 6-2 builds on the work of Graves and Corcoran by providing a depiction of the relationship of data, information, and knowledge. As data are transformed into information and information into knowledge, each level increases in complexity and requires greater application of human intellect. The X-axis in Figure 6-2 represents interactions within and between the concepts as one moves from data to wisdom; the Y-axis represents the increasing complexity of the concepts' increasing interrelationships.

Wisdom is defined as the appropriate use of knowledge to manage and solve human problems. It is knowing when and how to apply knowledge to deal with complex problems or specific human need (Nelson & Joos, 1989; Nelson, 2002). While knowledge focuses on what is known; wisdom focuses on the appropriate application of that knowledge. For example, a knowledge base may include several options for managing an anxious family, while wisdom would guide the decisions about which of these options are most appropriate with a specific family. As this example demonstrates the scope of NI is based on the scope of nursing practice and nursing science with a concentration on data, information and knowledge. It is not limited by the current technology. If the study of NI was limited to what the computer can process, the study of informatics could not fully appreciate the interrelationships that exist between nursing science/practice and information science/technology. NI must consider how nurses impact the technology and how the technology impacts nursing. An understanding of this interaction makes it possible to understand how nurses create knowledge and how they make use of that knowledge in their practices.

The appropriate use of knowledge involves the integration of empirical, ethical, personal and aesthetic knowledge in the process of implementing actions. The individual must apply a high level of empirical knowledge in understanding the current situation; apply a professional value system in considering possible actions, be able to predict the potential outcome of these actions with a high level of accuracy, and then to have the will power to carry out the selected action in the current environment. An example of applied wisdom demonstrating this integration in NI is the appropriate use of information management and technological tools to support effective nursing practice.

The addition of wisdom raises new and important research questions. This challenges the discipline to develop tools and processes for classifying, measuring and coding wisdom as it relates to nursing, NI and informatics education. These research avenues will help clarify the relationships between wisdom and the intuitive thinking of expert nurses. Such research will be invaluable in building information systems to support expert healthcare practitioners as well as support the decision process of more novice nurses.

Two interrelated forces have encouraged the expansion of the NI model to include wisdom. First, the initial work was limited to the types of objects processed by automated systems in the mid-1980s. However, NI is now concerned with the use of information technology to improve the access and quality of health care that is delivered to individuals, families and communities. The addition of the concept of wisdom expands the focus of the model from the technology and the processing of objects to include the interaction of the human with the technology and resultant outcome(s).

Nurses have been recognized as primary processors of information for over 40 years (Jydstrup & Gross, 1966; Zielstroff, 1981). Other authors have focused on the amount of time nurses actually spend administering direct care to patients or the time involved in documentation (Norrie, 1999; Jinks, 2000; Harrison, 2002). In fact, Jydstrup and Gross (1966) estimated in the 1960s that nurses in acute care spent 30 to 40% of their time in information processing activities. In her frequently cited article, titled, “How do nurses spend their time?” Hendrickson (1990) determined that nurses spend only 31% of their time with patients. Other aspects of the nursing role included information management with ancillary services.

Sciences Underpinning Nursing Informatics

A significant contribution of Graves and Corcoran (1989) was a description and definition of nursing informatics (NI) that was widely accepted in the field in the 1990's. It stated that NI is a combination of nursing science, information science, and computer science to manage and process nursing data, information, and knowledge to facilitate the delivery of health care. The central notion was that the application of these three core sciences was what made NI unique and differentiated it from other informatics specialties.

In addition to these three core sciences, other sciences may be required to solve informatics issues. James Turley expanded the model of NI to include cognitive science (1996). Certainly the cognitive aspect of humans is a critical piece for INSs and for INs to understand. However, other sciences may be equally as critical depending upon the issue at hand. For example, if the INS is dealing with a system's implementation in an institution, an understanding of organizational theory may be germane to successful implementation (Staggers & Thompson, 2002). As science evolves, it may be necessary to include other core sciences in future models.

Although the core sciences are foundational to the work in NI, the practice of the specialty is considered an applied science rather than a basic science. The combination of sciences creates a unique blend that is greater than the sum of its parts, a unique combination that creates the definitive specialty of NI. Further, informatics realizes its full potential within health care when it is grounded within a discipline; in this case, the discipline is nursing. Computer and information science applied in isolation will have less impact if not applied within a disciplinary framework. Through application, the science of informatics can solve critical health care issues of concern to a particular discipline.

Structured Language as a Tool for Nursing Informatics

Many of the tools used by the **informatics nurse** and **informatics nurse specialist** are based on metastructures and concepts that incorporate knowledge from nursing and other health and information sciences. Nursing knowledge is gained by the ability to extract data that specifically defines nursing phenomena. Many different languages and ways of organizing data, information and knowledge exist based on different concepts.

The creation of nursing taxonomies and nomenclatures has occurred over the past years allowing these iterations to occur. The ANA has formalized the recognition of these languages/vocabularies through a review process of the Committee on Nursing Practice Information Infrastructure (CNPII). For more information, see Table 6-1 and http://nursingworld.org/ npii/terminologies.htm. To promote the integration of standardized terminologies within information technology solutions, the ANA's Nursing Information and Data Set Evaluation Center (NIDSEC) conducts the following activities:

TABLE 6-1
ANA Recognized Terminologies and Data Element Sets

Program	Setting Where Developed	Content
Data Element Sets		
1. NMDS Nursing minimum data set currently recognized	All nursing	Clinical data elements
2. NMMDS Nursing management minimum data set currently recognized	All settings	Nursing administrative data elements
Interface Terminologies		
3. CCC Clinical care classification currently recognized	All nursing care	Diagnoses, interventions, and outcomes
4. ICNP International classification of nursing practice currently recognized	All nursing	Diagnoses, interventions, and outcomes
5. NANDA [North American Nursing Diagnosis Association] NANDA International currently recognized	All nursing	Diagnoses
6. NIC Nursing intervention classification currently recognized	All nursing	Interventions
7. NOC Nursing outcome classification currently recognized	All nursing	Outcomes
8. OMAHA system Omaha system currently recognized	Home care, public health, and community	Diagnoses, interventions, and outcomes
9. PCDS Patient care data set retired	Acute care	Diagnoses, interventions, and outcomes
10. PNDS Perioperative nursing data set currently recognized	Perioperative	Diagnoses, interventions, and outcomes
Multidisciplinary Terminologies		
11. ABC Alternative billing codes currently recognized	Nursing and other	Interventions

TABLE 6-1 ***(Continued)***
ANA Recognized Terminologies and Data Element Sets

Program	Setting Where Developed	Content
Data Element Sets		
12. LOINC Logical observation identifiers names and codes currently recognized	Nursing and other	Outcome and assessments
13. SNOMED CT Systematic nomenclature of medicine clinical terms currently recognized	Nursing and other	Diagnoses, interventions, and outcomes

- Develops and disseminates standards pertaining to information systems that support the documentation of nursing practice, and
- Evaluates voluntarily submitted information systems against these standards.

At a higher level of structure, several resources have developed to facilitate interoperability between different types of systems of concepts and nomenclature. For instance, the Systemized Nomenclature of Medicine (SNOMED CT) is considered a universal healthcare terminology and messaging structure. In nursing, SNOMED enables terminology from one system to be mapped to concepts from another, e.g., North American Nursing Diagnosis Association (NANDA), Nursing Intervention Classification (NIC) and Nursing Outcome Classification (NOC). On a larger scale, the Unified Medical Language System of the National Library of Medicine (UMLS; http://www.nlm.nih.gov/research/umls) incorporates the work of over one hundred vocabularies, including SNOMED (http://www.nlm.nih.gov/research/umls/metaa1.html). The INS must be aware of these tools, and may be called upon to understand the concepts of one or more languages, the relationships between related concepts, and integration into existing vocabularies for a given organization.

The importance of languages and vocabularies cannot be understated. INSs must seek a broader picture of the implications of their work, and the uses and outcomes of languages and vocabularies for end users. For instance, nurses working in mapping a home care vocabulary with an intervention vocabulary must see beyond the technical aspect of the work. They must understand that there may be a case manager for a multi-system health organization or a home care agency who will be developing knowledge of nursing acuity and case mix based on the differing vocabularies that they have integrated. The INS must attempt to envision the differing functions that may be used with the data, information and knowledge that have been created.

Concepts and Tools from Information Science and Computer Science

Informatics tools and methods from computer and information sciences are considered fundamental elements of NI, including:

- Information technology
- Information structures
- Information management
- Information communication

Information technology includes computer hardware, software, communication, and network technologies, derived primarily from computer science. The other three elements are derived primarily from information science. Information structures organize data, information, and knowledge for processing by computers. Information management is an elemental process within informatics in which one is able to file, store, and manipulate data for various uses. Information communication processes enable systems to send data, and to present information in a format that improves understanding. The use of information technology distinguishes informatics from more traditional methods of information management. Thus, NI incorporates the above four additional elements from computer and information science. Underlying all of these are human–computer interaction concepts discussed in the next section.

Human–Computer Interaction and Related Concepts

Human–computer interaction (HCI), usability and ergonomics concepts are of fundamental interest to the INS. Essentially, HCI deals with people, software applications, computer technology and the ways they influence each other (Dix, Finlay, Abowd, & Beale, 2004). Elements of HCI are rooted in psychology, social psychology and/or cognitive science. However, the design, development, implementation, and evaluation of applications derive from applied work in computer science, the specific discipline at hand (in this case nursing), and information science. For example, an INS would assess an application before purchase to determine whether the application design complements the way nurses cognitively process medication orders.

A related concept is **usability** which deals with specific issues of human performance during computer interactions for specific tasks within a particular context (Dix et al., 2004). Usability issues address the efficiency and effectiveness of an application. For example, an INS might study the ease of learning an application, the ease of using an application, or the speed of task completion and errors that occurred during application use when determining which system or application would be best utilized on a nursing unit.

The term **ergonomics** typically is used in the United States to describe the design and implementation of equipment, tools, and machines related to human safety, comfort, and convenience. Commonly, the term ergonomics refers to attributes of physical equipment or to principles of arrangement of equipment in the work environment. For instance, an INS may have a role in ensuring that good ergonomics principles are used in an intensive care unit to select and arrange various devices to support workflow for cross-disciplinary providers as well as patients' families.

HCI, usability, and ergonomics are related concepts typically subsumed under the rubric of human factors or how humans and technology relate to each other. The overall goal is better design for software, devices and equipment to promote optimal task completion in various contexts or environments. Optimal task completion includes the concepts of efficiency and effectiveness, including considerations about the safety of the user. These concepts are essential for the INS to understand for effective strategies to develop, select, implement, and evaluate information structures and informatics solutions.

The importance of human factors in health care was elevated with the Institute of Medicine's 2001 report (IOM, 2001). Before this, HCI and usability assessments and methods were being incorporated into health at a glacial speed. In the past 5 years the number of HCI and usability publications in health care has increased substantially. Vendors have installed usability laboratories and incorporated usability testing of their products into their systems lifecycles. The FDA has mandated usability testing as part of their approval process for any new devices (Medical Devices Today, 2007). Thus, HCI and usability are critical concepts for INs and INSs to understand. Numerous usability methods and tools are available, e.g., heuristics (rules of thumb), naturalistic observation and think aloud protocols. Readers are referred to HCI references and Chapter 5 to learn these methods.

Phenomena of Nursing

The metaparadigm of nursing comprises four key concepts: nurse, person, health, and environment. Nursing actions are based upon the inter-relationships between the concepts and are related to the values nurses hold relative to them. Nurses make decisions about interventions from their unique perspectives. Decision making is the process of choosing among alternatives. The decisions that nurses make can be characterized by both the quality of decisions and the impact of the actions resulting from those decisions. As knowledge workers, nurses make numerous decisions that affect the life and well-being of individuals, families, and communities. The process of decision making in nursing is guided by the concept of critical thinking. Critical thinking is the intellectually disciplined process of actively and skillfully using knowledge to conceptualize, apply, analyze, synthesize, and/or evaluate data and information as a guide to belief and action (Scriven & Paul, 1997).

Clinical wisdom is the ability of the nurse to add experience and intuition to a situation involving the care of a person (Benner, Hooper-Kyriadkidis, & Stannard, 1999). Wisdom in informatics is the ability of the NIS to evaluate the documentation drawn from a Health Information System (HIS) and the ability to adapt or change the system settings or parameters to improve the workflow of the clinical nurse.

Nurses' decision-making is described as an array of decisions that include specific behaviors, as well as cognitive processes surrounding a cluster of issues. For example, nurses use data transformed into information to determine interventions for persons, families, and communities. Nurses make decisions about potential problems presented by an individual and about appropriate recommendations for addressing those problems. They also make decisions in collaboration with other healthcare professionals such as physicians, pharmacists or social workers. Decisions also may occur within specific environments such as executive offices, classrooms, and research laboratories.

An information system collects and processes data and information. **Decision support systems** are computer applications designed to facilitate human decision-making processes. Decision support systems are typically rule-based, using a specified knowledge base and a set of rules to analyze data and information and provide recommendations. Other decision support systems are based upon knowledge models induced directly from data, regression or classification models that predict characteristics or outcomes. An **expert system** is a type of decision support system that implements the knowledge of one or more human experts. Recommendations take the form of alerts (for instance, calling user attention to abnormal lab results, potential adverse drug events) or suggestions, e.g., appropriate medications, therapies or other actions (Haug, Gardner, & Evans, 1999). Whereas control systems implement decisions without involvement of a user, decision support systems merely provide recommendations and rely upon the wisdom of the user for appropriate application of these provided recommendations. As Blum demonstrated in the mid-1980's, the concepts of data, information, knowledge and wisdom exemplify different levels of automated systems. The relationships among these concepts and information, decision support and expert systems are represented in Figure 6-3.

FIGURE 6-3
Levels and types of automated systems.

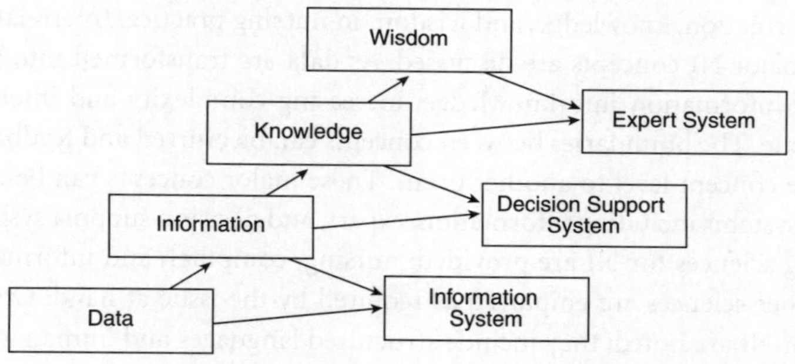

SOURCE: Reprinted from Englebardt, S. & Nelson, R. (2002). *Health care informatics: An Interdisciplinary approach* (Figure 1-5, page 14). St. Louis, MO: Elsevier. Reprinted with permission from Elsevier.

An INS must be able to navigate the complexity of the relationships between the following elements and understand how they facilitate decision making:

- Data, information, knowledge and wisdom
- Nursing science, information science, computer science and other sciences of interest to the issue at hand (e.g., cognitive science)
- Nurse, person, health, environment, and decision making
- Information structures, information technology, managing and communicating information

THE FUTURE OF NURSING INFORMATICS

The future of nursing informatics promises increased saturation of informatics concepts and solutions into mainstream nursing and healthcare practices. As informatics solutions become as common a tool as the stethoscope, each nurse may be considered, in part, an informatics nurse. New materials and concepts will evolve in the future. For example, **nanotechnology** promises to redefine the composition of nearly every man-made material and drastically alter biomedical applications (Alivisatos, 2001). How these new, microscopic materials generate data and information will be a fascination. A future outcome will be to determine how nanotechnology is incorporated into information systems (or become information systems themselves) to create knowledge. In another example, the concept of wisdom has just emerged as a key concept for nursing informatics. Its more detailed definition and measurement will be a part of the future. These are only two examples of the shape of nursing informatics in the future.

SUMMARY

In this chapter, the foundations of nursing informatics (NI) were outlined. The following definition for NI is offered: NI is a specialty that integrates nursing science, computer science, and information science to manage and communicate data, information, knowledge, and wisdom in nursing practice. Interrelationships among major NI concepts are discussed. As data are transformed into information and information into knowledge, increasing complexity and interrelationships ensue. The boundaries between concepts can be blurred and feedback loops from one concept level to another occur. These major concepts can be related to types of systems including information, expert, and decision support systems. The following sciences for NI are provided: nursing, computer, and information science. Other sciences are employed as required by the issue at hand. Critical elements for NI are noted; they include structured languages and human–computer interaction (HCI) concepts. Taxonomies and other current structured languages for nursing are listed. HCI concepts are briefly defined and discussed because they are critical to the success of informatics solutions. Last and importantly, the construct of decision making is added to the traditional nursing metaparadigms of nurse, person, health, and environment. Decision making is not only at the crux of nursing practice in all settings and roles; it is a fundamental concern of nursing informatics.

The most important thought we would like to leave you with is that nursing's work is centered in the following concepts of nursing informatics: data, information, knowledge, and wisdom. Information technology per se is not the focus; it is the information it conveys that is central. Nursing informatics is no longer the domain of experts in the field. More interestingly, one does not need technology to be performing informatics. The centerpiece of informatics is the manipulation of data, information, and knowledge, especially related to any decision making in any aspect of nursing or in any setting. In a way, all of us are already informatics nurses.

THOUGHT-PROVOKING Questions

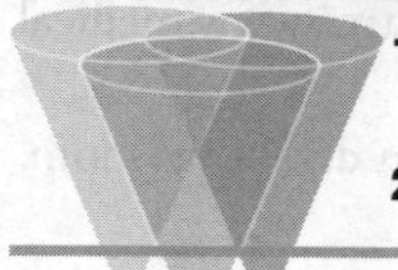

1. How is the concept of wisdom in nursing informatics like or unlike professional nursing judgment?
2. Think of a futuristic technology and explain its impact on nursing.

References

Alivisatos, A. P. (2001). Less is more in medicine: Sophisticated forms of nanotechnology will find some of the first real-world applications in biomedical research, disease diagnosis and possibly therapy. *Scientific American, 285*(3), 66–73.

Benner, P., Hooper-Kyriadkidis, P., & Stannard, D. (1999). *Clinical wisdom and interventions in critical care: A thinking-in-action approach.* Philadelphia: Saunders.

Blum, B. (1986). *Clinical information systems.* New York: Springer-Verlag.

Brennan, R. (2003). *One size doesn't fit all—Pedagogy in the online environment: Vol. 1.* Adelaide: National Centre for Vocational Education Research. Retrieved March 17, 2008, from http://www.ncver.edu.au/research/proj/nr0F05e.htm

Dix, A., Finlay, J., Abowd, G., & Beale, R. (2004). *Human–computer interaction.* Harlow, England: Pearson, Prentice Hall.

Graves, J., & Corcoran, S. (1989, winter). The study of nursing informatics. *Image, 21*(4), 227–230.

Harrison, L. (2002). Nursing activity in general intensive care. *Journal of Clinical Nursing, 11*(2), 158–167.

Haug, P., Gardner, R., & Evans, S. (1999). Hospital-based decision support. In E. S. Berner (Ed.), *Clinical decision support systems: Theory and practice* (pp. 77–104). New York: Springer-Verlag.

Hendrickson, G. (1990, March). How do nurses use their time? *Journal of Nursing Administration, 20*(3), 31–38.

IOM. (2001). *Crossing the quality chasm: A new health system for the 21st century.* Washington, DC: National Academies Press.

Jinks, A. M. (2000, September). What do nurses do? An observational survey of the activities of nurses on acute surgical and rehabilitative wards. *Journal of Nursing Management, 8*(5), 273–279.

Jydstrup, R. A., & Gross, J. J. (1966). Cost of information handling in hospitals. *Health Services Research, 1*(3), 235–271.

Medical Devices Today. (2007). *New usability standard aims to help firms institute human factors programs.* Retrieved March 17, 2008, from http://www.medicaldevicestoday.com/2007/04/new_usability_s.html

Nelson, R., & Joos, I. (1989, fall). On language in nursing: From data to wisdom. *PLN Vision*, p. 6.

Norrie, P. (1999). The parameters that cardiothoracic intensive care nurses use to assess the progress or deterioration of their patients. *Nursing Critical Care, 4*(3), 133–137.

Scriven, M. & Paul, R. (1997). *A working definition of critical thinking.* Retrieved March 17, 2008, from http://lonestar.texas.net/~mseifert/crit2.html

Staggers, N., & Thompson, C. B. (2002). The evolution of definitions for nursing informatics: A critical analysis and revised definition. *Journal of the American Medical Informatics Association (JAMIA), 33*(1), 75–81.

Turley, J. (1996, winter). Toward a model for nursing informatics. *Image: Journal of Nursing Scholarship, 28*(4), 309–313.

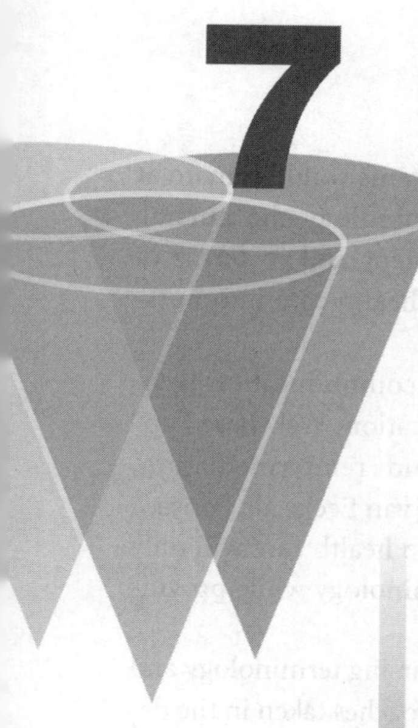

7 Developing Standardized Terminologies in Nursing Informatics

Nicholas Hardiker

Objectives

1. Explore the need and motivation behind the development of standardized terminologies for nursing.
2. Describe the different approaches to terminology development.
3. Assess initiatives seeking to exploit commonalities among terminologies and to ensure appropriate implementation and consistent use.

Key Terms

Accessibility
Archetypes
Enumerative approach
Longevity
Model of terminology use
Nursing terminology
Ontological approach
Ontology
Reusability
Standardized nursing terminology
Term
Terminology
Ubiquity

INTRODUCTION

Since the early 1970's, there has been a concerted effort to develop standardized terminologies for nursing. Work continues, driven by the following increasing demands placed on health-related information and knowledge:

- **Accessibility:** It should be easy to access the information and knowledge needed to deliver care or manage a health service.
- **Ubiquity:** With changing models of healthcare delivery, information and knowledge should be available anywhere.
- **Longevity:** Information should be usable beyond the immediate clinical encounter.
- **Reusability:** Information should be useful for a range of purposes.

Without a standardized nursing terminology, it would remain difficult to quantify nursing, the unique contribution and impact of nursing would go unrecognized, and the nursing component of electronic health record systems would remain at best rudimentary. Not least, without a standardized **terminology** the nursing knowledge base would suffer, both in terms of development and in terms of access, thereby delaying the integration of evidence-based health care into nursing practice.

The current and future landscape of information and communication technologies (e.g., connection anywhere, borderless communication, Web-based applications, collaborative working, disintermediation and reintermediation, consumerization, ubiquitous advanced digital content, etc. [van Eecke, da Fonseca Pinto, & Egyedi, 2007]) and their inevitable infiltration into health care will only serve to reinforce the need for a standardized nursing terminology while providing an additional sense of urgency.

This chapter explains what is meant by a standardized nursing terminology and lists several examples. It describes in detail the different approaches taken in the development of two example terminologies. It presents, in the form of an international technical standard, a means of ensuring consistency among the plethora of contemporary standardized nursing terminologies, with a view to harmonization and possible convergence. Finally, it provides a rationale for the shared development of models of terminology use; models that embody both clinical and pragmatic knowledge in order to ensure that contemporary nursing record systems reflect the best available evidence and fit comfortably with routine practice.

STANDARDIZED NURSING TERMINOLOGIES

A **term** at its simplest level is a word or phrase used to describe something concrete, e.g., leg, or abstract, e.g., plan. A **nursing terminology** is a body of the terms used in nursing. There are many nursing terminologies, formal and informal. Nursing terminologies allow us to capture, represent, access, and communicate nursing data, information, and knowledge. A **standardized nursing terminology**, therefore, is a nursing terminology that is in some way approved by an appropriate authority (*de jure* standardization) or by general consent (*de facto* standardization).

In North America, one such authority is the American Nurses Association (ANA), which operates a process of *de jure* standardization through its committee for nursing practice information infrastructure (CNPII) (http://www.nursinginsider.com/npii). While at the time there were obviously many more nursing terminologies in use around the world, in 2007, CNPII had recognized the following seven active (i.e., not retired) nursing terminologies (so-called interface terminologies):

1. Clinical care classification (CCC) (http://www.sabacare.com)—The clinical care classification (CCC) system consists of two interrelated terminologies

that cover nursing diagnoses, nursing outcomes, nursing interventions, and nursing actions. The two terminologies are linked by a common framework of care components.

2. International classification of nursing practice (ICNP) (http://www.icn.ch/icnp.htm)—ICNP is a compositional nursing terminology developed by the International Council of Nurses that covers nursing phenomena (i.e., diagnoses), nursing actions, and nursing outcomes. ICNP seeks to support the development of local terminologies and facilitate cross-mapping among terminologies.
3. North American Nursing Diagnosis Association International (NANDA-I) (http://www.nanda.org)—NANDA International maintains an agreed set of nursing diagnoses organized as a multiaxial taxonomy of domains and classes.
4. Nursing intervention classification (NIC) (http://www.nursing.uiowa.edu/excellence/nursing_knowledge/clinical_effectiveness/nic.htm)—The nursing interventions classification (NIC) is terminology that covers interventions performed by nurses and other providers. In common with NANDA, NIC interventions are organized into classes and domains.
5. Nursing outcomes classification (NOC) (http://www.nursing.uiowa.edu/excellence/nursing_knowledge/clinical_effectiveness/noc.htm)—The nursing outcomes classification (NOC) is a terminology that covers patient/client outcomes, presented as an alphabetical list.
6. Omaha Home Health Care system (http://www.omahasystem.org)—The Omaha system has three components: the problem classification scheme, the intervention scheme, and the problem rating scale for outcomes. These components provide both a terminology and a framework for documentation.
7. Perioperative nursing data set (PNDS) (http://www.aorn.org/PracticeResources/PNDS)—In contrast to the other terminologies listed here, which are intended for use in any setting and for any specialty, the perioperative nursing data set (PNDS) is a terminology that covers specifically the perioperative patient experience in terms of nursing diagnoses, nursing interventions, and nurse-sensitive patient outcomes.

In 2007 the CNPII had also recognized the retired nursing terminology patient care data set along with three multidisciplinary terminologies:

- Alternative billing codes (ABC) (http://www.alternativelink.com)
- Logical observation identifiers names and codes (LOINC) (http://www.loinc.org)
- Systematic nomenclature of medicine clinical terms (SNOMED CT) (http://www.snomed.org)

Finally, CNPII recognized two data element sets: nursing minimum data set (NMDS) and nursing management minimum data set (NMMDS). Work on a standardized data element set for nursing, which in the United States began in the 1980s with the NMDS (Werley & Lang, 1988), provided an additional catalyst for the development of many of the aforementioned terminologies listed—standardized nursing terminologies that could provide values (e.g., *chronic pain*) for particular data elements in the NMDS (e.g., *nursing diagnosis*). The data element sets provide a framework for the uniform collection and management of nursing data; the use of a standardized nursing terminology to represent that data serves to further enhance consistency.

APPROACHES TO NURSING TERMINOLOGY

From relatively humble beginnings, nursing terminologies have evolved significantly over the past several decades in line with best practices in terminology work, from simple lists of words or phrases to large, complex so-called **ontologies** (descriptions of entities within a domain and the relationships between them). This evolution has been facilitated by advances in knowledge representation, e.g., the refinement of the description logic that underpins many contemporary ontologies, and in their accompanying technologies, e.g., automated reasoners that can check consistency and identify equivalence and subsumption (i.e., subclass–superclass) relationships within those ontologies. The following section expands on two of the terminologies listed previously: NANDA and ICNP. These terminologies have been selected as examples to demonstrate the relative extremes of the terminological evolutionary path. No assumption should be made that either of the example terminologies is better than or worse than the other. Nor should any assumption be made that either of these terminologies is better than or worse than any other terminology. The examples merely represent different approaches that serve to complement one another, affording an opportunity for synergism.

Enumerative Approach

With the **enumerative approach,** words or phrases are represented in a list or a simple hierarchy. In NANDA, a nursing diagnosis has an associated name or label and a textual definition (NANDA International, 2005). Each nursing diagnosis may have a set of defining characteristics and related or risk factors. These additional features do not constitute part of the core terminology. Instead, they are intended to be used as an aid to diagnosis. As mentioned previously, NANDA's multiaxial taxonomy (i.e., taxonomy II) organizes nursing diagnoses into classes and domains. While taxonomy II provides an organizational framework for NANDA nursing diagnoses, it makes no attempt to organize nursing diagnoses among themselves; i.e., there are no hierarchical relationships among NANDA nursing diagnoses. Furthermore, there are no associative relationships apart from the implicit and global sibling relationship; i.e., every nursing diagnosis appears at the same level of indentation in the list, and there is no means to identify equivalent nursing diagnoses. However, what NANDA may lack in terms of hierarchical sophistication, it makes up for in terms of simplicity and potential ease of implementation and use.

Ontological Approach

The **ontological approach** is compositional in nature and a partial representation of the entities within a domain and the relationships that hold between them. ICNP takes the ontological approach—a different approach than NANDA. ICNP is described as a unified nursing language system. It seeks to provide a resource that can be used to develop local terminologies and to facilitate cross-mapping between terminologies in order to compare and combine data from different sources—the existence of a number of overlapping standardized nursing terminologies is problematic in terms of data comparison and aggregation (International Council of Nurses, 2005).

ICNP version 1.0 is an example of an ontology. The core of ICNP is represented in the Web ontology language (OWL), a recommendation of the World Wide Web Consortium (W3C) that is rapidly becoming the *de facto* standard language for representing ontologies (McGuiness & van Harmelen, 2004). The ICNP ontology comprises OWL classes and OWL properties. Classes are organized into a taxonomy. Properties link individuals (i.e., members of classes) together. A simplified graphical representation of chronic confusion showing the hasOnset property and the relationship that holds between individuals in the confusion and chronic classes is shown in Figure 7-1.

FIGURE 7-1
Simplified OWL representation of chronic confusion. Squares represent classes, while circles represent individuals with classes. The arrow represents a relationship along the hasOnset property.

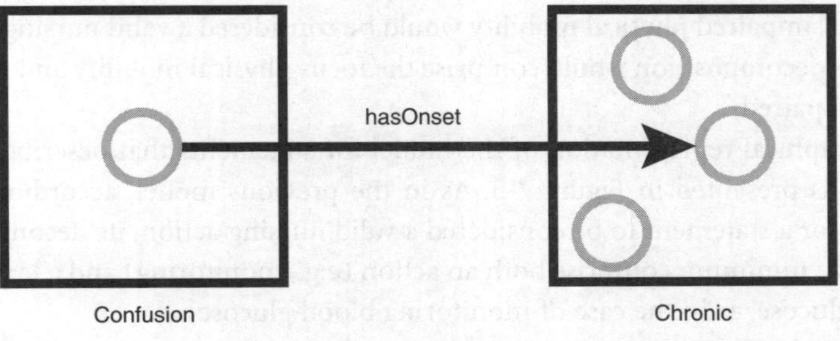

As it is underpinned by description logic, OWL permits the use of automated reasoners that can check consistency, identify equivalence, and support classification within the ICNP ontology. The result is a rigorously and predictably defined multiple hierarchy. The compositional nature of the ICNP ontology makes it well suited to support the development of local terminologies; the rich hierarchy (and the opportunity for automated reasoning) make it well suited to support cross-mapping between terminologies. However, ICNP is computer based—it may be more powerful than NANDA, but in its raw form it may also be more difficult to implement and use.

EXPLOITING COMMONALITY AMONG NURSING TERMINOLOGIES

There are many differences between NANDA and ICNP. However, they both purport at least to represent nursing diagnoses (ICNP also represents nursing actions and nursing outcomes); and they are both recognized by ANA (through CNPII) as interface terminologies that support nursing practice.

Indeed there are many differences between the broader set of standardized nursing terminologies in terms of scale, scope, structure, and intended use. But as with NANDA and ICNP there are many similarities, particularly concerning content. These similarities have been exploited in the development of an international technical standard: ISO 18104:2003 health informatics—integration of a reference terminology model for nursing (International Organization for Standardization, 2003). ISO 18104:2003 was developed through a consensus process that considered a number of standardized nursing terminologies in order to determine a model or schema that could outline the basic form of nursing statements (i.e., a reference terminology model for nursing).

At the heart of the standard are in fact two models—a model for nursing diagnosis and a model for nursing action. A graphical representation of the model for statements that describe nursing diagnoses is presented in Figure 7-2. According to this model, for a statement to be considered a valid nursing diagnosis, its decomposition must at minimum comprise both a focus and a judgment. For example, impaired physical mobility would be considered a valid nursing diagnosis as its decomposition would comprise the focus physical mobility and the judgment impaired.

A graphical representation of the model for statements that describe nursing actions is presented in Figure 7-3. As in the previous model, according to this model, for a statement to be considered a valid nursing action, its decomposition must as a minimum comprise both an action (e.g., monitoring) and a target (e.g., blood glucose, as in the case of monitoring blood glucose).

FIGURE 7-2
Model for nursing diagnosis.

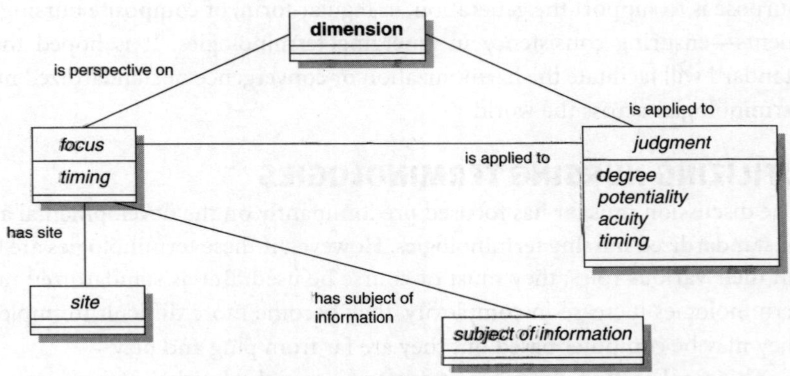

SOURCE: The terms and definitions taken from ISO 18104:2003 health informatics—integration of a reference terminology model for nursing are reproduced with the permission of the International Organization of Standardization (ISO). The standard can be obtained from any ISO member and from the Web site of the ISO central secretariat at the following address: http://www.iso.org. Copyright remains with ISO.

FIGURE 7-3
Model for nursing action.

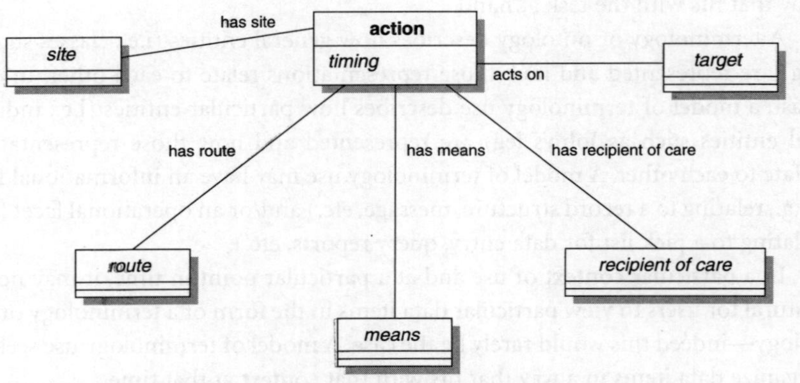

SOURCE: The terms and definitions taken from ISO 18104:2003 health informatics—integration of a reference terminology model for nursing are reproduced with the permission of the International Organization of Standardization (ISO). The standard can be obtained from any ISO member and from the Web site of the ISO central secretariat at the following address: http://www.iso.org. Copyright remains with ISO.

One of the main purposes cited by ISO 18104:2003 is to facilitate the systematic evaluation and refinement of existing terminologies—discovering anomalies within nursing terminologies through noncompliant decompositions. Another purpose is to support the generation, in regular form, of composite nursing statements—ensuring consistency in emerging terminologies. It is hoped that the standard will facilitate the harmonization or convergence of standardized nursing terminologies across the world.

UTILIZING NURSING TERMINOLOGIES

The discussion thus far has focused predominantly on the developmental aspects of standardized nursing terminologies. However, if these terminologies are to fulfill their various roles, they must of course be used. But as standardized nursing terminologies increase in complexity, they become more difficult to implement; they may be computer based but they are far from plug and play.

This final section describes attempts to ease the burden of implementation through the development of models of terminology use. Terminologies help us to convey our understanding of the world. Models of terminology use help us to structure information for particular purposes. For example, a restaurant menu lists all of the dishes we might wish to order—this represents the terminology. The menu organizes the dishes in a way that encourages us to select dishes, and allows us to select dishes according to our shared view of the world (e.g., appetizer, followed by main course, followed by dessert)—this represents the **model of terminology use**. The menu encourages us to make use of the terminology while delivering it in a way that fits with the task at hand.

A terminology or ontology describes how general entities (i.e., classes such as leg) are represented and how those representations relate to each other. In contrast, a model of terminology use describes how particular entities (i.e., individual entities such as John's leg) are represented and how those representations relate to each other. A model of terminology use may have an informational facet (e.g., relating to a record structure, message, etc.) and/or an operational facet (e.g., relating to a pick list for data entry, query reports, etc.).

In a particular context of use and at a particular point in time, it may not be natural for users to view particular data items in the form of a terminology or ontology—indeed this would rarely be the case. A model of terminology use seeks to organize data items in a way that fits with that context at that time.

Previously the onus had been on the developers of end-user applications to determine their own models of terminology use. The nursing terminologies were standardized, but the models of terminology use were not. These were often embedded within applications, and it would not be possible to share the valuable clinical and pragmatic knowledge they contained. There had been much duplication of effort, with the developers of end-user applications and their prospective users working towards the same goal, but in parallel streams. This situation provided a major motivation for further standards development—standards that might support the shared development of shareable models of terminology use. Examples of a shareable model of terminology use include archetypes, care information models, clinical statements, templates, clinical elements, etc. Archetypes will be used as an example to illustrate the common principles that underpin many of these initiatives.

An **archetype** is "a computable expression of a domain content model in the form of structured constraint statements, based on a reference (information) model" (Beale & Heard, 2007, p. 8). In routine general clinical practice, a blood pressure observation usually comprises, at a minimum, a systolic blood pressure and a diastolic blood pressure. Without an explicit model of terminology use, these would either remain as separate terms in a terminology or ontology, or they would need to be linked together within individual end-user applications. Archetypes capture this knowledge along with appropriate terminological bindings and other nonterminological details such as associated units (e.g., mm Hg, minimum value e.g. 0, etc.). Thus archetypes provide a means of defining explicitly clinical and pragmatic knowledge apart from the applications that might use it.

SUMMARY

This chapter has described the need for and motivation behind the development of standardized terminologies for nursing. It has described different approaches to terminology development and introduced initiatives that seek to exploit commonalities among today's terminologies and to ensure their appropriate implementation and consistent use.

The most important thought I would like to leave you with is that standardized nursing terminologies (and the structures and systems that support their implementation and use) are merely a means to an end; they do not obviate the need to think and work creatively, to do right by the people in our care and to continue to advance nursing.

THOUGHT-PROVOKING Questions

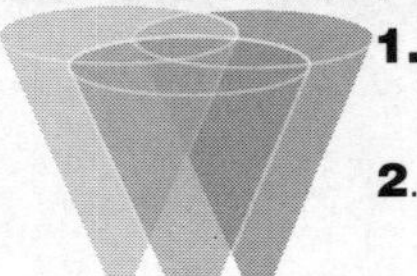

1. What do you believe are the advantages and disadvantages of having a single shared consensus-driven model of terminology use?
2. How can a single agreed-upon model of terminology use (with linkages to a single terminology) help to integrate knowledge into routine clinical practice?

References

Beale, T., & Heard, S. (Eds.). (2007). *Archetype definitions and principles.* Revision 1.0. [online]. The *open*EHR Foundation. Retrieved March 17, 2008, from http://svn.openehr.org/specification/TRUNK/publishing/architecture/am/archetype_principles.pdf

International Council of Nurses. (2005). *International classification for nursing practice. Version 1.0.* Geneva, Switzerland: International Council of Nurses.

International Organization for Standardization. (2003). *International standard ISO 18104:2003 health informatics—integration of a reference terminology model for nursing.* Geneva, Switzerland: International Organization for Standardization.

McGuiness, D. L., & van Harmelen, F. (Eds.). (2004). *OWL Web ontology language overview* [online]. World Wide Web Consortium. Retrieved October 5, 2007, from http://www.w3.org/TR/owl-features

NANDA International. (2005). *Nursing diagnoses: Definitions & classification 2005–2006.* Philadelphia, PA: NANDA International.

van Eecke, P., da Fonseca Pinto, P., & Egyedi, T., for the European Commission. (2007). *EU study on the specific policy needs for ICT standardisation.* [Final report]. Retrieved October 5, 2007, from http://ec.europa.eu/enterprise/ict/policy/doc/2007-ict-std-full-rep.pdf

Werley, H. H., & Lang, N. M. (Eds.). (1988). *Identification of the nursing minimum data set.* New York: Springer Publishing Company.

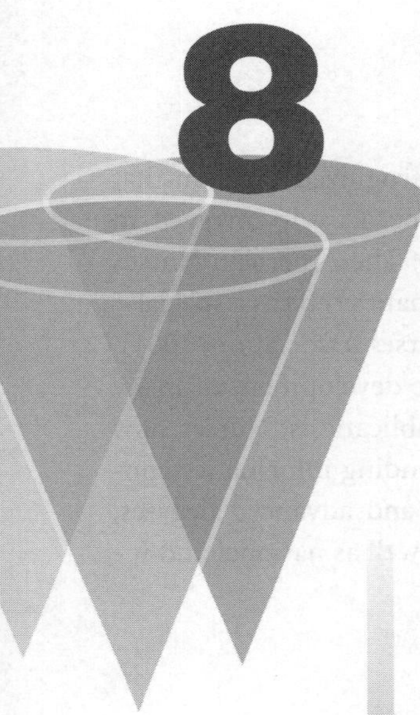

8 Nursing Informatics Roles, Competencies, and Skills

Julie A. Kenney and Ida Androwich

Objectives

1. Provide an overview of nursing informatics' historical development.
2. Explore the concept of nurses as knowledge workers.
3. Discuss the evolving roles and competencies of nursing informatics practice.

Key Terms

Advocate/policy developer
Certification
Cognitive activity
Consultant
Continuous learner
Core sciences
Data
Data gatherer
Decision support/ outcomes manager
Educator
Entrepreneur
Industrial Age
Informatics
Informatics innovator
Informatics nurse specialist
Information
Information Age
Information user
Informatique
Interdisciplinary knowledge team
Knowledge
Knowledge builder
Knowledge user

INTRODUCTION

The world has witnessed an unprecedented number of technological advances during the last 100 years. The early 20th century witnessed the invention of the car and the airplane. These modes of transportation drastically changed how people work and play. The entertainment world was dramatically altered by the invention of radio and television. The introduction of the computer altered the way data and information were viewed and utilized and changed the way business was conducted. The computer is now changing nursing and health care.

Nurses have historically gathered and interpreted data. Florence Nightingale was the first nurse to use data to change the way she cared for her patients. While serving in the Crimean War, she began to gather data regarding the conditions in which the patients were living and the diseases they contracted and from which they expired. This data was later used to improve patient conditions at both city and military hospitals (O'Connor & Robertson, 2003).

Today, nurses are able to access information quickly and easily. Accessing the information via the Internet or the electronic health record (EHR) allows the nurse to

Key Terms *Continued*
Knowledge worker
Medical informatics
Nursing informatics (NI) competencies
Product developer
Project manager
Researcher
Technologist
TIGER initiative

provide the best possible patient care. Nursing recognized early on that computers would change health care and became actively involved in shaping how computers were used in health care. The American Nurses Association (ANA) first recognized nursing informatics (NI) as a specialty in 1992 (Saba & McCormick, 2006; American Nurses Association, 2001). The introduction of this specialty has spurred the development of many informatics jobs as well as organizations and publications. Nurses now have the ability to further their education by attending informatics conferences, reading journals, obtaining certificates and advanced degrees, and participating in numerous hospital-based, as well as national and international informatics committees and groups.

WHAT IS NURSING INFORMATICS?

Definitions

The term **informatics** was derived from the French term informatique, which means to refer to the computer milieu (Saba, 2001). The Health Information and Management Systems Society (HIMSS) defines informatics as "the discipline concerned with the study of information and manipulation of information via computer-based tools" (2006, p. 44). The definition for medical informatics was the first connection between informatics and health care. **Medical informatics** is described as collected informational technologies that affect the medical decisions made regarding patient care (Hannah, Ball, & Edwards, 2006).

NI has been defined numerous times over the years. One of the most widely cited definitions was by Graves and Corcoran (1989). Their definition moved away from the earlier definitions that tended to put a greater emphasis on technology and moved toward a more conceptually based definition. Graves and Corcoran define NI as a "combination of computer science, information science and nursing science designed to assist in the management and processing of nursing data, information and knowledge to support the practice of nursing and the delivery of nursing care" (p. 227). In 2001, ANA published an updated NI definition as well as an updated scope and practice. The 2001 ANA definition of nursing informatics was:

> A specialty that integrates nursing science, computer science, and information science to manage and communicate data, information, and knowledge in nursing practice. Nursing informatics facilitates the integration of data, information, and knowledge to support patients, nurses, and other providers in their decision-making in all roles and settings. This support is accomplished through the use of information structures, information processes, and information technology. (p. vii)

In 2008, the ANA updated the definition and scopes and standards.

Staggers and Thompson (2002) believed that there were too many definitions for NI, which was causing the specialty to grow without a solid foundation. They believed that without this foundation it was difficult to build a solid informatics practice or the needed educational base for this specialty practice. Staggers and Thompson performed a critical analysis of the definitions, which resulted in a new definition. The new definition is as follows:

> Nursing informatics is a specialty that integrates nursing science, computer science, and information science to manage and communicate data, information, and knowledge in nursing practice. Nursing informatics facilitates the integration of data, information, and knowledge to support patients, nurses, and other providers in their decision making in all roles and settings. This support is accomplished through the use of information structures, information processes, and information technology. (p. 260)

One theme that flows throughout these definitions is the combining of nursing, computer, and information science. The ANA (2001) calls these the **core sciences** of NI. These core sciences differentiate NI from other informatics specialties. NI may incorporate other sciences to solve informatics issues. An example would be an informatics nurse who was working on a system implementation project. This informatics nurse would need to be able to apply the three core sciences, as well as organizational science and change management, to the project. The ANA points out that even though NI is based on science, it is an applied science and not a basic science.

A second theme that flows through these definitions is the use of data, information, and knowledge by an informatics nurse. Graves and Corcoran (1989) and the ANA (2001) both believe that data, information, and knowledge are key components of NI practice. **Data** is defined by Graves and Corcoran as a single entity that has been described objectively and not interpreted. An example of data would be a single blood pressure. **Information** is defined as data that has been interpreted, organized, or structured (ANA). An example of information is a nurse beginning to notice trends in the patient data. Knowledge is defined as information that has been synthesized so that relationships are identified and formalized (ANA). An example of this would be realizing that the increased temperature, heart, and respiratory rate and the dropping blood pressure are probably the result of sepsis, which would require certain medical treatments in order for the patient to improve. Data, information, knowledge, and the core sciences, when combined, represent the foundation of NI practice.

History

In order to understand NI, one must understand its history. Health care began to use computers in the 1950s. Computers, in this era, were typically used in the business office (Saba & McCormick, 2006). In the 1970s, nursing began to realize the importance of computers to the nursing profession and became involved in the design, purchase, and implementation of information systems (Saba & McCormick). In the 1980s, medical and nursing informatics specialties emerged. The personal computer was introduced, which allowed for flexibility in how these clinical systems were used. It also brought to everyone's attention that not just NI specialists, but all healthcare personnel, would need to know about these systems (Hannah et al., 2006; Saba & McCormick). The first certification exam for NI was taken in 1995 (Saba & McCormick). The post-2000 era saw an unprecedented explosion in the number and sophistication of both computer hardware and software. Electronic patient records became an integral part of clinical information systems. Telemedicine became possible and was recognized as a specialty in the late 1990s (Saba & McCormick). NI has experienced rapid growth in the last 40 years, and it does not appear to be slowing. It will be interesting to see what will happen over the next 40 years.

Goal of Nursing Informatics

In 2001, ANA published the *Scope and Standards of Nursing Informatics Practice.* ANA lists the goal of NI as:

> The goal of NI is to improve the health of populations, communities, families, and individuals by optimizing information management and communication. This includes the use of technology in the direct provision of care, establishing effective administrative systems, managing and delivering education experiences, supporting life-long learning, and supporting nursing research. (p. 17)

ANA updated the scope and standards for nursing informatics in 2008.

THE NURSE AS A KNOWLEDGE WORKER

It has been established that nurses use data and information. This information is then converted to knowledge. The nurse then acts upon this knowledge by initiating a plan of care, updating an existing one or maintaining status quo. Does this use of knowledge make the nurse a knowledge worker? This section will focus on the definition of a knowledge worker as well as the history of the term and how it is utilized in health care and business. This chapter will examine how nursing relates to the term of knowledge worker as well as the effect a knowledge worker has on health care.

Definitions

Knowledge can be defined as "the distillation of information that has been collected, classified, organized, integrated, abstracted, and value added" (HIMSS,

2006, p. 49). A worker is "one that works especially at manual or industrial labor or with a particular material" (Merriam-Webster, 2007). The term **knowledge worker** was first coined by Peter Drucker in his 1959 book, *Landmarks of Tomorrow* (Drucker, 1994). Knowledge work is defined as nonrepetitive, nonroutine work that entails a significant amount of **cognitive activity** (Sorrells-Jones & Weaver, 1999a). Drucker (1994) describes a knowledge worker as one who has advanced formal education and is able to apply theoretical and analytical knowledge. According to Drucker, the knowledge worker must be a **continuous learner** and a specialist in a field.

Knowledge Worker Concept

The world is transitioning from the **Industrial Age** to the **Information Age** (Snyder-Halpern, Corcoran-Perry, & Narayan, 2001; Sorrells-Jones & Weaver, 1999a). The early 1900s workforce consisted predominantly of farmers. After World War I, the workforce began to become predominantly blue collar. This occurred when many farmers and domestic help moved to the cities to take jobs at factories. The industrial worker is slowly being replaced by the technologist (Drucker, 1994). The **technologist** is adept at using both mind and hand. Many industrial workers are finding it more and more difficult to obtain jobs as they do not have the educational base or mind set required of knowledge workers (Drucker). The technologist is no longer trained on the job as were the industrial workers, which can cause significant problems for the industrial worker who does not have the education required to transition to a knowledge worker position (Drucker; Sorrells-Jones & Weaver, 1999a).

Knowledge workers are innovators, and the work they produce is the foundation for organizational sustainability and growth. Knowledge workers are specialized, have advanced education, and typically have a high degree of autonomy and control over their own work environments (Davenport, Thomas, & Cantrell, 2002; Sorrells-Jones & Weaver, 1999a). Knowledge workers are most efficient when they are working in a multidisciplinary team. The teams are typically composed of members whose knowledge bases are complementary. The team members possess problem-solving and decision-making skills as well as advanced interpersonal skills. All members of the team are considered equal and are there to contribute their expertise. Leadership will shift and change as the team tackles different parts of the project, with the topic expert taking the lead. A well-functioning team will consistently outperform an individual (Sorrells-Jones & Weaver, 1999b). Many of these teams become focused and passionate about the project.

A key impediment to an effective team is a lack of understanding between team members as well as a lack of respect for each other's knowledge and experience

(Sorrells-Jones & Weaver, 1999a). Another barrier to the efficient multidisciplinary team is the individual knowledge worker who does not want to give up his own identity even though he may be swayed by other professional opinions. Professionals have a more difficult time adjusting to working in a team than do non-professionals. Professionals fail very few times in their lives, which results in their not being able to learn from their failures (Sorrells-Jones & Weaver, 1999b). Knowledge workers tend to be resistant to change, which results in them digging in their heels and refusing to adapt to changes that the management has implemented to improve the work process or work flow (Davenport et al., 2002).

Companies that employ knowledge workers have had to change their management structure to support the knowledge workers. Management no longer commands but inspires the workers to produce the best product (Drucker, 1992). These companies have come to the realization that the machines are unproductive without the knowledge of a knowledge worker. Loyalty is no longer purchased with a paycheck, but is earned by giving the knowledge workers the ability to use their knowledge effectively and innovatively (Drucker, 1992). The physical environment and workplace arrangements have been adjusted in order to maximize the work flow of the knowledge workers (Davenport et al., 2002). Many of these changes have occurred in the business world but have been slow to be adopted in health care.

Knowledge Workers and Health Care

The healthcare industry is firmly rooted in the Industrial Age. This is resulting in an industry that is not conducive to support the knowledge workers that represent the vast majority of the workforce (Sorrells-Jones & Weaver, 1999a; Wickramasinghe & Ginzberg, 2001). Sorrells-Jones & Weaver (1999a) state that "healthcare institutions are among the most rigidly bureaucratic and hierarchical, discipline-fragmented organizations in the U.S." (p. 16). This is evidenced by multiple administrative levels that manage a single function unit. Corporate values reflect the desire for employees to be loyal and compliant, to avoid risk, and to see failure as negative instead of positive. Senior leadership keeps information tightly controlled and fails to see the need to bring in external intelligence and influence. Rewards are based on individual rather than team performance and a significant pay difference exists between those at the top and those that produce the product (Weaver & Sorrells-Jones, 1999).

Health care needs to begin making the transition from the Industrial Age to the Information Age. This transition will be challenging due to the success healthcare institutions have had using the current management methods. This success will make it difficult to abandon the old in order to learn the new. Health care can begin this transition by adopting a new philosophy that recognizes that employees are mature, self-reliant, independent-thinking adults who function as partners in carrying out the work of the organization. The organization needs to view the employee as an asset and supply the resources, tools, information, and power they need to self-manage their work. Innovation needs to be supported, especially when it meets the customers' needs, desires, and wishes (Weaver & Sorrells-Jones, 1999).

Currently, there is a management trend to use flatter management styles with fewer layers of administration. Organizations are beginning to switch to a clinical product or service line format. This format is typically designed with the physician as the content expert and the nurse as the patient care expert. Unfortunately, this format does not represent a significant change from the way things are currently being done (Weaver & Sorrells-Jones, 1999). Management needs to understand and support the knowledge work and nonknowledge work that is performed daily in health care. Both types of work are integral to caring for patients safely (Weaver & Sorrells-Jones, 1999). Organizations must switch from measuring the number of tasks completed to measuring the outcomes obtained by knowledge workers (Sorrells-Jones & Weaver, 1999b). This trend is becoming more evident with the posting of hospital report cards that demonstrate how effectively the hospital is caring for certain types of patients.

Nurses as Knowledge Workers

The question to ask is, "Are nurses knowledge workers?" See Table 8-1 for a comparison of nursing to the characteristics of a knowledge worker. When nursing characteristics are compared to the knowledge worker's characteristics, nursing does meet the criteria to be a knowledge worker. Nursing entails a significant amount of knowledge and nonknowledge work. Knowledge work would include such things as interpreting trends in labs and symptoms. Nonknowledge work would include such items as calling the lab to check on lab results or making beds. Nurses, on a daily basis, rely on their extensive clinical information and specialized knowledge in order to implement and evaluate the processes and outcomes related to patient care (Snyder-Halpern et al., 2001, 2001).

Snyder-Halpern et al., 2001 (2001) have identified the following four tasks that are associated with human information processing: data gathering, information use, creative application of knowledge to clinical practice, and generation of new knowledge. These four tasks are associated with four roles that nursing takes on as a knowledge worker. These roles are the data gatherer, information user, knowledge user, and knowledge builder.

Nurses are **data gatherers** by nature. Nurses collect and record objective clinical data on a daily basis (Snyder-Halpern et al., 2001, 2001). These may include such things as patient history information, vital signs, and patient assessment

TABLE 8-1
A Comparison of Knowledge Worker Characteristics and Nursing Characteristics

Knowledge Worker Characteristics	Nursing Characteristics
Advanced formal education	• All nurses have college degrees ranging from AND to PhD
Able to apply theoretical and analytical knowledge	• Nurses are educated on nursing theory and how to apply it in patient situations
Continuous learner	• Obtain advanced degrees • Attend seminars • Earn contact hours
Specialized	• Nursing specialties are as numerous as medical specialties
Innovator	• Nurses become innovative when they do not have proper equipment to care for the patients or they feel that current products are inadequate
Team member	• Have been a member of the interdisciplinary team for a significant amount of time

data. Data gatherers transition to **information users**. This transition occurs when nurses begin to interpret the data that they have collected and recorded. The information users then structure the clinical data into information that can be used to guide patient care decisions (Snyder-Halpern et al., 2001). An example of this is when the nurse notices that the patient's blood pressures have been elevated. Information users transition to **knowledge users** when they begin to notice trends in a patient's clinical data and determine if the clinical data falls within or outside of the normal data range. Nurses will transition from knowledge users to **knowledge builders** when they examine clinical data and trends across groups of patients. These trends are interpreted and compared to current scientific data to determine if this data would improve the nursing knowledge domain. An example of the transition to knowledge builder would be an observation of medication compliance rates over a specified time period for patients diagnosed with chronic high blood pressure, and then comparing these rates to evidence-based literature to determine if this information would improve the nursing knowledge base (Snyder-Halpern et al., 2001).

Snyder-Halpern et al. (2001) found that as nurses assumed each of these roles, they required different types of decision support processes to support their knowledge needs. The data gatherer requires a system that will capture and store data accurately and reliably and allow the data to be readily accessed. The majority of current healthcare decision support systems (DSSs) support the nurse in this role (Snyder-Halpern et al., 2001). The information user role requires a system that can transform clinical data into a format that allows for easy recognition of patterns and trends. This data recognizes the trend and displays it for the nurse, who in turn uses it to adjust the plan of care (POC) for the patient. The information user role is generally well supported by current DSSs (Snyder-Halpern et al., 2001). The knowledge user role is the least supported role, and many systems are currently looking at ways to support the nurses in this role. One advantage of these decision support systems is their ability to bring knowledge to nurses so that they will not have to retrieve the information themselves, which allows them to adjust the patient's POC in a more efficient and timely manner. The knowledge builder role is typically seen in conjunction with the nurse researcher role and quality management roles. These roles typically look at aggregated data that has been captured over time and from numerous patients and is then compared to clinical variables and interventions, which then results in the development of new domain knowledge (Snyder-Halpern et al., 2001). The knowledge needs of nurses will continue to improve as the systems improve.

The Challenge of Nurses as Knowledge Workers

In order for nurses to be treated as knowledge workers, nurses must first be recognized as knowledge workers (Snyder-Halpern et al., 2001). Nurses have been part of the interdisciplinary team for years, but are nurses ready to become part of the **interdisciplinary knowledge team**? Nursing may be ready to take that step, but are other members of the healthcare team ready to acknowledge nurses as a respected member of the team (Sorrells-Jones & Weaver, 1999a)? One reason that acceptance may be difficult is the fact that nurses tend to be the least educated member of the interdisciplinary knowledge team (Sorrells-Jones & Weaver, 1999b). Another reason is that nurses, historically, have had a difficult time being an active member of the interdisciplinary team (Sorrells-Jones & Weaver, 1999b). Nursing still has a long way to go before being accepted as an equal participant in the interdisciplinary knowledge team. In order for nurses to be an accepted member of the interdisciplinary knowledge team, a major attitude change toward nursing will need to take place. In addition, nurses must become better educated and more involved in the interdisciplinary knowledge team.

THE KNOWLEDGE NEEDS AND COMPETENCIES OF NURSES

In the early days of medicine, all medical knowledge fit into a single volume. Today, the amount of information available is vast and expanding exponentially, which makes the healthcare industry the most knowledge-intense environment (Snyder-Halpern, Corcoran-Perry, & Narayan, 2001). Computers, technology, and the informatics fields are assisting healthcare workers in dealing with this information explosion.

Knowledge Needs

Nurses deal with a vast amount of information and knowledge every day, which they use to care for their patients. Nurses rely on an extensive amount of clinical information and specialized knowledge in order to evaluate the processes they have implemented and measure the corresponding outcomes (Snyder-Halpern, Corcoran-Perry, & Narayan, 2001). Nurses rely on their own knowledge, but there are times when this is not adequate and they must access information in order to provide safe patient care. A national survey was conducted and found that consulting a peer was the most frequent way that information was obtained. The survey also found that most of those surveyed did not utilize information resources to gather practice information, and that only approximately 25% had been trained on how to use an electronic database (Barton, 2005). If a peer does not have the information the nurse is seeking, the nurse will turn to a hospital policy, a journal, a textbook, a drug book, an online resource, the EHR, or many other possible sources.

For this information to be beneficial to the nurse and the patient, it must be reliable and credible. The resource must be easily accessible and packaged in such a way that the nurse is able to find the necessary information quickly and with a minimal amount of difficulty. One way this can be accomplished is by implementing a decision support system (DSS), which is designed to support the nurses in their decision-making activities. DSSs may be incorporated into the EHR.

Nursing Informatics Competencies

One challenge that health care is currently facing is the vast differences in computer literacy and information management skills that healthcare workers possess (McNeil, Elfrink, Beyea, Pierce, & Bickford, 2006). Barton (2005) feels that new nurses should have the following critical skills:

- Use e-mail
- Operate Windows applications
- Search databases
- Know institution-specific nursing software that is used for charting and medication administration

These skills should not be limited to just new nurses but should be required of all nurses and healthcare workers.

Staggers, Gassert, & Curran (2001) believe that nursing students and practicing nurses should be educated on core **NI competencies**. Many authors have devised lists of NI competencies, but none agree on how to incorporate this information into curricula or educate the practicing nurses. Information technology and informatics concepts need to be incorporated into nursing school curriculum, but progress has been slow (Staggers et al., 2001). In the 1980s, a nursing group of the International Medical Informatics Association (IMIA) convened to develop the first level of nursing competencies. While developing these competencies, the nursing group found that nurses fell in to one of the following three categories: user, developer, or expert. These categories have since been expanded upon.

Staggers et al. (2001) decided that the NI competencies developed in the 1980s were inadequate and needed to be updated. Staggers et al. reviewed 35 NI competency articles and 14 job descriptions, which resulted in 1,159 items that were sorted into three broad categories:

1. Computer skills
2. Informatics knowledge
3. Informatics skills

These items were placed in a database where redundant items were removed. When this process was completed, 313 items remained. These items were then further subdivided, and this was when Staggers and colleagues, along with the American Medical Informatics Association (AMIA) work group, realized that these competencies were not universal to all nurses, and before it could be determined if the competency was an NI competency, nursing skill levels would need to be defined. This group determined that practicing nurses fell into the following four categories:

1. Beginning nurse
2. Experienced nurse
3. Informatics nurse specialist
4. **Informatics innovator**

Each of these skill levels would need to be defined before Staggers et al. (2001) could determine which level was the most appropriate for that skill set. See Table 8-2 for the definition criteria of each skill level. Once the levels were defined, the group determined that 305 items were NI competencies and placed them into appropriate categories.

Staggers, Gassert, & Curran (2002) conducted a Delphi study to validate the placement of the competencies into the correct skill level. Of the 305 original competencies identified, 281 achieved an 80% approval rating for both importance as a competency and placement in the correct practice level. Staggers et al.

TABLE 8-2
Definitions of Four Levels of Practicing Nurses

Beginning Nurse

- Has basic computer technology skills and information management skills
- Uses institution's information systems and the contained information to manage patients

Experienced Nurse

- Proficient in a specialty
- Highly skilled in using computer technology skills and information management skills to support his or her specialty area of practice
- Pulls trends out of data and makes judgments based on this information
- Uses current systems, but will collaborate with informatics nurse specialist regarding concerns or suggestions provided by staff

Informatics Nurse Specialist

- RN with advanced education who possesses additional knowledge and skills specific to computer technology and information management
- Focuses on nursing's information needs, which include education, administration, research, and clinical practice
- Application and integration of the core informatics sciences: information, computer, and nursing science
- Uses critical thinking, process skills, data management skills, systems life cycle development, and computer skills

Informatics Innovator

- Conducts informatics research and generates informatics theory
- Vision of what is possible
- Keen sense of timing to make things happen
- Creative in developing solutions
- Leads the advancement of informatics practice and research
- Sophisticated level of skills and understanding in computer technology and information management
- Cognizant of the interdependence of systems, disciplines, and outcomes, and is able to finesse situations to obtain the best outcome

SOURCE: Staggers, N., Gassert, C., & Curran, C. (2001). Informatics competencies for nurses at four levels of practice. *Journal of Nursing Education, 40*(7), 303–316.

(2002) stress that this is a comprehensive list and that for a nurse to enter a skill level, that nurse does not have to have mastered every item listed in the skill level. To access the entire list of competencies by skill level, visit http://www.nurs.utah.edu/informatics/competencies.htm. See Table 8-3 for a modified version of the list.

In 2004, a group of nurses came together after attending a national informatics conference to ensure that nursing was equally recognized in the national informatics movement. They were called the Technology Informatics Guiding Education Reform (TIGER) team. This group determined that utilizing informatics was a core competency for all healthcare workers. They also determined that many nurses lack IT skills, which limits their ability to access evidence-based information that could be incorporated into their daily practice. This group is currently working on a plan to incorporate informatics courses into all levels of nursing education, and then they will look at how to get the information out to

TABLE 8-3
Nursing Informatics Competencies by Skill Level

Beginning Nurse

- Uses e-mail
- Uses Internet to locate and download information of interest
- Uses computerized patient monitoring systems
- Identifies the basic components of a computer system
- Recognizes that a computer program has limitations due to its design and capacity of the computer

Experienced Nurse

- Defines the impact of computerized information management on the role of the nurse
- Applies monitoring system appropriately according to the data needed
- Performs basic troubleshooting in applications
- As a clinician, participates in the selection process, design, implementation, and evaluation of systems
- Assesses the accuracy of health information on the Internet

Informatics Nurse Specialist

- Demonstrates fluency in informatics and nursing terminologies
- Implements and evaluates application/system training programs for users and clients
- Determines projected impacts to users and organizations when changing to computerized information management
- Applies human factors and ergonomics to the design of the computer screen, location and design of devices, and design of software
- Consults in the design or enhancements to integrated patient information, management, educational, or research systems

Informatics Innovator

- Develops models for simulation purposes
- Evaluates the performance and impact of information management technologies on clinical practice, education, administration, and/or research
- Develops new methods of organizing data to enhance research capacities
- Applies advanced analysis and design concepts to the system life cycle process
- Applies sophisticated educational design and research evaluation concepts to the use of innovative computer-based education techniques

NOTE: A complete list of NI competencies is available at http://www.nurs.utah.edu/informatics/competencies.htm

SOURCE: Staggers, N., Gassert, C., & Curran, C. (2002). A Delphi study to determine informatics competencies for nurses at four levels of practice. *Nursing Research*, *51*(6), 383–390.

practicing nurses who are not currently enrolled in an academic program (TIGER Initiative, 2006). Many of the items identified as lacking in both nursing students and practicing nurses are items that Staggers et al. (2002) determined to be NI competencies. To learn more about the **TIGER initiative**, please visit https://www.tigersummit.com/Home_Page.html.

WHAT IS NURSING INFORMATICS SPECIALTY PRACTICE?

NI is an established and ever-evolving profession that began when computers were introduced into health care (Belanger, 2006). Those choosing NI as a career will find it full of numerous and varied opportunities. Until recently, most nurse informaticists entered the field by showing an understanding and enthusiasm for working with computers. Now, nurses have many educational opportunities available to become formally trained in the field of NI. This section of the chapter will explore the scope and standards of NI, NI roles, education and specialization, rewards of working in the field, and organizations and professional journals of the nursing informatics specialist (NIS).

Nursing Contributions to Healthcare Informatics

Nursing has been involved in the purchase, design, and implementation of information systems (IS) since the 1970s (Saba & McCormick, 2006). One of the first health information system (HIS) vendors studied how nurses managed patient care and realized that nursing activity was the core of patient activity and needed to be the foundation of the HIS. As a result of the study, he designed the Technicon HIS, which is now called Ecylypsis (Saba, 2001). Nursing has been instrumental in designing a standard language to be used in the HIS, which was discussed in depth earlier in this chapter. Nursing is involved heavily in the design of educational materials for practicing nurses, student nurses, other healthcare workers, and patients. Computers have revolutionized the way patients access information and have also revolutionized the educational process (Saba).

Scopes and Standards

NI is important to nursing and health care as it focuses on representing nursing data, information, and knowledge. NI does the following for the health informatics (ANA, 2001; Brennan, 1994):

- Provides a nursing perspective
- Showcases nursing values and beliefs
- Provides a foundation for nurses in NI
- Produces unique knowledge
- Distinguishes groups of practitioners
- Emphasizes the interest for nursing
- Provides needed nursing language and word context

In 2001, ANA published a revised *Scope and Standards of Nursing Informatics Practice*, which, as previously mentioned, was revised again in 2008. The publication includes the **informatics nurse specialist** standards of practice as well as the informatics nurse specialist standards of professional performance. The three overarching standards of practice are (ANA, p. 33):

1. Incorporate theories, principles, and concepts from appropriate sciences into informatics practice.

TABLE 8-4
Informatics Nurse Specialist Standards of Practice

Standard I. Identify the issue or problem
Standard II. Identify alternatives
Standard III. Choose and develop a solution
Standard IV. Implement the solution
Standard V. Evaluate and adjust solutions

SOURCE: American Nurses Association (ANA). (2001). *Scope and standards of nursing informatics practice.* Washington, DC: American Nurses Publishing.

TABLE 8-5
Informatics Nurse Specialist Standards of Professional Performance

Standard I. Quality of nursing informatics practice
Standard II. Performance appraisal
Standard III. Education
Standard IV. Collegiality
Standard V. Ethics
Standard VI. Collaboration
Standard VII. Research
Standard VIII. Resource utilization
Standard IX. Communication

SOURCE: American Nurses Association (ANA). (2001). *Scope and standards of nursing informatics practice.* Washington, DC: American Nurses Publishing.

2. Integrate ergonomics and human–computer interaction (HCI) principles into informatics solution design, development, selection, implementation, and evaluation.
3. Systematically determine the social, legal, and ethical impact of an informatics solution within nursing and health care.

The standards of practice and the standards of professional performance for an informatics nurse specialist are listed in Tables 8-4 and 8-5, respectively.

Nursing Informatics Roles

NI has become a viable and essential nursing specialty with the introduction of computers and the EHR to health care. Many nurses entered the NI field because of their natural curiosity and their dedication to being a lifelong learner. Nurses who enter this field may have done so by accident because they were comfortable working with computers and their coworkers used them as a resource for computer-related questions. The introduction of the EHR has strained clinicians to learn this new technology and incorporate it into their already busy days. It has been estimated that nurses spend as little as 15% of their days with their patients and as much as 50% of their day documenting (HIMSS Nursing Informatics Awareness Task Force, 2007). Assisting nurses to incorporate this new technology into their daily workflow is one of many challenges that the NIS may tackle. The roles that the NIS may engage in are numerous. One position that nurses do quite well in is the role of the project manager, which is a result of their ability to manage multiple complex situations at one time (HIMSS Nursing Informatics Awareness Task Force). Because of the breadth of the NI field, many NISs find that they will need to further specialize. The following list includes some typical NIS positions. This list is far from comprehensive, as this field changes as rapidly as technology (ANA, 2001; Thede, 2003). For a listing of NI positions with job descriptions, visit http://www.amia.org/mbrcenter/wg/ni/roles.asp.

Project Manager—In the **project manager** role, the NIS will be responsible for the planning and implementing of an informatics project. The NIS will utilize communication, change management, process analysis, risk assessment, scope definition, and team building. This role acts as the liaison between clinicians, management, IS, vendors, and all other interested parties.

Consultant—The NI who takes on the **consultant** role will provide her expert advice, opinions, and recommendations based on her area of expertise. Flexibility, good communication skills, excellent interpersonal skills, and extensive clinical and informatics knowledge are highly desirable skills sets needed by the NI consultant.

Educator—The success or failure of an informatics solution can be directly related to the education that was provided. The NIS who chooses the **educator** role will develop and implement educational materials and educational sessions as well as provide education about the system to new employees or during an implementation or an upgrade.

Researcher—The **researcher** role entails conducting research to create new informatics knowledge. Research may range from basic informatics research to developing clinical decision support tools for nurses.

Product Developer—An NIS in the **product developer** role will participate in the design, production, and marketing of new informatics solutions. An understanding of business and nursing is essential in this role.

Decision Support/Outcomes Manager—Nurses assuming the role of **decision support/outcomes manager** will use tools to maintain data integrity and reliability. Contributing to the development of a nursing knowledge base is an integral component of this role.

Advocate/Policy Developer—NISs are key to developing the infrastructure of health policy. Policy development on a local, national, and international level is an integral part of the **advocate/policy developer** role.

System Specialist—NISs may work at varying levels and serve as a link between nursing and information services.

Entrepreneur—Those involved in the **entrepreneur** role analyze nursing information needs and develop and market solutions.

Specialty Education and Certification

Many nurses who entered into NI did so without any formal education. These nurses were the unit resource for computer or program questions. Many of these nurses acquired their skills with on-the-job training and/or by attending classes. This still holds true today, but now there are formal ways of acquiring these skills. The NIS may obtain an advanced degree or a post-master's certificate. The first two graduate NI programs were introduced at the University of Maryland and the University of Utah in 1989. The first doctoral program was offered in 1991 at the University of Maryland (Duke University School of Nursing, n.d.). NISs may attend informatics conferences and obtain contact hours or continuing education units. See Table 8-6 for a list of colleges and universities that offer advanced degrees or certificates in NI. This is not a comprehensive list; new programs are being developed. Local colleges and universities should be researched to see which may have added informatics programs.

Nurses who choose to specialize have two **certifications** available to them. The first is through the American Nurses Credentialing Center (ANCC). The ANCC exam is specific for the informatics nurse. The applicant must be a licensed registered nurse (RN) with at least 2 years of recent experience and have a baccalaureate degree in nursing (BS/BSN). The applicant must have completed 30 contact hours of continuing education in informatics. The applicant must meet one of the following criteria:

- 2,000 hours practicing as an informatics nurse
- 1,000 hours practicing as an informatics nurse and 12 semester hours of graduate academic credit towards a nursing informatics degree
- Completion of a nursing informatics degree that included at least 200 supervised practicum hours

TABLE 8-6
Formal Nursing Informatics Educational Programs

Graduate Degree Programs

- Duke University: http://onlineinformatics.com
- Excelsior College: https://www.excelsior.edu/portal/page?_pageid=57,570971&_dad=portal&_schema=PORTAL
- Loyola University Chicago: http://www.luc.edu/schools/nursing/majorsprograms/healthsysman.html
- New York University: http://www.nyu.edu/nursing/academicprograms/masters/programs/informatics.html
- University of Alabama at Birmingham: http://main.uab.edu/sites/nursing/programs/msn/9053
- University of Colorado at Denver: http://www.uchsc.edu/nursing/informatics.htm
- University of Iowa: http://www.nursing.uiowa.edu/academic_programs/graduate/msn/programs.htm#msn8
- University of Kansas: http://www2.kumc.edu/son/academicinformation/healthcareinformatics.html
- University of Maryland: http://nursing.umaryland.edu/programs/ms/informatics.htm
- University of Nebraska Medical Center: http://app1.unmc.edu/nursing/conweb/view_content.cfm?lev1=progs&lev2=msn&lev3=hsns&web=pub
- University of North Carolina at Chapel Hill: http://nursing.unc.edu/degree/msn/hcs.html
- University of Pittsburgh: http://www.pitt.edu/~nursing/informatics
- University of Utah: http://www.nurs.utah.edu/programs/informatics/study_inform.htm
- University of Washington: http://www.son.washington.edu/eo/cipct
- Vanderbilt University: http://www.mc.vanderbilt.edu/nursing/msn/ni.html

Certificate Programs

- Eastern University: http://www.eastern.edu/academic/accel/sps/undg/rntobsn/online/nursing_informatics.shtml
- Loyola University Chicago: http://www.luc.edu/schools/nursing/majorsprograms/healthsysman.html
- Northeastern University: http://www.bouve.neu.edu/programs/nuradmin/index.php
- Slippery Rock University of Pennsylvania: http://www.sru.edu/pages/2265.asp
- University of Arizona: http://www.nursing.arizona.edu/PostMastCert.htm#HCI
- University of Iowa: http://www.nursing.uiowa.edu/academic_programs/certificate/NursingInformaticsCertificate.htm
- University of Washington: http://www.son.washington.edu/eo/cipct

For further information on this certification exam, visit http://www.nursecredentialing.org/cert/eligibility/informatics.html. This Web site includes the aforementioned criteria as well as information about test eligibility, fees, exam context, exam locations, study materials, and practice tests.

The second certification exam is sponsored by HIMSS. Candidates who successfully pass this exam will carry the designation of certified professional in healthcare information and management systems (CPHIMS). This exam is open to any candidate who is involved in healthcare informatics. Candidates must hold positions in the following fields: administration/management, clinical information systems, e-health, information systems, or management engineering. Candidates may include any of the following: CEOs, CIOs, chief operating officers (COOs), senior executives, senior managers, IS technical staff, physicians, nurses, consultants, attorneys, financial advisors, technology vendors, academicians, management engineers, and students. The candidates must meet the following criteria in order to be eligible to sit for the exam:

- Baccalaureate degree plus 5 years of associated information and management systems experience; 3 of those years in health care.
- Graduate degree plus 3 years of associated information and management systems experience; 2 of those years in health care.

The information discussed in this text and additional information about the exam can be found by visiting http://www.himss.org/ASP/certification_cphims.asp.

Rewards of NI Practice

NI is a nursing specialty that does not focus on direct patient care but instead focuses on how to improve patient care and safety as well as on improving the workflow and work processes of nurses and other healthcare workers. The NIS is instrumental in designing the electronic healthcare records that healthcare workers use on a daily basis. The NIS is responsible for designing tools that allow healthcare workers to access patient information more efficiently than they have been able to in the past. Watching these changes take place brings great satisfaction to the NIS.

Change is a factor that an NIS deals with on a daily basis. This is probably the most difficult aspect of the position because people deal with change differently. Understanding change and how it affects people allows the NIS to develop strategies to allow the healthcare workers to accept changes and become proficient in informatics solutions that are implemented. Seeing the change adopted with a minimal amount of discord is very rewarding to the NIS.

The NIS participates in informatics organizations that allow NISs to network and share experiences with each other. This allows them to bring these new solutions back to their respective organizations and improve informatics issues. Attending professional conferences allows the NIS to stay abreast of changes in the industry. Continuing education allows the NIS to improve a process or workflow within the hospital or to change the way a system upgrade is rolled out.

NI Organizations and Journals

One of the first informatics organizations founded was the Healthcare Information and Management Systems Society (HIMSS). HIMSS was founded in 1961 with offices in Chicago, Washington, D.C., Brussels, Belgium, and other locations located throughout the United States and Europe. HIMSS currently represents 20,000 individuals and 300 corporations. HIMSS offers local as well as national chapters. HIMSS has many work groups associated with it, one of them is a nursing informatics work group. HIMSS is well known for its development of industry-wide policies and its educational and professional development initiatives, which all lead to the one goal of ensuring safe patient care. HIMSS offers many advantages for its members. Membership includes numerous weekly and monthly publications, as well as a scholarly journal, *The Journal of Healthcare Information Management*. There are many educational programs offered, including virtual expos, which allow participants to experience the expo without having to travel. These educational opportunities allow participants to network with colleagues and peers, which is a valuable asset in this field. To find out more about HIMSS, visit their homepage at http://www.himss.org/ASP/index.asp.

The American Medical Informatics Association (AMIA) was founded in 1990 when three health informatics associations merged. AMIA currently has over 3,000 members who reside in 42 countries. AMIA's focus is the development and application of biomedical and healthcare informatics. Members include physicians, nurses, dentists, pharmacists, health information technology professionals, biomedical engineers, and many others. AMIA offers many benefits to its members. Membership includes weekly and monthly publications as well as a scholarly journal, *JAMIA—The Journal of the American Medical Informatics Association*. Members may join a working group that is specific to their specialty, which includes a nursing informatics work group. AMIA offers multiple educational opportunities as well as many opportunities for networking with colleagues. To view this information and to see what else AMIA offers, visit http://www.amia.org/ index.asp (AMIA, 2007).

The American Nursing Informatics Association (ANIA) was established in 1992 to provide an opportunity for southern California informatics nurses to meet. It has since grown to a national organization whose members include healthcare professionals who work with clinical information systems, educational applications, data collection/research applications, administrative/decision support systems, and those who have an interest in the field of nursing informatics. Membership benefits include an electronic quarterly newsletter. Members receive a discounted rate for *CIN: Computers, Informatics, Nursing,* as well as for attendance at the annual conference. Members enjoy networking opportunities as well as access to informatics job opportunities. To view this information and learn more about ANIA, visit http://www.ania.org/ (ANIA, 2007).

The Alliance of Nursing Informatics (ANI) is a collaboration of NI groups that represents 3,000 nurses and 20 distinct nursing informatics groups in the United States. The membership represents local, national, and international nursing informatics members and groups. These individual groups have developed organizational structures and have established programs and publications. ANI functions as the link between nursing informatics organizations and the general nursing and healthcare communities. ANI provides the united voice of nursing informatics. To view this information and learn more about ANI visit http://www.allianceni.org (ANI, 2007).

TABLE 8-7
Nursing Informatics Web Sites and Corresponding Journals

Alliance for Nursing Informatics (ANI)

Web site: www.allianceni.org

American Health Information Management Association (AHIMA)

Web site: www.ahima.org
Journal: *Journal of AHIMA & Perspectives in Health Information Management* [online]

American Medical Informatics Association (AMIA)

Web site: www.amia.org
Journal: *JAMIA—Journal of the American Medical Informatics Association*
NI Web site: http://www.amia.org/mbrcenter/wg/ni

American Nursing Informatics Association (ANIA)

Web site: www.ania.org
Resources link: http://www.ania.org/Resources.htm
Journal: *CIN: Computers, Informatics, Nursing*

Capital Area Roundtable on Informatics in Nursing (CARING)

Web site: www.caringonline.org
Newsletter: *CARING,* available at http://www.caringonline.org/mc/page.do?orgId=car&sitePageId=27887

Health Information and Management Systems Society (HIMSS)

Web site: www.himss.org
Chapter Web sites: http://www.himss.org/ASP/chaptersHome.asp
Journal: *The Journal of Healthcare Information Management*
NI Web site: http://www.himss.org/asp/topics_nursingInformatics.asp

International Medical Informatics Association (IMIA)

Web site: www.imia.org
Journal: *International Journal of Medical Informatics*
NI Web site: http://www.imia.org/ni

Online Journal of Nursing Informatics (OJNI)

Web site: http://www.ojni.org

These groups have been instrumental in establishing the informatics community. There are many informatics groups that have not been covered here. For additional groups, please see Table 8-7 for a list of organizations and the publications produced by each group.

SUMMARY

Nursing informatics is a relatively new nursing specialty that combines nursing science, information science, and computer science. Informatics practices support nurses to effectively and safely care for their patients as the information that they need is made more readily available. Nurses have been actively involved in this field since computers were introduced to health care. With the advent of EHRs, it became apparent that nursing needed to develop its own language. NI was instrumental in assisting in nursing language development.

The healthcare industry employs the largest number of knowledge workers. This is resulting in the realization that healthcare administrators must begin to change the way that they look at their employees. The nurses and physicians are bright, highly skilled, and dedicated to giving the best patient care. Administrators who tap into this wealth of knowledge will begin to find they have happier employees and find that the patients' care will become safer and more efficient.

NI is a specialty that is governed by the standards that have been established by the ANA. NI is a very diverse field, which results in many NISs becoming specialized in one segment of the field. NI is a recognized specialty, but it affects all nurses. Nursing informatics competencies have been developed to ensure that all entry-level nurses will be ready to enter a field that is becoming more technologically advanced. The competencies may be used to determine the educational needs of current staff members. The growth of the NI field has resulted in the formation of numerous NI organizations or subgroups of the medical informatics organizations. Nurses no longer have to enter the field as a fluke but can obtain an advanced degree in NI at many well established universities throughout the country. The NIS may continue learning by attending one of numerous conferences offered. NI has grown tremendously as a specialty since its inception and looks to continue growing. It will be interesting to see where technology takes health care in the future.

The Future of Nursing Informatics

NI is in its infancy, as is the technology that the NIS uses on a daily basis. NI will continue to influence the development of the EHR. The EHR will continue to improve and will one day accurately capture the care nurses give to their patients. This will be a formidable challenge as much of the care provided by nurses is intangible. The EHR will provide data to the NIS to be used to improve nursing workflow as well as determine if current practices are the most efficient and beneficial to the patient. Nursing and health care are on a roller-coaster ride that looks to prove very interesting. New technology is being introduced at a breakneck speed and nursing and healthcare must be ready to ride this roller coaster. Programs will need to be developed to keep nurses and healthcare workers abreast of the new technological changes as they occur. Educating new nurses as well as current nurses presents a significant challenge to the NIS. The NIS's future looks very promising and rewarding.

The most important thought I would like to leave you with is that NI is a field that many have fallen into by accident. That is exactly what happened to me. Since becoming a nurse, I have always had a knack for using machines. Any time that someone was having trouble with a machine, they came and found me to assist them with the problem. I was one of the few nurses who could enter orders into the computer, as most were too afraid to try. In 1999, the labor and delivery unit I was working on was installing a new computerized fetal monitoring system. The unit was in need of staff members to be trainers. I was volunteered because I was good with our unit computer. A year later, the system manager moved and I was given her position because I was one of the few who could function comfortably in the system. I was in charge of educating new nurses as well as modifying the system as needed. This was my introduction into NI. Six years later, the hospital implemented a housewide documentation system. I was again elected to be a trainer. I was in charge of training all the labor and delivery nurses as well as the obstetrics nurses. Shortly after the go-live date, I changed positions and became the primary educator for my current hospital's EHR. This entailed educating all new employees on the system, serving as a resource for the system, and educating the current staff when new upgrades were implemented. I decided to take the plunge and went back to school to obtain an MSN in health systems management with an emphasis in informatics. Now I am an official informatics nurse. I plan on taking at least one if not both of the certification exams that are available to informatics nurses. I really look forward to seeing where my degree and informatics take me.

Those looking to enter the field should have a general knowledge of computers and not be afraid of working with them. Change plays a significant part in this role and those interested in NI must embrace and enjoy change. They must also be good at enticing others to embrace change. NI candidates must realize that with change comes resistance. They must also be ready to leave the bedside because nurses entering into this field will no longer be working at the bedside. NI is a very challenging but very rewarding field to those who choose to enter.

THOUGHT-PROVOKING Questions

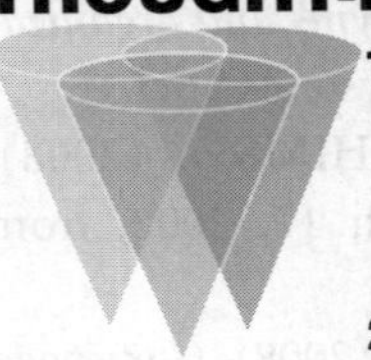

1. Hospital C is looking to implement an EHR. It has been suggested that an NIS be hired. This position does not involve direct patient care and the administration is struggling with how to justify the position. How can this position be justified?
2. This chapter discusses the fact that nurses are knowledge workers. How does nursing move from measuring the tasks completed to measuring the final outcome of the patient?

References

Alliance of Nursing Informatics (ANI). (2007). *Homepage.* Retrieved September 15, 2007, from http://http://www.allianceni.org

American Medical Informatics Association (AMIA). (2007). *Homepage.* Retrieved September 9, 2007, from http://www.amia.org/index.asp

American Nurses Association (ANA). (2001). *Scope and standards of nursing informatics practice.* Washington, DC: American Nurses Publishing.

American Nursing Informatics Association (ANIA). (2007). *Homepage.* Retrieved September 9, 2007, from http://www.ania.org

Barton, A. J. (2005). Cultivating informatics competencies in a community of practice. *Nursing Administration Quarterly, 29*(4), 323–328.

Belanger, J. (2006, February). Nursing informatics on the move. *Online Journal of Nursing Informatics (OJNI), 10*(1) [Online]. Retrieved August 4, 2007, from http://ojni.org/10_1/index.html

Brennan, P. F. (1994). On the relevance of discipline to informatics. *Journal of the American Medical Informatics Association, 1*(2), 200–201.

Davenport, T. H., Thomas, R., & Cantrell, S. (2002). The mysterious art and science of knowledge worker performance. *MIT Sloan Management Review, 44*(1), 23–30.

Drucker, P. F. (1992). The new society of organizations. *Harvard Business Review, 70*(5), 95–104.

Drucker, P. F. (1994). The age of social transformation. *The Atlantic Monthly, 274*(5), 52–80.

Duke University College of Nursing. (n.d.). Retrieved September 3, 2007, from http://www.duke.edu/~goodw010/AMIA

Graves, J. R., & Corcoran, S. (1989). The study of nursing informatics. *IMAGE: Journal of Nursing Scholarship, 21*(4), 227–231.

Hannah, K. J., Ball, M. J., & Edwards, M. J. A. (2006). *Introduction to nursing informatics* (3rd ed.). New York: Springer.

Health Information and Management Systems Society (HIMSS). (2006). *HIMSS dictionary of healthcare information technology terms, acronyms and organizations.* Chicago: Healthcare Information and Management Systems Society.

Health Information and Management Systems Society (HIMSS). (2008). *CPHIMS: HIMSS CPHIMS certification.* Retrieved March 17, 2008, from http://www.himss.org/ASP/certification_cphims.asp

Health Information and Management Systems Society (HIMSS). (2008). *Homepage.* Retrieved March 17, 2008, from http://www.himss.org/ASP/ index.asp

HIMSS Nursing Informatics Awareness Task Force. (2007). An emerging giant: Nursing informatics. *Nursing Management, 13*(10), 38–42.

McNeil, B. J., Elfrink, V., Beyea, S. C., Pierce, S., & Bickford, C. J. (2006). Computer literacy study: Report of qualitative findings. *Professional Nursing, 22*(1), 52–59.

Merriam-Webster Online. (2007). Retrieved August 5, 2007, from http://mw1.merriam-webster.com/dictionary/worker

O'Connor, J. J., & Robertson, E. F. (2003). *Florence Nightingale biography.* Retrieved August 5, 2007, from http://www-history.mcs.st-andrews.ac.uk/Biographies/Nightingale.html

Saba, V. K. (2001). Nursing informatics: Yesterday, today, and tomorrow. *International Nursing Review, 48*(3), 177–187.

Saba, V. K., & McCormick, K. A. (Eds.). (2006). *Essentials of nursing informatics* (4th ed.). New York: McGraw-Hill.

Snyder-Halpern, R., Corcoran-Perry, S., & Narayan, S. (2001). Developing clinical practice environments supporting the knowledge work of nurses. *Computers in Nursing, 19*(1), 17–26.

Sorrells-Jones, J., & Weaver, D. (1999a). Knowledge workers and knowledge-intense organizations, Part 1: A promising framework for nursing and health-care. *Journal of Nursing Administration, 29*(7/8), 12–18.

Sorrells-Jones, J., & Weaver, D. (1999b). Knowledge workers and knowledge-intense organizations, Part 3: Implications for preparing healthcare professionals. *Journal of Nursing Administration, 29*(10), 14–21.

Staggers, N., Gassert, C., & Curran, C. (2001). Informatics competencies for nurses at four levels of practice. *Journal of Nursing Education, 40*(7), 303–316.

Staggers, N., Gassert, C., & Curran, C. (2002). A Delphi study to determine informatics competencies for nurses at four levels of practice. *Nursing Research, 51*(6), 383–390.

Staggers, N., & Thompson, C. B. (2002). The evolution of definitions for nursing informatics. *Journal of the American Medical Informatics Association, 9*(3), 255–261.

Thede, L. Q. (2003). *Informatics and nursing: Opportunities & challenges* (2nd ed.). Philadelphia: Lippincott Williams & Wilkins.

The TIGER Initiative. (2006). *Welcome to TIGER!* Retrieved August 26, 2007, from http://www.umbc.edu/tiger/index.html

Weaver, D., & Sorrells-Jones, J. (1999). Knowledge workers and knowledge-intense organizations, Part 2: Designing and managing for productivity. *Journal of Nursing Administration, 29*(9), 19–25.

Wickramasinghe, N., & Ginzberg, M. J. (2001). Integrating knowledge workers and the organization: Role of IT. *International Journal of Health Care Quality Assurance, 14*(6), 245–253.

McNeil, B. J., Elfrink, V., Beyea, S. C., Pierce, S., & Bickford, C. J. (2006). Computer literacy study: Report of qualitative findings. *Journal of Professional Nursing, 22*(1), 52–59.

Merriam-Webster Online. (2007). Retrieved August 5, 2007, from http://www.merriam-webster.com/dictionary/worker

O'Connor, J. J., & Robertson, E. F. (2003). *Florence Nightingale biography*. Retrieved August 5, 2007, from http://www-history.mcs.st-andrews.ac.uk/Biographies/Nightingale.html

Saba, V. K. (2001). Nursing informatics: Yesterday, today, and tomorrow. *International Nursing Review, 48*(3), 177–187.

Saba, V. K., & McCormick, K. A. (Eds.). (2006). *Essentials of nursing informatics* (4th ed.). New York: McGraw-Hill.

Snyder-Halpern, R., Corcoran-Perry, S., & Narayan, S. (2001). Developing clinical practice environments supporting the knowledge work of nurses. *Computers in Nursing, 19*(1), 17–26.

Sorrells-Jones, J., & Weaver, D. (1999a). Knowledge workers and knowledge-intense organizations, Part 1: A promising framework for nursing and healthcare. *Journal of Nursing Administration, 29*(7/8), 12–18.

Sorrells-Jones, J., & Weaver, D. (1999b). Knowledge workers and knowledge-intense organizations, Part 3: Implications for preparing healthcare professionals. *Journal of Nursing Administration, 29*(10), 14–21.

Staggers, N., Gassert, C. A., & Curran, C. (2001). Informatics competencies for nurses at four levels of practice. *Journal of Nursing Education, 40*(7), 303–316.

Staggers, N., Gassert, C. A., & Curran, C. (2002). A Delphi study to determine informatics competencies for nurses at four levels of practice. *Nursing Research, 51*(6), 383–390.

Staggers, N., & Thompson, C. B. (2002). The evolution of definitions for nursing informatics. *Journal of the American Medical Informatics Association, 9*(3), 255–261.

Thede, L. Q. (2003). *Informatics and nursing: Opportunities & challenges* (2nd ed.). Philadelphia: Lippincott Williams & Wilkins.

The TIGER Initiative. (2006). *Welcome to TIGER*. Retrieved August 26, 2007, from http://www.umbc.edu/tiger/index.html

Weaver, D., & Sorrells-Jones, J. (1999). Knowledge workers and knowledge-intense organizations, Part 2: Designing and managing for productivity. *Journal of Nursing Administration, 29*(9), 19–25.

Wickramasinghe, N., & Ginzberg, M. J. (2001). Integrating knowledge workers and the organization: Role of IT. *International Journal of Health Care Quality Assurance, 14*(6), 245–253.

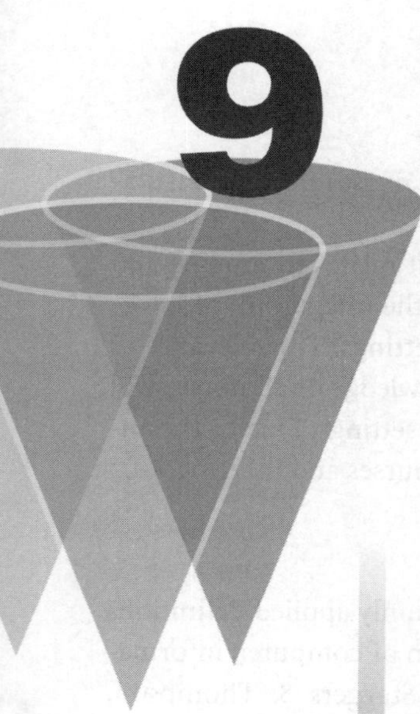

9 Information and Knowledge Needs of Nurses in the 21st Century

Lynn M. Nagle

Objectives

1. Describe the goal of nursing informatics.
2. Assess the nurse as knowledge worker.
3. Explore how nurses create clinical knowledge.
4. Evaluate how nurses use clinical knowledge.
5. Explain clinical decision support.

Key Terms

Clinical decision support (CDS)
Clinical information system (CIS)
Evidence-based practice (EBP)
Nursing informatics (NI)
Nursing knowledge
Research utilization (RU)

INTRODUCTION

The information and knowledge informing the 21st century of healthcare delivery has been growing at an unprecedented pace in recent years. Research in particular has been propelling our understanding of the efficacy of various clinical practices, treatment regimes, and interventions. Extended and expanded access to clinical research findings and decision support tools has been significantly influenced by the advent of computerization and the Internet. Indeed, the conduct of research itself has been accelerated by virtue of ubiquitous computing. Working in environments of increasingly complex clinical care and contending with the management of large volumes of information, nurses need to avail themselves of the technological tools that can support quality practice that is optimally safe, informed, and knowledge based. While the increased deployment of information technologies within healthcare settings presumes that nurses and other health professionals will be proficient in the use of computing devices, the processes and potential outcomes associated with informatics are yet to be fully realized or understood. But suffice it to say that nurses need to participate in the creation of those possibilities.

This chapter will address the goals of informatics as it relates to nursing and more specifically address the benefits to be derived from the integration of information and communication technologies into practice settings. The relevance of informatics to support and advance the practice and knowledge of all nurses will be discussed in the context of today's healthcare delivery settings. Finally, the author will provide a contemplative view of the future for nurses and informatics.

INFORMATICS DEFINED

While varied and evolving over the years, the most commonly applied definitions of **nursing informatics (NI)** describe it as the intersection of computer, information, and nursing science (Graves & Corcoran, 1989; Staggers & Thompson, 2002). Readers may find Staggers and Thompson's definitional review particularly helpful in understanding the different foci of those most widely cited in years past. They suggested that earlier definitions were primarily one of three orientations: (1) information technology, (2) conceptual, or (3) role focused. Building upon the work of others (Graves & Corcoran, 1989; Hannah, Ball, & Edwards, 1984; Schwirian, 1986; Turley, 1996), they attempted to capture all of these elements in advancing the following definition:

> A specialty that integrates nursing science, computer science, and information science to manage and communicate data, information, and knowledge in nursing practice. Nursing informatics facilitates the integration of data, information, and knowledge to support patients, nurses, and other providers in their decision-making in all roles, and settings. This support is accomplished through the use of information structures, information processes, and information technology. (p. 260)

In general, this definition reflects the work of nurse informaticists, the emergence of patients as active participants in their own care, and the key concepts intersecting nursing and informatics (Staggers & Thompson, 2002). Nurses in identified informatics roles typically focus their efforts on articulating meaningful clinical nursing data and information structures that can be codified and processed; identifying the information processes associated with nurses' work; and determining ways in which information and communication technologies can be most effectively utilized to support the capture, retrieval, and use of data, information, and knowledge. Nevertheless, for nurses in other roles, the term *informatics* remains substantively obscure and misunderstood, if at all, as does the relevance and importance of the associated work.

WHAT IS THE GOAL OF INFORMATICS?

Although already in use for a number of decades, the term *informatics* is typically viewed by the broader nursing community as the use of computers by nurses. But informatics experts are quick to identify that computer literacy is but one dimension of the latter. Hence, one might surmise that the goal of informatics is even less understood and in greater need of clear articulation. According to Staggers and Thompson (2002), the goal of nursing informatics is:

> to improve the health of populations, communities, families, and individuals by optimizing information management and communication. This includes the use of information and technology in the direct provision of care, in establishing effective administrative systems, in managing and delivering educational experiences, in supporting lifelong learning, and in supporting nursing research. (p. 260)

This goal statement reflects the breadth of the potential impact on nurses no matter what their specific role or practice setting. We might also consider that with minor modifications this statement could be applied to the broader concept of health informatics. To this end, there are some nurse authors beginning to deemphasize the notion of nursing informatics and discussing the role of nurses and their work processes in the context of health informatics (Hannah, 1995). Health informatics has been described as "knowledge of health services delivery, technology, applications, information, methodologies, and data management processes" (Kathryn Hannah cited in Thede, 2006, p. 244). The umbrella of health informatics suggests that the informatics work being done by nurses must fit within the context of the whole system. Furthermore, nurses in informatics roles are contributing to the foundation of information technology solutions and clinical processes that will support and inform interprofessional care that is *client* rather than *discipline* centric.

More timely access to data and information, clinical and financial, has been identified as a necessity in the climate of 21st-century healthcare delivery (Hannah, 1995). Health service organizations, societies, and governments throughout the industrialized world are obsessed with assuring that healthcare delivery is safer, knowledge-based, cost effective, seamless, and timely. Beyond these deliverables are also expectations of improved efficiency and quality, as well as the active engagement of consumers in their care. Several national studies have highlighted the criticality of information technology (IT) in achieving each of these goals (Institute of Medicine, 2001; Kirby, 2002; Romanow, 2002).

An additional challenge within the nursing profession is the pending human resource crisis and dire projections of imminent shortages. Consequently, nursing's focus on IT has been elevated as a central means by which nurses can be sufficiently supported in their work environments. Most importantly, IT has the potential to reduce the waste of valuable nursing resources by reducing the time spent in the care and feeding of patient records. Having more time for direct client care that is supported by ready access to information and knowledge translates into the provision of safer, quality care. Thus nurses need to be appropriately equipped with the tools to effectively and efficiently manage data, information, and knowledge. The work of nurse informaticists has become germane to the future of all nurses' work!

NURSE AS KNOWLEDGE WORKER

Nurses definitely fall into the category of knowledge workers. In fact, studies have identified that depending upon the setting, nurses spend anywhere between 25 and 50% of their day managing and recording clinical information and seeking knowledge to inform their practice (Gugerty et al., 2007). Nurses gather atomic-level data (e.g., blood pressure, pulse, blood glucose, pallor), aggregate data to derive information (e.g., impending shock), and apply knowledge (e.g., lowering head of bed to minimize the potentially deleterious effects of impending shock). Over the years, these data have been recorded into individuals' hard copy health records, chronicling findings, actions, and outcomes; this is data and information forever lost unless extracted for research purposes.

As the evidence to support nursing practice continues to be uncovered by researchers and integrated into healthcare delivery, attention must be given to the tools that will afford ready and easy access to same. It could be suggested that as knowledge workers, nurses are also, albeit unwittingly, informaticians to a large extent. With the advent of **clinical information systems (CISs)**, specifically electronic documentation and **clinical decision support (CDS)** applications, every nurse has the capacity to be contributing to the advancement of nursing knowledge on many different levels. Imagine the use of IT solutions to not only capture discrete, quantifiable data, but also the nurse's experiential and intuitive personal knowledge not typically captured in paper records. Further to that, add family history, culture, environment and social factors, past experiences, and perspectives from patients and families into the mix—the possibilities for generating new understandings within populations and across the life span and care continuum are endless.

CREATING CLINICAL KNOWLEDGE

Graves and Corcoran (1989) suggest that **nursing knowledge** is "simultaneously the laws and relationships that exist between the elements that describe the phenomena of concern in nursing (factual knowledge) and the laws or rules that the nurse uses to combine the facts to make clinical nursing decisions" (p. 230). In their view, not only does knowledge support decision making, but it also leads to new discoveries. Thus, we might think about the future creation of nursing knowledge as being the discovery of new laws and relationships that can continue to advance nursing practice.

New technologies have made the capture of multifaceted data and information possible through the use of technologies like digital imaging (e.g., photography to support wound management). Now part of the clinical record, such images add a new dimension to the assessment, monitoring, and treatment of illness and the maintenance of wellness. Beyond the use of computer keyboards, input devices are being integrated with CIS and utilized to gather data and information for the following clinical and administrative purposes:

- Biometrics (e.g., facial recognition, security)
- Voice and video recordings (e.g., client interviews and observations, diagnostic procedures—ultrasounds)
- Voice-to-text files (e.g., voice recognition for documentation)
- Medical devices, (e.g., infusion pumps, ventilators, hemodynamic monitors)
- Bar-code technologies (e.g., medication administration)
- Telehome monitoring (e.g., for use in diabetes and other chronic disease management)

These are but a few of the emerging capabilities that will allow for numerous data inputs to be transposed—combined, analyzed, and displayed to provide information and views of clinical situations currently not possible in a world dominated by hard copy documentation. With the use of information and communication technologies to support the capture and processing (i.e., interpretation, organization, and structuring) of all relevant clinical data, relationships can be identified and formalized into new knowledge. This transformational process is at the core of generating new nursing knowledge at a rate never experienced before, and in the context of our current research paradigms, the same relationships would likely take years to uncover.

Many renowned nurse authors have described the knowledge used by nurses (Benner, 1983; Carper, 1978; Schultz & Meleis, 1988). Carper's landmark paper on the fundamental patterns of knowing was the genesis of many subsequent papers and analyses. Although it is beyond the scope of this chapter, a revisiting of Carper's four ways of knowing gives a context for considering the capture, retrieval, and generation of knowledge through the use of information technology and the possibilities for the future. The four patterns of knowing she addressed included "(1) empirics, the science of nursing; (2) esthetics, the art of nursing; (3) personal knowledge; and (4) ethics, the moral knowledge of nursing" (p. 14). If we fundamentally agree with Carper that …

> nursing … depends on the scientific knowledge of human behavior in health and in illness, the esthetic perception of significant human experiences, a personal understanding of the unique individuality of the self and the capacity to make choices within concrete situations involving particular moral judgements (p. 22)

… then imagine the information system possibilities for each of the following:

1. *Empirics*—access to factual knowledge derived from repositories of aggregated clinical research findings and integrated with the CIS. A nurse assesses a stroke patient for signs of skin breakdown, photographs and documents early ulcerations, and submits the photos and documentation to CIS. The nurse receives an option to review the best practices for care of the patient and to submit consult to a wound management specialist. Clinical findings, treatment, and response are logged and aggregated with similar cases contributing to the knowledge base related to nursing and care of the integumentary system.
2. *Esthetics*—access to multicultural practices and beliefs. A client expresses concerns with her prescribed dietary treatment and expresses a preference for a female care provider. With a query to the CIS for the client's history and sociocultural background, the nurse derives an explanation from the patient's religious, cultural background, and makes a notation to carry forward for future admissions.
3. *Personal*—access to a personal repository of clinical experiences and reactions. A nurse is finding it difficult to interact with a pregnant client with a known history of alcohol abuse. While reflecting on her negativity, she submits a query to the CIS of her past assignments to identify related clinical cases. Upon reviewing the results, she identifies a painful past experience she had with a child who succumbed to the effects of fetal alcohol syndrome. She has heightened sensitivity to her potential negative reactions to this client and recognizes that she may not be optimally therapeutic in this situation.
4. *Ethics*—access to standards of ethical practice, but also access to experts in the field of moral reasoning to guide interaction. An ICU team is having difficulty dealing with the family of a patient with a brain tumor and extensive metastatic disease. They are requesting lifesaving measures at any cost. The team seeks consultation from a bioethicist and seeks out relevant case examples from the ethics CDS system to guide their discussions.

In each and every instance of interacting with the CIS, a nurse will add further to these repositories of knowledge on the basis of his or her daily clinical challenges and queries. The continued expansion and aggregation of knowledge about clients and populations; their personal, cultural, physical, and clinical presentations; and our own experiences and guidance from others will only serve to enhance the personalization and knowledge base of care provided.

There will come a day when all nurses become generators of new knowledge by virtue of CISs that embed machine learning and case-based reasoning methods within their core functionality. Imagine the power of having access to systems that aggregate the same data elements and information garnered from multiple clinical situations and provide a probability estimate of the likely outcome for individuals of a certain age, with a specific diagnosis and comorbid conditions, medication profile, symptoms, and interventions. How much more rapidly would our understanding of the efficacy of clinical interventions be elucidated? Historically, some knowledge might have taken years of research to discover—e.g., that long-standing practices are sometimes more harmful than beneficial! A case in point is the long-standing practice of instilling endotracheal tubes with normal saline prior to suctioning (O'Neal, Grap, Thompson, & Dudley, 2001). Based upon the evidence gathered through several studies, we are now aware of the potentially deleterious effects of this practice. Conceivably a meta-analysis approach to clinical studies will be expedited by converging large clinical data repositories across care settings, reflecting the collective contributions of health professionals and longitudinal outcomes for individuals, families, and populations.

USING CLINICAL KNOWLEDGE

Evidence-based practice (EBP) and **research utilization (RU)** are concepts that have been widely addressed in the nursing literature. Although the benefits of integrating research into practice may be viewed as self-evident, Estabrooks (1999) suggested that we know little as yet about what factors influence the adoption of clinical research findings into practice. She reported that nurses infrequently sourced out research journals to support and guide clinical practice decisions. She also posed a number of questions, such as how will we synthesize and incorporate different research findings that result from different methodological, and sometimes epistemological, research traditions? What will be the role of synthesized research findings? Are we presently equipped to synthesize all forms of research findings? These questions, in the context of the preceding discussion, may have answers in the design of the CIS of the future.

Best practice guidelines hold much promise for the future, but again in their typical form of paper volumes and oft unsearchable online versions, these resources will not realize significant adoption by an already stressed and stretched nursing workforce. To achieve the goals inherent in the notions of EBP and RU, the profession needs to assure that CIS solutions have the capacity for integrated access to nursing knowledge resources. To this end, nurses need to be engaged in the design of CIS tools that support access to and the generation of nursing knowledge. Of particular importance to the future design of CIS is the adoption of clinical data standards. Although this is beyond the scope of this chapter, there has been at least 2 decades of work effort directed to the articulation of standardized data elements that reflect nursing practice. The profession has been steadily moving towards consensus on the adoption of data standards, and recent work suggests that we are achieving significant strides (Bickford & Hunter, 2006; Delaney, 2006). Consider that as CISs are widely implemented, as standards for nursing documentation and reporting are adopted, and as healthcare IT solutions continue to evolve, the potential to synthesize findings from a variety of methods and worldviews becomes much more probable.

CLINICAL DECISION SUPPORT

Clinical decision support tools have evolved beyond the previously prevailing notion of accessible reference texts and written resource materials like policies and procedures. In the world of clinical computing, the capability to link various information sources and present a clinician with immediate guidance and support has begun to net benefits for safer care and improved clinical outcomes. Osheroff and colleagues (2007) defined clinical decision support as tools that: "provide(s) clinicians, staff, patients, or other individuals with knowledge and person-specific information, intelligently filtered or presented at appropriate times, to enhance health and health care" (p. 141).

Most available CDS for nursing practice, although promising, is simplistic and in early development. Typically, CDS includes tools such as (1) computerized alerts and reminders (e.g., medication due, patient has an allergy, potassium level abnormal); (2) clinical guidelines (e.g., best practice for prevention of skin breakdown); (3) online information retrieval (e.g., CINAHL, drug information); (4) clinical order sets and protocols; and (5) online access to organizational policies and procedures. In the future, these tools will be possibly expanded to include applications with embedded case-based reasoning.

CHALLENGES IN GETTING THERE

Leadership

The field of nurse leaders in health informatics has markedly grown in the past 2 decades. However, a significant knowledge gap needs addressing within our nursing leadership community. Many of our nurse leaders need to acquire a new set of skills and knowledge to understand and advance the adoption of information tools and technologies to support the delivery of clinical care. For several years, nurse informaticians have advocated for the need for all nursing leaders to become knowledgeable and engaged in setting the direction for informatics in the profession (Nagle, 2005; Simpson, 2000).

Strategies:

1. Identify the informatics education needs of nurse leaders.
2. Develop mentorship programs for the acquisition of informatics leadership skills.
3. Assure enrollment of nurse leaders as sponsors for electronic health records initiatives.

Clinical Practice

Despite many valiant efforts to implement comprehensive CIS throughout North American healthcare settings, there are still many provider organizations with limited online functionality available to nurses. As indicated by numerous studies and reports of the state of IT adoption, many providers are still in the early phases of acquisition and implementation (Eggert & Protti, 2006). Ironically, this is probably good news for nursing. There is an opportunity for nurses to immerse themselves in the developmental work of IT solutions to support practice.

Over the years, nurses have been on the receiving end of systems that either did not add value to their work or by virtue of poor design created additional work. The opportunity to avoid future installations of IT solutions that do nothing to benefit and support the clinical practice of nurses and healthcare teams is upon us now. It behooves nurses to be engaged in the acquisition, design, implementation, and evaluation of CIS to assure the realization of benefits for clinical care and outcomes.

It is equally important to consider that due to the average age of a majority of practicing nurses, many have yet to develop a comfort level with the use of computers in their work settings. In order to minimize the anxiety associated with expected IT use, particular attention needs to be given to the issue of computer literacy. If nurses lack a solid footing in computer use, expectations for integration of informatics will be difficult, if not impossible to realize.

Strategies for Nurses

1. Be encouraged and supported to participate in the acquisition, design, implementation, and evaluation phases of CIS.
2. Demand the adoption of IT solutions that support the delivery of safe, quality care.

3. Be provided with material and people resources to support their acquisition of informatics competencies.

Education

Over the years, numerous efforts have been undertaken to identify the core informatics competencies needed by nurses. These efforts have encompassed attempts to articulate core competencies for all nurses, from novice to expert (Hebert, 2000) as well as competencies for informatics experts (Hersh, 2006). In recognizing nursing informatics as a specialty, the American Nurses Association (2001) has articulated scope and standards of nursing informatics practice. What remains clear is that while progress has been made in the preparation of nursing informatics experts, there is still much work to be done at the grassroots level of nursing education.

Recent studies of schools of nursing indicate that few basic nursing education programs have embedded the concepts and processes associated with informatics within the core curricula (Carty & Rosenfeld, 1998; Nagle & Clarke, 2004). The primary obstacles to realizing curricula with embedded informatics concepts have been cited to include a lack of faculty capacity, constraints of clinical practice environments (e.g., lack of student access to clinical information systems), and limited funding. These barriers need to be addressed to assure that graduates of the future are prepared for settings utilizing information technology to support clinical care.

The core concepts and competencies of informatics are particularly well suited to a model of interprofessional education. Ideally, when emulating clinical settings, informatics knowledge should be integrated with the processes of interprofessional teams and decision making. As simulation laboratories are becoming increasingly common fixtures in the delivery of health professional education, they provide a perfect opportunity to incorporate EHR applications including access to CDS. The learning laboratory will then more closely approximate the IT-enabled clinical settings that are emerging.

A presumption is often made that future graduates will be more computer literate than nurses currently in practice. Although this is likely true, computer comfort does not equate to an understanding of the facilitative and transformative role that IT will have in the future. It is essential that the future curricula of basic nursing programs embed the concepts of the role of information technology in supporting clinical care delivery.

Strategies:

1. Need to share prototypes of informatics integration among schools of nursing.

2. Consider interprofessional education opportunities in addressing informatics concepts and competencies.
3. Nursing faculty need to be obligated and supported in the attainment of basic informatics competencies.
4. Seek and allocate funding for the development of innovative curricular models and associated technological support.
5. Incorporate accreditation criteria that necessitate an integration of informatics core concepts *and competencies in all basic nursing programs.*

A VIEW TO THE FUTURE

Overall, it is fair to say that a majority of nurses have yet to embrace the notion of informatics and understand its meaning and relevance to their work. There is an emerging global focus on information technology to support clinical care and the potential benefits for clinicians and patients. The future holds a landscape yet to be understood as technology evolves with a rapidity and unfolding that is rich with promise and potential peril. Anticipate that in the future, we will have the computing power to aggregate and transform additional multidimensional data and information sources (e.g., historical, multisensory, experiential, and genetic sources) into CIS. With the availability of such rich repositories, there will be opportunities to do the following:

- Further enhance the training of health professionals
- Advance the design and application of CDSs
- Deliver care that is informed by the most current evidence
- Engage with individuals and families in ways yet unimagined

The basic education of all health professions will evolve over the next decade to incorporate core informatics competencies. In general, the clinical care environments will be connected, and information will be integrated across disciplines to the benefit of care providers and citizens alike. The future of health care will be highly dependent upon the use of CIS and CDS to achieve the systems' global aspirations of safer, quality care for all citizens.

SUMMARY

In this chapter, the author has advanced a view that every nurse's practice will make contributions to new nursing knowledge in dynamically interactive CIS environments. Afforded with the right tools to support the management of data, complex information processing and ready access to knowledge, nursing will be positioned to lay valid claims to EBP and RU. The core concepts and competencies associated with informatics will be embedded in the practice of every nurse, whether administrator, researcher, educator, or practitioner. Informatics will be prominent in the knowledge work of nurses, yet it will be a subtlety because of its eventual fulsome integration with clinical care processes. Clinical care will be substantially supported by the capacity and promise of technology—today and tomorrow.

The most important thought that I would like to leave with you is not to limit the possibilities for the future by focusing on the world of practice as we know it today. Information technology is not a panacea, but it will provide the profession with unprecedented capacity to more rapidly generate and disseminate new knowledge. Realizing the possibilities necessitates that all nurses understand and leverage the informatician within and contribute to the future that awaits.

THOUGHT-PROVOKING Questions

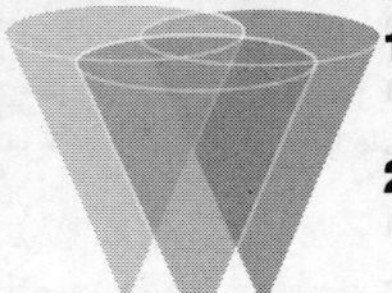

1. What are the possibilities to accelerate the generation and uptake of new nursing knowledge?
2. What should be the areas of priority for the advancement of informatics in nursing?

References

American Nurses Association. (2001). *Scope and standards of nursing informatics practice.* Washington, DC: ANA.

Benner, P. (1983). Uncovering the knowledge embedded in clinical practice. *Image: The Journal of Nursing Scholarship, 15*(2), 36–41.

Bickford, C. J., & Hunter, K. M. (2006). Theories, models, and frameworks. In V. K. Saba & K. A. McCormick (Eds.), *Essentials of nursing informatics* (4th ed., pp. 265–278). New York: McGraw Hill.

Carper, B. A. (1978). Fundamental patterns of knowing in nursing. *Advances in Nursing Science, 1*(1), 13–23.

Carty, B., & Rosenfeld, P. (1998). From computer technology to information technology. Findings from a national study of nursing education. *Computers in Nursing, 16*(5), 259–265.

Delaney, C. W. (2006). Nursing minimum data set systems. In V. K. Saba & K. A. McCormick (Eds.), *Essentials of nursing informatics* (4th ed., pp. 249–261). New York: McGraw Hill.

Eggert, C., & Protti, D. (2006). Clinical electronic communications: A new paradigm that is here to stay? *Electronic Healthcare, 5*(2), 88–96.

Estabrooks, C. (1999). Will evidence-based practice make practice perfect? *Canadian Journal of Nursing Research, 30*(4), 273–294. Retrieved August 27, 2007, from http://cjnr.mcgill.ca/archive/30/30_4_estabrooks.html

Graves, J. R., & Corcoran, S. (1989). The study of nursing informatics. *Image: The Journal of Nursing Scholarship, 21*(4), 227–231.

Gugerty, B., Maranda, M. J., Beachley, M., Navarro, V. B., Newbold, S., Hawk, W., et al. (2007). *Challenges and opportunities in documentation of the nursing care of patients.* Baltimore: Documentation Work Group, Maryland Nursing Workforce Commission. Retrieved August 27, 2007, from http://www.mbon.org/commission2/documentation_challenges.pdf

Hannah, K. J. (1995). Transforming information: Data management support of healthcare reorganization. *Journal of the American Medical Informatics Association, 2*(3), 147–155.

Hannah, K. J., Ball, M. J., & Edwards, M. J. A. (1984). *Introduction to nursing informatics.* New York: Springer-Verlag.

Hebert, M. (2000). A national education strategy to develop nursing informatics competencies. *Canadian Journal of Nursing Leadership, 13*(2), 11–14.

Hersh, W. (2006). Who are the informaticians? What we know and should know. *Journal of the American Medical Informatics Association, 13*(2), 166–170.

Institute of Medicine. (2001). *Crossing the quality chasm: A new health system for the 21st century.* Washington, DC: National Academy Press.

Kirby, M. J. L. (2002). *Final report: The health of Canadians—The federal role.* Ottawa, Ontario, Canada: Queen's Printer.

Nagle, L. M. (2005). Dr. Lynn Nagle and the case for nursing informatics. *Canadian Journal of Nursing Leadership, 18*(1), 16–18.

Nagle, L. M., & Clarke, H. F. (2004). Assessing informatics in Canadian schools of nursing. *Proceedings 11th World Congress on Medical Informatics.* San Francisco. [CD].

O'Neal, P. V., Grap, M. J., Thompson, C., & Dudley, W. (2001). Level of dyspnea experienced in mechanically ventilated adults with and without saline instillation prior to endotracheal suctioning. *Intensive Critical Care Nursing, 17*(6), 356–363.

Osheroff, J. A., Teich, J. M., Middleton, B., Steen, E. B., Wright, A., & Detmer, D. E. (2007). A roadmap for national action on clinical decision support. *Journal of the American Medical Informatics Association, 14*(2), 141–145.

Romanow, R. J. (2002). *Building on values: The future of healthcare in Canada.* Ottawa, Ontario, Canada: Queen's Printer.

Schultz, P. R., & Meleis, A. I. (1988). Nursing epistemology: Traditions, insights, questions. *Image: The Journal of Nursing Scholarship, 20*(4), 217–221.

Schwirian, P. (1986). The NI pyramid: A model for research in nursing informatics. *Computers in Nursing, 4*(6), 134–136.

Simpson, R. L. (2000). Need to know: Essential survival skills for the Information Age. *Nursing Administration Quarterly, 25*(1), 142–147.

Staggers, N., & Thompson, C. B. (2002). The evolution of definitions for nursing informatics: A critical analysis and revised definition. *Journal of the American Medical Informatics Association, 9*(3), 255–261.

Thede, L. Q. (2006). Top drawer. *Computers, Informatics, Nursing, 24*(5), 243–245.

Turley, J. (1996). Toward a model for nursing informatics. *Image: Journal of Nursing Scholarship, 28*, 309–313.

section

Nursing Informatics Applications: Nursing Administration and Nursing Practice

Nursing informatics (NI) and information technology (IT) have invaded nursing, and some nurses are happy with the capabilities afforded by this specialty. Others remain convinced that changes wrought by information technology are nothing more than a nuisance. In the past, nursing administrators have found the implementation of technology tools to be an expensive venture with minimal rewards. This is likely related to their lack of knowledge about NI, which caused nursing administrators to listen to vendors or other colleagues—in essence, it was decision making based on limited and biased information. There were at least two reasons for the experience of limited rewards. One was the failure to include nurses in the testing and implementation of products designed for nurses and nursing tasks. Second, the new products they purchased had to interface with old, legacy systems and were not at all compatible or seemed compatible until the glitches arose. The glitches caused frustration for clinicians and administrators alike. They purchased tools that should have made the nurses happy, but instead all they did was grumble. The good news is that we have changed our approaches as a result of the difficult lessons we learned in the early forays into technology tools. Nursing personnel are involved both at the agency level as well as the vendor level, in the decision making and development of new systems and products charged with enhancing the practice of nursing. Older legacy systems are being replaced with newer systems that have more capacity to interface with other systems. Nurses and administrators have become more astute in the realm of NI. Having said that, however, we caution that we still have a long way to go!

The electronic health record (EHR) initiative has moved many healthcare agencies into the information age. Clinical information systems (CIS) have traditionally been designed for use by one unit or department within an institution. However, because clinicians working in other areas of the organization need access to this information, this data and information is generally used by more than one area. The new initiatives arising with the development of the EHR place institutions in the position of striving to manage their CIS through the EHR. Currently, there are many CISs, including nursing, laboratory, pharmacy, monitoring, and order entry, plus additional ancillary systems to meet the individual institutions' needs. Each organization must determine who can access and use their information systems. The information systems, electronic documentation, and the EHR are changing the way nurses and physicians practice. It is also changing how patients enter and receive data and information. Some institutions are permitting patient access to their own records electronically via the Internet. Confidentiality and privacy issues loom with the new electronic systems. HIPAA regulations and professional ethics principles must remain at the forefront when we interact electronically with intimate patient data and information.

Administrators need information systems that facilitate their administrative role, and they particularly need systems that provide financial, risk management, quality assurance, human resources, payroll, patient registration, acuity, communication, and scheduling functions. The administrator must be open to learning about all of the tools available to them. One of the most important tasks that an administrator can oversee and engage in is data mining, or the extraction of data and information from sizeable data sets collected and warehoused. Data mining helps to identify patterns in aggregate data, gain insights, and ultimately discover and generate knowledge applicable to nursing science. Nursing administrators must become astute informaticists—knowledge workers who harness the information and knowledge at their fingertips to facilitate the practice of their clinicians, improve patient care, and advance the science of nursing.

Nursing information systems must support nurses enacting their roles to deliver quality patient care. The system must be responsive to their needs, allowing them to manage their data and information as they need to as well as providing access to necessary references, literature sources, and other networked departments. Nurses have always practiced in a field where they have had to use their ingenuity, resourcefulness, creativity, initiative, and skills. These clinicians as knowledge workers also need to apply these same abilities and skills to become astute users of the information systems available to them to improve patient care and advance the science of nursing.

FIGURE III-1
Foundation of Knowledge model. (Designed by Alicia Mastrian.)

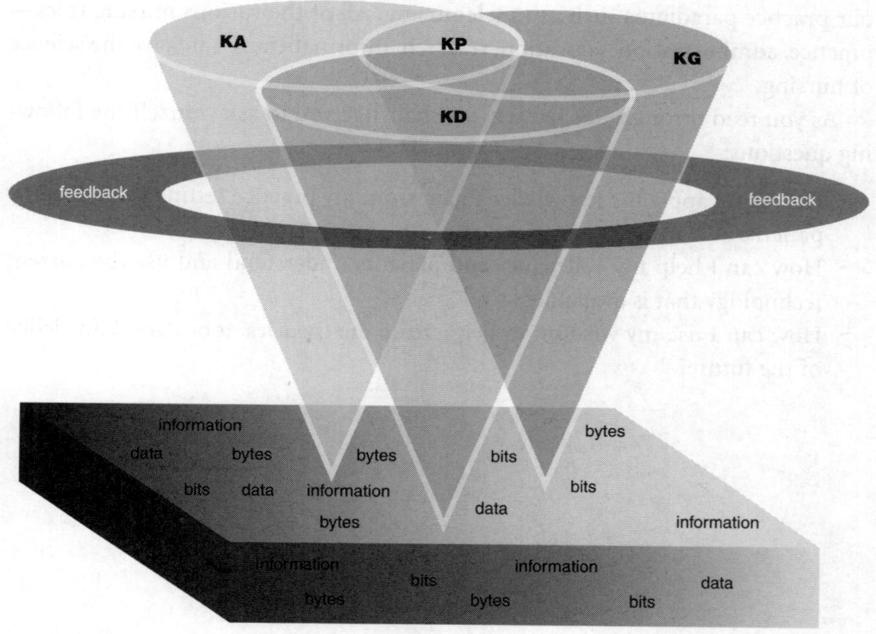

KA- Knowledge Acquisition
KD- Knowledge Dissemination
KG- Knowledge Generation
KP- Knowledge Processing

In this section you will learn about ethics, HIPAA, securing information, clinical practice tools, EHR, administrative and clinical information systems, consumer information and education needs, population and community health, telehealth, and telenursing. Many of the chapters in this section were contributed by informatics experts from around the world. While there may occasionally be some similarities in the information presented, we believe that it is important to preserve the perspective provided by our expert contributors.

As you are aware, the material within this book is placed within the context of the Foundation of Knowledge model (see Figure III-1) to meet healthcare delivery systems', organizations', patients', and nurses' needs. Continue to assess where you are in the model. The Foundation of Knowledge model reflects that knowledge is powerful, and for that reason, nurses focus on information as a key resource. This section addresses the information systems that administrators and clinicians interact with in their healthcare environments that are affected by legislation, professional codes of ethics, consumerism, and reconceptualization of our practice paradigms such as in telenursing. All of the various nursing roles—practice, administration, education, research, informaticians—involve the science of nursing.

As you read through this section, we challenge you to ask yourself the following questions:

- How can I apply the knowledge I gain from my practice setting to benefit my patients and enhance my practice?
- How can I help my colleagues and patients understand and use the current technology that is available?
- How can I use my wisdom to help create the theories, tools, and knowledge of the future?

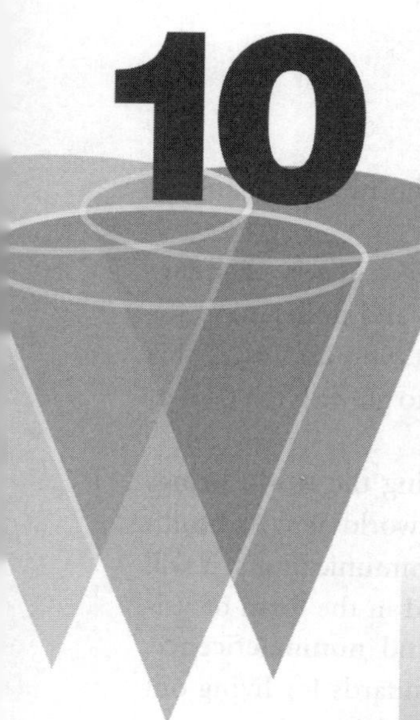

10 Ethical Applications of Informatics

Kathleen Mastrian, Dee McGonigle, and Nedra Farcus

Objectives

1. Recognize ethical dilemmas in nursing informatics.
2. Examine ethical implications of nursing informatics.
3. Evaluate professional responsibilities for the ethical use of healthcare informatics technology.
4. Explore the ethical model for ethical decision making.
5. Analyze practical ways of applying the ethical model for ethical decision making to manage ethical dilemmas in nursing informatics.

Key Terms

Alternatives
Antiprinciplism
Autonomy
Beneficence
Bioethics
Bioinformatics
Care ethics
Casuist approach
Confidentiality
Consequences
Courage
Decision making
Decision support
Duty
Ethical decision making
Ethical dilemma
Ethical, social, and legal implications (ESLI)
Ethicist
Ethics
Eudaemonistic
Fidelity
Good
Harm
Justice
Liberty

INTRODUCTION

As we followed the actual events or were entertained by the movie *Apollo 13* (Howard, 1995), we all watched the astronauts trying against all odds to bring their crippled spaceship back to Earth. The speed of their travel was incomprehensible to most of us, and the task of bringing that spaceship back to Earth seemed nearly impossible. They were experiencing a crisis never imagined by the experts at NASA, and they were making up their survival plan moment by moment. What brought them back to Earth safely? Surely we must give credit to the technology and the spaceship's ability to withstand the trauma it experienced. But what amazed us most were the traditional nontechnological tools, skills, and supplies that were used in new and different ways to stabilize the spacecraft's environment and keep the astronauts safe while traveling toward their uncertain future.

This sense of constancy in the midst of change serves to stabilize our experience in many different life events and contributes to our survival of crisis and change. This rhythmic process is also vital to the healthcare

Key Terms *Continued*
Moral dilemmas
Moral rights
Morals
Negligence
Nicomachean
Nonmaleficence
Principlism
Privacy
Rights
Security
Self-control
Standard
Truth
Uncertainty
Values
Veracity
Virtue
Virtue ethics
Wisdom

system's stability and survival in the presence of the rapidly changing events of the Information Age.

No one can dispute the fact that the Information Age is changing health care in ways that will not be fully recognized and understood for years. The change is paradigmatic and every expert who addresses this change reminds healthcare professionals of the need to go with the flow of rapid change or be left behind.

As with any paradigm shift, a new way of viewing the world brings with it some of the enduring **values** of the previous worldview. As health care journeys into the brave new world of digital communications, it will bring along some familiar tools and skills recognized in the form of values, such as **privacy**, **confidentiality**, autonomy, and **nonmaleficence.** While these basic values remain unchanged, the standards for living out these values will take on new meaning as health professionals are confronted with new and different **moral dilemmas. Ethical decision-making** frameworks will remain constant, but the context for examining these **moral** issues or **ethical dilemmas** will become increasingly complex.

This brief overview will provide you with some familiar ethical concepts to take with you on your challenging journey into the increasingly complex future of healthcare informatics. We will briefly define ethics and bioethics and examine the evolution of ethical approaches from the Hippocratic ethic era through principlism and to the current antiprinciplism movement of ethical decision making. We encourage you to read more about these approaches as you review the cases presented in this text and as you venture further into the unfolding era of healthcare informatics.

ETHICS

Ethics is a process of systematically examining varying viewpoints related to moral questions of right and wrong. **Ethicists** have defined the term in a variety of ways, with each reflecting a basic theoretical philosophical perspective. Beauchamp and Childress (1994) refer to ethics as a generic term for various ways of understanding and examining the moral life. Ethical approaches to this examination may be normative, presenting standards of right or good action; descriptive, reporting what people believe and how they act; or explorative, analyzing the concepts and methods of ethics. Husted and Husted (1995) emphasize a practice-based ethics, stating "… ethics examines the ways men and women can exercise their power in order to bring about human benefit—the ways in which one can act in order to bring about the conditions of happiness" (p. 3). Velasquez, Andre, Shanks, and Myer (1987) posed the question, *What is* *ethics?* and answered this question with the following two-part response: "First, ethics refers to well-based standards of right and wrong that prescribe what humans ought to do, usually in terms of rights, obligations, benefits to society, fairness, or specific virtues" (¶ 10); and "Secondly, ethics refers to the study and development of one's ethical standards" (¶ 11). Regardless of the theoretical definition, common characteristics regarding ethics are its dialectical, goal-oriented approach to answering questions that have the potential of multiple acceptable answers.

BIOETHICS

Bioethics is defined as the study and formulation of healthcare ethics. Bioethics takes on relevant ethical problems experienced by healthcare providers in the provision of care to individuals and groups. Husted and Husted (1995) state the fundamental background of bioethics that forms its essential nature is "1. The nature and needs of humans as living, thinking beings; 2. The purpose and function of the healthcare system in a human society; and 3. An increased cultural awareness of human beings' essential moral status" (p. 7). Bioethics arose in the 1970s as health care began to change its focus from a mechanistic approach of treating disease to a more holistic approach of treating people with illnesses. As technology advances increased, recognition and acknowledgment of **rights** and the needs of individuals and groups receiving this high-tech care also increased.

ETHICAL DILEMMAS AND MORALS

Ethical dilemmas arise when moral issues raise questions that cannot be answered with a simple, clearly defined rule, fact, or authoritative view. **Morals** refer to social convention about right and wrong human conduct that are so widely shared that they form a stable (although usually incomplete) communal consensus (Beauchamp & Childress, 1994). Moral dilemmas arise with **uncertainty** as is the case when the evidence we are confronted with indicates an action is morally right and other evidence indicates that this action is also morally wrong. Uncertainty is stressful and in the face of inconclusive evidence on both sides of the dilemma, causes the person to question what he or she should do. There are times when the individual concludes that based on his or her moral beliefs, he or she cannot act. Uncertainty also arises from unanticipated effects or unforeseeable behavioral responses to actions or the lack of action. Adding uncertainty to the situational factors and personal beliefs that must be considered creates a need for an ethical decision making model to help one choose the best action.

ETHICAL DECISION MAKING

Ethical **decision making** refers to the process of making informed choices about ethical dilemmas based on a set of standards differentiating right from wrong. The decision making reflects an understanding of the principles and standards of ethical decision making, as well as philosophical approaches to ethical decision making, and it requires a systematic framework for addressing the complex and often controversial moral questions.

THINK ABOUT THIS . . .

As we delve into the high-speed era of digital communications, the rights and the needs of individuals and groups will be of utmost concern to all healthcare professionals. The changing meaning of *communication* alone will bring with it new concerns by healthcare professionals for protecting patients' rights of confidentiality, privacy, and autonomy. The concept of nonmaleficence, or do no **harm**, will be broadened to include those individuals and groups we may never see in person, but with whom we will enter into a professional relationship of trust and care. Systematic and flexible ethical decision-making abilities will be essential for all healthcare professionals.

THEORETICAL APPROACHES TO HEALTHCARE ETHICS

Theoretical approaches to healthcare ethics have evolved in response to societal changes. In a 30-year retrospective article for the *Journal of the American Medical Association,* Pellegrino (1993) traced the evolution of healthcare ethics from the Hippocratic ethic through **principlism** and into the current **antiprinciplism** movement.

The Hippocratic tradition emerged from relatively homogenous societies where beliefs were similar and the majority of societal members shared common values. The emphasis was on **duty**, virtue, and gentlemanly conduct.

Principlism arose as societies became more heterogeneous and members began experiencing a diversity of incompatible beliefs and values. Principlism emerged as a foundation for ethical decision making. Principles were expansive enough to be shared by all rational individuals, regardless of their background and individual beliefs. This approach continued into the 20th century and was popularized by two bioethicists, Beauchamp and Childress (1977, 1994), in the last quarter of the century. Principles are considered as broad guidelines that provide us with guidance or direction but leave substantial room for our case-specific judgment. From principles, we are able to develop more detailed rules and policies. Beauchamp and Childress (1994) proposed four principles, including respect for autonomy, nonmaleficence, beneficence, and **justice**. Nonmaleficence asserts an obligation not to inflict harm intentionally and forms the framework for the **standard** of due care to be met by any professional. Obligations of nonmaleficence are obligations of not inflicting harm and not imposing risks of harm. **Negligence**, a departure from the standard of due care toward others, includes intentionally posing risks that are unreasonable as well as unintentionally but carelessly imposing risks. **Autonomy** refers to the individual's freedom from controlling interferences by others and from personal limitations that prevent meaningful choices, such as adequate understanding. The following two conditions are essential for autonomy: **liberty**, the independence from controlling influences; and the individual's capacity for intentional action. **Beneficence** refers to actions performed that contribute to the welfare of others. There are two principles of beneficence, which are: positive beneficence requires the provision of benefits, and utility requires that benefits and drawbacks be balanced. One must avoid negative beneficence that occurs when there are constraints on activities that, even though might not be unjust, could in some situations cause detriment or harm to others. Justice refers to the fair, equitable, and appropriate treatment in light of what is due or owed to a person. Distributive justice refers to fair, equitable, and appropriate distribution in society determined by justified norms that structure the terms of social cooperation. Beauchamp and Childress also suggest three types of rules for guiding actions (rules are more restrictive in scope than principles are and are more specific in content). Substantive rules are rules of truth telling, confidentiality, privacy, **fidelity**, and those pertaining to the allocation and rationing of health care, omitting treatment, physician-assisted suicide, and informed consent. Authority rules are those rules regarding who may and should perform actions. Procedural rules establish procedures to be followed.

The antiprinciplism movement has emerged with the expansive technological changes and the tremendous rise in ethical dilemmas accompanying these changes. Opponents of principlism include those who claim that its principles do not represent a theoretical approach and those who claim that its principles are too far removed from the concrete particularities of everyday human existence; the principles are too conceptual, intangible, or abstract; or they disregard or do not take into account a person's psychological factors, personality, life history, sexual orientation, or religious, ethnic, and cultural background. We will briefly explore different approaches to making ethical decisions, providing you with an understanding of the varied methods professionals may use to arrive at an ethical decision.

The **casuist approach** to ethical decision making grew out of the concern for more concrete methods of examining ethical dilemmas. Casuistry is a case-based ethical reasoning method that analyzes the facts of a case in a sound, logical, and ordered or structured manner. The facts are compared to the decisions arising out of consensus in previous paradigmatic or model cases. One casuist proponent, Jonsen (1991), prefers particular and concrete paradigms and analogies over the universal and abstract theories of principlism.

The Husted bioethical decision-making model centers on the healthcare professional's implicit agreement with patient/client (Husted & Husted, 1995), and is based on six contemporary bioethical standards: autonomy, freedom, **veracity**, privacy, beneficence, and fidelity.

The **virtue ethics** approach emphasizes the virtuous character of individuals who make the choices. A **virtue** is any characteristic or disposition we desire in others or ourselves. It comes from the Greek word *aretai*, meaning excellence, and it refers to what we expect of ourselves and others. Virtue ethicists emphasize the ideal situation and attempt to identify and define ideals. Virtue ethics dates back to Plato and Socrates. When asked "whether virtue can be taught or whether virtue can be acquired in some other way, Socrates answers that if virtue is knowledge, then it can be taught. Thus, Socrates assumes that whatever can be known can be taught" (Scott, 2002, ¶ 9).

Thus, the cause of any moral weakness was not a matter of character flaws but of ignorance. A person acts immorally because he does not know what is really good for him. A person can be overpowered by immediate pleasures and forget to consider the long-term **consequences**. Plato emphasized that to lead a moral life and not succumb to immediate pleasures and gratification, one must have a moral vision. He identified four cardinal virtues: **wisdom**, **courage**, **self-control**, and justice. Aristotle's **Nicomachean** principles (Aristotle, 350 BC) also contribute to virtue ethics. Virtues are connected to will and motive since the intention is what determines if one is acting virtuously or not. Ethical considerations, according to his **eudaemonistic** principles, address the question, "What is it to be an excellent person?" For Aristotle this ultimately means acting in a temperate manner according to a rational mean between extreme possibilities.

Virtue ethics has seen a resurgence recently (Healthcare Ethics, 2007). Two of the most influential moral and medical authors, Pellegrino and Thomasma (1993), have maintained that virtue theory should be related to other theories within comprehensive philosophy of the health professions. They argued that moral events are composed of four elements—the agent, the act, the circumstances, and the consequences—and that a variety of theories must be interrelated to account for different facets of moral judgment.

Care ethics is responsiveness to the needs of others that dictates providing care, preventing harm, and maintaining relationships. This viewpoint has been in existence for some time. Engster (n.d.) states that "Carol Gilligan's *In a Different*

Voice (1982) established care ethics as a major new perspective in contemporary moral and political discourse" (p. 2). The relationship between care and virtue is complex and Benjamin and Curtis (1992) base their framework on care ethics; they propose that "critical reflection and inquiry in ethics involves the complex interplay of a variety of human faculties, ranging from empathy and moral imagination on the one hand to analytic precision and careful reasoning on the other" (p. 12). Care ethicists are less guided by rules and focus on the needs of others and one's responsibility to meet those needs. The central focus is responsiveness to the needs of others that dictates providing care, preventing harm, and maintaining relationships. As opposed to the aforementioned theories that focused on the individual's rights, an ethic of care emphasizes a personal part of an interdependent relationship that affects how decisions are made. In this theory, the specific situation and context in which the person is embedded becomes a part of the decision-making process.

The consensus-based approach to bioethics was proposed by Martin (1999). Martin claims that American bioethics harbors a variety of ethical methods that emphasize different ethical factors, including principles, circumstances, character, interpersonal needs, and personal meaning. Each method reflects an important aspect of ethical experience, adds to the others, and enriches the ethical imagination. Thus, working with these methods provides the challenge and the opportunity necessary for the perceptive and shrewd bioethicist to transform them into something new with value through the process of building ethical consensus. Diverse ethical insights can be integrated to support a particular bioethical decision, and that decision can be understood as a new, ethical whole.

APPLYING ETHICS TO INFORMATICS

With the Information Age has come global closeness or the ability to reach around the globe instantaneously through technology. Language barriers are being broken through technological translators to enhance our interaction and exchange of data and information. Informatics practitioners are bridging continents, and international panels, committees, and organizations are beginning to establish standards and rules for the implementation of informatics. This international perspective must be taken into consideration as we ethically examine informatics dilemmas, since they will influence the development of ethical approaches that begin to accept that we are working within international networks and must recognize, respect, and regard the diverse political, social, and human factors within informatics ethics.

The ethical approaches can be used to help healthcare professionals make ethical decisions in all areas of practice. The focus of this text is on informatics. Since informatics theory and practice has continued to grow at a rapid rate, it is infiltrating every area of our professional lives. New applications and ways of performing our skills are being developed daily. Therefore, education in informatics ethics is extremely important.

Typically, situations are analyzed using our past experience and in collaboration with others. Each situation warrants its own deliberation and unique approach, since each individual patient seeking or receiving care has his/her own preferences, quality of life, and healthcare needs in a situational milieu framed within financial, provider, setting, or institutions, and social context issues. Clinicians must take into consideration all of these factors when they make ethical decisions.

The use of expert systems, **decision support** tools, evidence-based practice, and artificial intelligence in the care of our patients provides challenges as to who should use these tools, how they are implemented, and how they are tempered with clinical judgment. All clinical situations are not the same, and even though the result of interacting with these systems and tools is enhanced information and knowledge, the clinician must weigh this information in light of the patient's unique clinical circumstances including their beliefs and wishes. Our patients demand access to quality care and the information necessary to control their lives. Clinicians need to analyze and synthesize the parameters of each distinctive situation using a specific decision-making framework that helps them make the best decisions. Getting it right the first time has a tremendous impact on the expected patient outcomes. The focus needs to remain on patient outcomes while we ethically incorporate the informatics tools available.

Facing ethical dilemmas on a daily basis and struggling with unique client situations cause many clinicians to question their own actions as well as the actions of their colleagues and patients. We must realize that our colleagues and patients may reach very different decisions than we do, but that does not mean anyone is wrong. Instead, everyone reaches their ethical decision based on their individual review of the situational facts and understanding of ethics. As we deal with diversity among our patients, colleagues, and administrators, we must constantly strive to use our ethical imaginations to reach ethically competent decisions. Balancing the needs of society, her/his employer, and patients could cause the clinician to continually face ethical challenges. Society expects judicious use of the finite healthcare resources. Employers have their own policies, standards, and practices that at times can inhibit the practice of the clinician. Each patient is unique and has life experiences that affect his/her healthcare perspective, choices, motivation, and adherence. Combine all of this with the challenges of informatics, and it is clear that the evolving healthcare arena calls for an informatics-competent, politically active, consumer-oriented, business-savvy, ethical clinician to rule this ever-changing landscape we know as health care.

The goal of any ethical system should be that a rational, justifiable decision was reached. Ethics is always there to help us decide what is right. Indeed, the measure of an adequate ethical system or theory or approach is in part its ability to be useful in novel contexts. A comprehensive, robust theory of ethics should be up to the task of addressing a broad variety of new applications and challenges at the intersection of informatics and health care.

The information concerning an ethical dilemma must remain in the context of the dilemma in order to be useful. **Bioinformatics** could gather, manipulate, classify, analyze, synthesize, retrieve, and maintain databases related to ethical cases, the effective reasoning applied to various ethical dilemmas, and the resulting ethical decisions. This would be potent but the resolution of dilemmas cannot be had from just examining relevant cases from this database. Clinicians must assess each situational context, the patient's specific situation and needs, and make their ethical decisions based on all of the information they have at hand.

Ethics is exciting, and competent clinicians need to know about ethical dilemmas and solutions in their professions. Ethicists have been thought of as experts in the arbitrary, ambiguous, and ungrounded judgments of other people. Ethicists know that they make the best decision they can based on the situation and stakeholders at hand. Just as we try to make the best decisions with and for our patients, ethically we must do the same. We must critically think through the situation to arrive at the best decision.

In order to make ethical decisions about informatics technologies and patients' intimate healthcare data and information, we must be informatics competent. To the extent that information technology is reshaping healthcare practices or promises to improve patient care, then healthcare professionals must be trained and be competent in the use of these tools. This competency needs to be evaluated by instruments developed by professional groups or societies; this will help with consistency and quality. In order for the healthcare professional to be a patient advocate, it is necessary for the professional to understand how information technology impacts the patient and the subsequent delivery of care. Information science and its effect on health care are both interesting and important. It follows that IT and its **ethical, social, and legal implications** (**ESLI**) should be incorporated into all levels of professional education. The need for confidentiality was perhaps first articulated by Hippocrates, so if anything is different it is in the ways it can be violated. It might be that the use of computers for clinical decision support and data mining in research raise new ethical issues. Ethical dilemmas associated with the integration of informatics must be examined to provide an ethical framework that considers all of the stakeholders. Patients' rights must be protected in the face of a healthcare provider's duty to his or her employer and society at large when initiating care and assigning finite healthcare resources. An ethical framework is necessary to help guide healthcare providers in reference to the ethical treatment of electronic data and information during all stages of collection, storage, manipulation, and dissemination.

These new approaches and means come with their own ethical dilemmas. Many times, they are dilemmas we have not yet faced if we are on the cutting edge of these technologies. You have just learned about ethics and varied ethical approaches; it is now time to help you synthesize what you have learned in order to make judicious ethical decisions in your practice. Just as we use processes and models to diagnose and treat our patients in practice, we can also apply a model in the analysis and synthesis of ethical dilemmas or cases. The ethical model for ethical decision making (see Box 10-1) facilitates our ability to analyze the dilemma and synthesize the information into a plan of action (McGonigle, 2000). It is based on the letters in the word *ethical*. Each letter guides and prompts us to critically think (think and rethink) through the situation presented. The model is a tool since, in the final analysis, it allows us to objectively ascertain the essence of the dilemma and develop a plan of action.

BOX 10-1

Ethical Model for Ethical Decision Making

Examine the ethical dilemma (conflicting values exist).
Thoroughly comprehend the possible alternatives available.
Hypothesize ethical arguments.
Investigate, compare, and evaluate the arguments for each alternative.
Choose the alternative you would recommend.
Act on your chosen alternative.
Look at the ethical dilemma and examine the outcomes while reflecting on the ethical decision.

Applying the Ethical Model

Examine the ethical dilemma.

- Use your problem-solving, decision-making, and critical-thinking skills.
- What is the dilemma you are analyzing? Collect as much information about the dilemma as you can, making sure to gather the relevant facts that clearly identify the dilemma. You should be able to describe the dilemma you are analyzing in detail.
- Ascertain exactly what must be decided.
- Who should be involved in the decision-making process for this specific case?

BOX Continued
10-1

- Who are the interested players or stakeholders?
  - Reflect on the viewpoints of these key players as well as their value systems.
  - What do you think each of these stakeholders would like you to decide as a plan of action for this dilemma?
  - How can you generate the greatest good?

Thoroughly comprehend the possible alternatives available.

- Use your problem-solving, decision-making, and critical-thinking skills.
- Create a list of the possible alternatives. Be creative when developing your alternatives. Be open minded; there is more than one way to reach a goal. Compel yourself to discern at least three alternatives.
- Clarify the alternatives available and predict the associated consequences, good and bad, of each potential alternative or intervention.
- For each alternative, ask the following questions:
- Do any of the principles or rules, such as legal, professional, or organizational, automatically nullify this alternative?
- If this alternative is chosen, what do you predict as the best-case and worst-case scenarios?
  - Do the best-case outcomes outweigh the worst-case outcomes?
  - Could you live with the worst-case scenario?
  - Will anyone be harmed? If so, how will they be harmed?
- Does the benefit obtained from this alternative overcome the risk of potential harm that it could cause to anyone?

Hypothesize ethical arguments.

- Use your problem-solving, decision-making, and critical-thinking skills.
- Determine which of the five approaches apply to this dilemma.
- Identify the moral principles that can be brought into play to support a conclusion as to what ought to be done ethically in this case or similar cases.
- Ascertain whether the approaches generate converging or diverging conclusions about what ought to be done.

Investigate, compare, and evaluate the arguments for each alternative.

- Use your problem-solving, decision-making, and critical-thinking skills.
- Appraise the relevant facts and assumptions prudently.
  - Is there ambiguous information that must be evaluated?
  - Are there any unjustifiable factual or illogical assumptions or debatable conceptual issues that must be explored?
- Rate the ethical reasoning and arguments for each alternative in terms of their relative significance.
  - 4 = extreme significance
  - 3 = major significance
  - 2 = significant
  - 1 = minor significance

BOX *Continued*

10-1

- Compare and contrast the alternatives available against the values of the key players involved.
- Reflect on these alternatives:
  - Does each alternative consider all of the key players?
  - Does each alternative take into account and reflect an interest in the concerns and welfare of all of the key players?
  - Which alternative will produce the greatest good or the least amount of harm for the greatest number of people?
- Refer to your professional codes of ethical conduct. Do they support your reasoning?

Choose the alternative you would recommend.

- Use your problem-solving, decision-making, and critical-thinking skills.
- Make a decision about the best alternative available.
  - Remember the Golden Rule—does your decision treat others as you would want to be treated?
  - Does your decision take into account and reflect an interest in the concerns and welfare of all of the key players?
  - Does your decision maximize the benefit and minimize the risk for everyone involved?
  - Become your own critic; challenge your decision as you think others might. Use the ethical arguments you predict they would use and defend your decision.
  - Would you be secure enough in your ethical decision-making process to see it aired on national television or sent out globally over the Internet?
  - Are you secure enough with this ethical decision that you could have allowed your loved ones to observe your decision-making process, your decision, and its outcomes?

Act on your chosen alternative.

- Use your problem-solving, decision-making, and critical-thinking skills.
- Formulate an implementation plan delineating the execution of the decision.
  - This plan should be designed to maximize the benefits and minimize the risks.
  - This plan must take into account all of the resources necessary for implementation, including personnel and money.
- Implement the plan.

Look at the ethical dilemma and examine the outcomes while reflecting on your ethical decision.

- Use your problem-solving, decision-making, and critical-thinking skills.
- Monitor the implementation plan and its outcomes. It is extremely important to reflect on specific case decisions and evaluate their outcomes in order to develop your ethical decision-making ability.

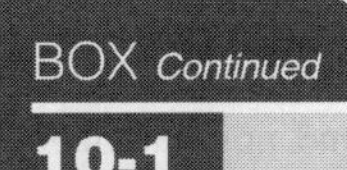

- If new information becomes available, the plan must be reevaluated.
- Monitor and revise the plan as necessary.

Source: The ethical model for ethical decision making was developed by Dr. Dee McGonigle and is the property of Educational Advancement Associates (EAA). The permission for its use in this text has been granted by Mr. Craig R. Goshow, vice president, EAA.

The following case study will help you to learn how to apply the ethical model. Review the model and then read through the case. You could try to apply the model to this case or follow along as we implement the model. You are challenged to determine your decision in this case and then compare and contrast your response with the decision the authors reached. There are several more case studies presented for you to practice implementing the ethical model for ethical decision making on this book's companion Web site (http://nursing.jbpub.com/informatics).

Case Analysis Demonstration

Allison is a charge nurse on a busy medical surgical unit. She is expecting the clinical instructor from the local university at 2 p.m. to review and discuss potential patient assignments for the nursing students scheduled for the following day. Just as the university professor arrives, one of the patients on the unit develops a crisis requiring Allison's attention. In order to expedite the student nurse assignments for the following day, Allison gives her electronic medical record access password to the instructor.

Examine the Ethical Dilemma

Allison made a commitment to meet with the university instructor to develop student assignments at 2 p.m. The patient emergency that developed prevented Allison from living up to that commitment. Allison had an obligation to provide patient care during the emergency and a competing obligation to the professor. She solved the dilemma of competing obligations by providing her electronic medical record access password to the university professor. By sharing her password, Allison most likely violated hospital policy related to the **security** of healthcare information. She may also have violated the American Nurses Association code of ethics in that nurses must judiciously protect information of a confidential nature. Since the university professor was also a nurse and had a legitimate interest in the protected healthcare information, there might not be an ANA code of ethics violation.

Thoroughly Comprehend the Possible Alternatives Available

1. Allison could have asked the professor to wait until the patient crisis was solved.
2. Allison could have delegated another staff member to assist the university professor.
3. Allison could have logged on to the system for the professor.

Hypothesize Ethical Arguments

The utilitarian approach applies to this situation. An ethical action is one that provides the greatest good for the greatest number; the principles are beneficence and nonmaleficence. The rights to be considered are: right of individual to choose for her/himself (autonomy), right to **truth** (veracity), right of privacy (ethical right to privacy avoids conflict and like all rights, promotes harmony), right not to be injured, and right to what has been promised (fidelity). Does the action respect the **moral rights** of everyone? The principles to consider would be autonomy, veracity, and fidelity. As for the fairness or justice, how fair is an action? Does it treat everyone in the same way, or does it show favoritism and discrimination? The principles to consider would be justice and distributive justice. Thinking about the common good assumes one's own good is inextricably linked to good of the community; community members are bound by pursuit of common values and goals and ensure that the social policies, social systems, institutions, and environments on which we depend are beneficial to all. Examples are affordable health care, effective public safety, a just legal system, and an unpolluted environment. The principle of distributive justice is considered. Virtue assumes there are certain ideals toward which we should strive that provide for the full development of our humanity. Virtues are attitudes or character traits that enable us to be and to act in ways that develop our highest potential; examples are honesty, courage, compassion, generosity, fidelity, integrity, fairness, self-control, and prudence. Like habits, they become a characteristic of the person. The virtuous person is the ethical person. Ask yourself, what kind of person should I be? What will promote the development of character within myself and my community? The principles considered would be fidelity, veracity, beneficence, nonmaleficence, justice, and distributive justice.

In this case, there is a clear violation of institutional policy designed to protect the privacy and confidentiality of medical records. However, the professor had a legitimate interest in the information and a legitimate right to the information. Allison trusted that the professor would not use the system password to obtain information outside the scope of the legitimate interest. However, Allison cannot be sure that the professor would not access inappropriate information. Further, Allison is responsible for how her access to the electronic system is used. Balancing the rights of everyone—the professor's right to the information, the patients' rights to expect that their information is safeguarded, and the right of the patient in crisis to expect the best possible care—is important and is the crux of the dilemma. Does the patient care obligation outweigh the obligation to the professor? Yes, probably. Allison did the right thing by caring for the patient in crisis. By giving out her system access password, Allison compromised the rights of the other patients on the unit to expect that their confidentiality and privacy would be safeguarded.

Virtue ethics suggests that individuals use power to bring about human benefit. One must consider the needs of others and the responsibility to meet those needs. Allison has to provide care, prevent harm, and maintain professional relationships all at the same time.

Allison may want to effect a long-term change in hospital policy for the common good. It is reasonable to assume that this is not an isolated incident and that the problem may recur in the future. Can institutional policy be amended to include professors in the access to medical records system? As suggested in the HIPAA administrative guidelines, the professor could receive the same staff training regarding appropriate and inappropriate use of access and sign the agreement to safeguard the records. If the institution has tracking software, the access could be monitored to watch for inappropriate use.

Identify the moral principles that can be brought into play to support a conclusion as to what ought to be done ethically in this case or similar cases. The International Council of Nurses code of ethics states that "The nurse holds in confidence personal information and uses judgment in sharing this information" (p. 4). The code also states, "The nurse uses judgment in relation to individual competence when accepting and delegating responsibilities" (p. 5). Both of these statements apply to the current situation.

Ascertain whether the approaches generate converging or diverging conclusions about what ought to be done. From the analysis, it is clear that the best immediate solution is to delegate assisting the professor with assignments to another nurse on the unit.

Investigate, Compare, and Evaluate the Arguments for Each Alternative

Review and think through the items listed in Table 10-1.

Choose the Alternative You Would Recommend

The best immediate solution is to delegate another staff member to assist the professor. The best long-tem solution is to change the hospital policy to include access for professors as described above.

Act on Your Chosen Alternative

Allison should delegate another staff member to assist the professor in making assignments.

TABLE 10-1
Detailed Analysis of Alternative Actions

Alternative	Good Consequences	Bad Consequences	Do Any Rules Nullify	Expected Outcome	Potential Benefit > Harm
1. Wait until crisis was solved	No policy violation Patient rights safeguarded	Not the best use of the professor's time	No	Best: Crisis will require a short time Worst: Crisis may take a long time	Patient rights protected Collegial relationship jeopardized Patient rights may take precedence
2. Delegate to another staff member	No policy violated	Other staff may be equally busy or might not be as familiar with all patients	No	Best: Assignments will be completed Worst: May not have benefit of expert advice	Confidentiality of record is assured May compromise student learning Patient rights may take precedence
3. Log on to the system for the professor	Professor can begin making assignments	May still be a violation of policy regarding system access	Rules regarding access to medical record	Best: Assignments can be completed Worst: Abuse of access to information	Potential compromise of records Patient in crisis is cared for

Look at the Ethical Dilemma and Examine the Outcomes While Reflecting on the Ethical Decision

As already indicated in the **alternative** analyses, delegation may not be an ideal solution since the staff nurse who is assigned to assist the professor may not possess the same extensive information about all of the patients as the charge nurse. It is, however, the best immediate solution to the dilemma and certainly safer than compromising computer system integrity. As noted above, Allison may want to pursue a long-term solution to a potentially recurring problem by helping the professor gain legitimate access to the computer system with the professor's own password. This way the system administrator may have the ability to track who used the system and what types of information were accessed during the use.

This case analysis demonstration provides you with the authors' perspective of this case and the ethical decision they made. If your decision varied, what was the basis for the difference of opinion? If you worked through the model, you might reach a different decision given your individual background and perspective. This does not make your decision right or wrong. Your decision should reflect the best decision you could make given your review, reflection, and critical thinking about this specific situation.

There are six additional cases provided in the online *Learner's Manual* for your review. Apply the model for each case study and discuss these with other colleagues or fellow classmates.

The most important point we'd like to leave you with is: as a healthcare professional, we must not be affected by conflicting loyalties; nothing should interfere with judicious, ethical decision making. As we navigate the technologically charged waters of health care, we have to hone a solid foundation of ethical decision making.

SUMMARY

As science and technology advances and policy makers and healthcare providers continue to shape healthcare practices including information management, it is paramount that ethical decisions are made. Healthcare professionals are typically honest, trustworthy, and ethical and understand that they are duty bound to focus on the needs and rights of their patients. At the same time, their day-to-day work is conducted in a world of changing healthcare landscapes consisting of new technologies, diverse patients, varied healthcare settings, and changing policies set by their employers, insurance companies, and providers. Healthcare professionals need to juggle all of the balls simultaneously, often resulting in far too many gray areas or ethical decision-making dilemmas with a lack of a clear right course of action. Patients rely on the ethical competence of their healthcare providers, believing that their situation is unique and will be respected and evaluated based on their own needs, abilities, and limitations. The healthcare professional cannot allow conflicting loyalties to interfere with judicious, ethical decision making. Just as in the opening example of the Apollo mission, we are not sure where this technologically heightened information era will take us, but if we have a solid foundation of ethical decision making, our duties and rights will be judiciously and ethically fulfilled.

THOUGHT-PROVOKING Questions

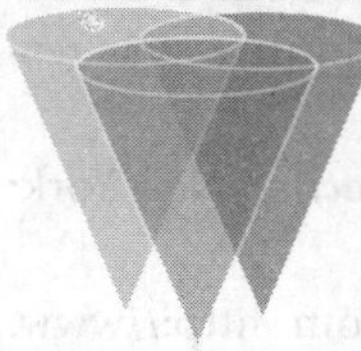

1. Identify moral dilemmas in healthcare informatics that would best be approached with the use of an ethical decision-making framework.
2. Discuss the evolving healthcare ethics traditions within their social and historical context.
3. Differentiate among the theoretical approaches to healthcare ethics as they relate to the theorists' perspectives of individuals and their relationships.
4. Select one of the healthcare ethics theories and support its use in examining ethical issues in healthcare informatics.
5. Select one of the healthcare ethics theories and argue against its use in examining ethical issues in healthcare informatics.

References

Aristotle. (350 BC). Nichomachean ethics. Book I. (W. D. Ross, Trans.). Retrieved March 28, 2008 from http://www.constitution.org/ari/ethic_00.htm

Beauchamp, T. L., & Childress, J. F. (1977). *Principles of biomedical ethics.* New York: Oxford University Press.

Beauchamp, T. L., & Childress, J. F. (1994). *Principles of biomedical ethics* (4th ed.). New York: Oxford University Press.

Benjamin, M., & Curtis, J. (1992). *Ethics in nursing* (3rd ed.). New York: Oxford University Press.

Engster, D. (n.d.). *Can care ethics be Institutionalized? Toward a Caring natural law theory.* Retrieved March 28, 2008 from http://www.csus.edu/org/wpsa/pisigmaalphaaward.pdf

Healthcare Ethics. (2007). *Virtue ethics.* Retrieved March 28, 2008 from http://www.ascensionhealth.org/ethics/public/issues/virtue.asp

Howard, R. (Director). (1995). *Apollo 13* [Motion picture]. Universal City, CA: MCA Universal Studios.

Husted, G. L., & Husted, J. H. (1995). *Ethical decision-making in nursing* (2nd ed.). New York: Mosby, Inc.

International Council of Nurses (ICN). (2006). *The ICN code of ethics for nurses.* Retrieved March 28, 2008 from http://www.icn.ch/icncode.pdf

Jonsen, A. R. (1991). Casuistry as methodology in clinical ethics. *Theoretical Medicine 12,* 295–307.

Martin, P. A. (1999). Bioethics and the whole: Pluralism, consensus, and the transmutation of bioethical methods into gold. *Journal of Law, Medicine & Ethics, 27*(4), 316–327.

McGonigle, D. (2000). The ethical model for ethical decision making. *Inside Case Management, 7*(8), 1–5.

Pellegrino, E. D. (1993). The metamorphosis of medical ethics: A thirty-year retrospective. *JAMA, 269,* 1158–1162.

Pellegrino, E., & Thomasma, D. (1993). *The virtues in medical practice.* New York: Oxford University Press.

Scott, A. (2002). *Plato's Meno.* Retrieved March 28, 2008 from http://www.angelfire.com/md2/timewarp/plato.html

Velasquez, M., Andre, C., Shanks, T., & Myer, M. (for the Markkula Center for Applied Ethics). (1987). *What is ethics?* Retrieved January 15, 2008, from http://www.scu.edu/SCU/Centers/Ethics/practicing/decision/whatisethics.shtml

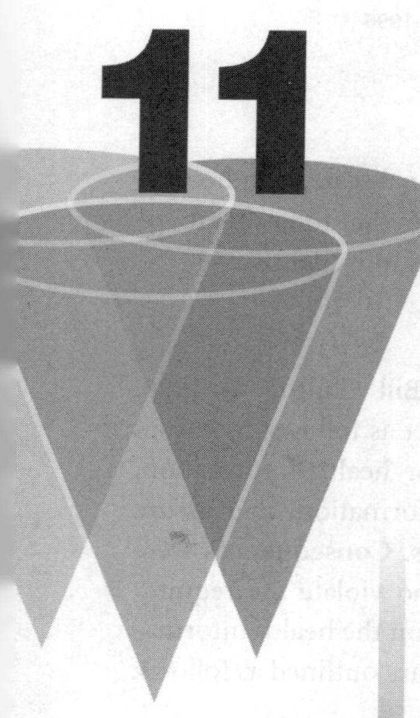

Overview of the Health Insurance Portability and Accountability Act of 1996

Dee McGonigle, Kathleen Mastrian, and Nedra Farcus

Objectives

1. Describe the Health Insurance Portability and Accountability Act (HIPAA) of 1996.
2. Determine how HIPAA applies to your practice and setting.
3. Explore the relationship among ANSI, HL7, ISO, and HIPAA.
4. Assess how other countries around the globe are addressing security and privacy.

Key Terms

American National Standards Institute (ANSI)
Center for Medicare and Medicaid Services (CMS)
Confidentiality
Consequences
Electronic data interchange (EDI)
Electronic health record (EHR)
Extensible markup language (XML)
Gramm-Leach-Bliley Act (GLBA)
Health Information Portability and Accountability Act (HIPAA)
Health information technology (HIT)
Health Level 7 (HL7)
Information technology (IT)
International Standards Organization (ISO)

INTRODUCTION

As informatics and healthcare technologies continue to evolve, we are constantly reexamining the role of intelligent machines, computers, information systems, and cognitive science in the collection, storage, analysis, synthesis, diagnosis, and transmission or dissemination and disposal of intimate patient information. The age-old healthcare issue seems to have remained the same—how can we best protect the patient's **privacy** and **confidentiality**? The debate continues in light of the Information Age and the speed at which data and information are shared, as well as the varied formats this information assumes. Recognizing the need to safeguard information in this tumultuous age, nationwide regulations, years in the making, were introduced under the **Health Insurance Portability and Accountability Act (HIPAA)** signed into law in 1996. However, what seemed

Key Terms *Continued*
National provider identifier (NPI)
Open systems interconnection (OSI)
Privacy
Protected health information (PHI)
Regional health information organizations (RHIOs)
Rights
Sarbanes-Oxley (SOX) Act
Security
Standard generalized markup language (SGML)
Standards-developing organizations (SDOs)

to be a good plan to handle information on a national scale soon became the target of much debate and criticism. In the years that followed, it appeared that the delays in implementation might lead to its demise.

OVERVIEW OF HIPAA

The HIPAA was signed into law by President Bill Clinton in 1996. Hellerstein (1999) summarized the intent of the act as follows: to curtail healthcare fraud and abuse, enforce standards for health information, guarantee the security and privacy of health information, and assure health insurance portability for employed persons. **Consequences** were put into place for institutions and individuals who violate the requirements of this act. For this text, we will concentrate on the health information security and privacy aspects of HIPAA, which are outlined as follows:

> The privacy provisions of the federal law, the Health Insurance Portability and Accountability Act of 1996 (HIPAA), apply to health information created or maintained by healthcare providers who engage in certain electronic transactions, health plans, and healthcare clearinghouses. The Department of Health and Human Services (HHS) has issued the regulation, "Standards for Privacy of Individually Identifiable Health Information," applicable to entities covered by HIPAA. The Office for Civil Rights (OCR) is the Departmental component responsible for implementing and enforcing the privacy regulation. (See the Statement of Delegation of Authority to the Office for Civil Rights, as published in the Federal Register on December 28, 2000 (U.S. Department of Health and Human Services, 2006, ¶ 1).

Guaranteeing the security and privacy of health information has been the focus of numerous debates. To date, comprehensive standards for the implementation of this portion of the act are finalized. In August of 1998, the U.S. Department of Health and Human Services released a set of proposed rules addressing health information management. Proposed rules specific to health information privacy and security were released in November of 1999. The purpose of the proposed rules is to balance patients' rights to privacy and providers' needs for access to information (Hellerstein, 2000).

One of the biggest stumbling blocks to implementation of comprehensive standards for privacy was the associated cost. The administrative simplification portion of the HIPAA calling for standardized forms for claims, medical records, lab reports, insurance forms, etc., was expected to save up to $250 billion after the initial conversion costs. Compliance with the proposed security and privacy rules was projected to be $6.7 billion by the Department of Health and Human Services. Not everyone agreed with the Health and Human Services estimate; in fact a study conducted by Blue Cross/Blue Shield and reported by Egger (2000) projected the costs would be closer to $43 billion over 5 years. An overview of the proposed standards helps to illustrate why implementation was estimated to be so costly.

Hellerstein (2000) summarized the proposed privacy rules. The rules do the following:

- Define **protected health information (PHI)** as "information relating to one's physical or mental health, the provision of one's healthcare, or the payment for that health care, that has been maintained or transmitted electronically and that can be reasonably identified with the individual it applies to" (Hellerstein, 2000, p 2).
- Propose that authorization by patients for release of information is not necessary when the release of information is directly related to treatment and payment for treatment. Specific patient authorization is not required for research, medical or police emergencies, legal proceedings, and collection of data for public health concerns. All other releases of health information require a specific form for each release and only information pertinent to the issue at hand is allowed. All releases of information must be formally documented and accessible to the patient upon request.
- Establish patient ownership of the healthcare record and allow for patient-initiated corrections and amendments.
- Mandate administrative requirements for the protection of healthcare information. All healthcare organizations are required to have a privacy official and an office to receive privacy violation complaints. A specific training program for employees that includes a certification of completion and a signed statement by all employees that they will uphold privacy procedures must be developed and implemented. All employees must re-sign the agreement to uphold privacy every 3 years. Sanctions for violations of policy must be clearly defined and applied.
- Mandate that all outside entities that conduct business with healthcare organizations (e.g., attorneys, consultants, auditors) must meet the same standards as the organization for information protection and security.
- Allow protected health information to be released without authorization for research studies. Patients may not access their information in blinded research studies because this access may affect the reliability of the study outcomes.
- Propose that protected health information may be deidentified before release in such a manner that the identity of the patient is protected. The healthcare organization may code the deidentification so that the information can be reidentified once it has been returned.
- Apply only to health information maintained or transmitted by electronic means.

As the concern mounted but deadlines loomed, the healthcare arena prepared to enact the requirements of the law. The administrative simplification portion of this law is intended to decrease the financial and administrative burdens by standardizing the electronic transmission of certain administrative and financial transactions. This section also addresses the security and privacy of healthcare data and information for the covered entities of healthcare providers who transmit any health information in electronic form in connection with a covered transaction, health plans, and healthcare clearinghouses. For more information, visit http://aspe.os.dhhs.gov/admnsimp/ (U.S. Department of Health and Human Services, 2007a).

The privacy requirements went into effect on April 14, 2003, and limit the release of PHI without the patient's knowledge and consent. Covered entities must comply with the requirements. Among the necessary rules they must comply with, they must dedicate a privacy officer, adopt and implement privacy procedures, educate their personnel, and secure their electronic patient records. We are all familiar with the need to notify patients of their privacy practice, since we all have signed forms upon interacting with our healthcare providers.

According to the U.S. Department of Health and Human Services (2002), there are certain **rights** provided to patients by the privacy rule. Some of the rights include the following: the right to request restrictions to access of the health record; the right to request an alternate method of communication with a provider; the right to receive a paper copy of the notice of privacy practices; the right to file a complaint if one believes his or her privacy rights were violated; the right to inspect and copy one's health record; the right to request an amendment to the health record; and the right to see an account of disclosures of one's health record. This places the burden on the healthcare system and not the patient.

On October 16, 2003, the electronic transaction and code set standards became effective. This does not require electronic transmission but mandates that if transactions are conducted electronically, they must comply with the required federal standards for electronically filed healthcare claims. "The Secretary has made the **Centers for Medicare & Medicaid Services (CMS)** responsible for enforcing the electronic transactions and code sets provisions of the law" (*Guidance on Compliance with HIPAA Transactions and Code Sets*, 2003, ¶ 3).

The security requirements went into effect on April 21, 2005 and require the covered entities to put safeguards that protect the confidentiality, integrity, and availability of protected health information when stored and transmitted electronically into place. According to Savage (2006), "After HIPAA's security requirements went into effect, many organizations in the healthcare industry continue to improve their security" (¶ 5). Some have had to engage in enormous amounts of resource expenditures involving people, time, and money. Savage states that "While the HIPAA rules have driven security improvements, their lack of specifics and a dearth of enforcement leaves much room for interpretation, making compliance hard to gauge" (¶ 5). Since it is believed that the pursuit of a perfect security system is a wild goose chase, the journey should be reflective of the needs of the organization and their unique requirements in relation to their obligations to the patients they serve while addressing the demands of HIPAA. The safeguards that are addressed are administrative, physical, and technical. The administrative safeguards refer to the documented formal policies and procedures that are used to manage and execute the security measures. They govern the protection of healthcare data and information and the conduct of the personnel. The physical safeguards refer to the policies and procedures that must be in place to limit physical access to electronic information systems. Technical safeguards are the policies and procedures used to control access to healthcare data and information. Safeguards need to be in place to control access whether the data and information are at rest, residing on a machine or storage medium, being processed, or in transmission, such as being backed up to storage or disseminated across a network.

Even though it is more than a decade after the act was signed into law, the concerns and ambiguity of implementation continue to exist and are evidenced by the Fifteenth National HIPAA Summit: Special Edition (2007) that was held from December 10–14 in 2007. There were special sessions on healthcare privacy, security and transactions, code sets, and identifiers. The following sessions were held:

- The Ten Key Privacy Issues That Must be Addressed in Order to Become a Successful and Effective Healthcare Privacy Professional
- What It Means to Be a Privacy Professional
- What Are the Key HIPAA Privacy Compliance Challenges Today and in the Future?
- How Broader Privacy Policy Issues Impact Healthcare
- Information Security in a Health Care Environment
- Questions HHS May Ask in a HIPAA Audit: Critical Steps for HIPAA Compliance
- Security Audit Survivor—How to Remain "On The Island" in the Wake of the Piedmont Audit
- Coordinating and Balancing Privacy, Security and Practical Operations
- Case Study: Building and Sustaining an Information Security Program
- Healthcare Security Professional Advanced Problem Solving Roundtable
- Overview of Healthcare Privacy Laws, Regulations and Guidance: HIPAA, Gramm-Leach-Bliley (GLBA), and State Law

- Organizing a Privacy Program: Administrative Infrastructure and Reporting Relationships
- Managing Your Institution-Specific HIPAA Compliance Policies and Procedures: Cutting Edge Issues
- State of the Art Workforce Training and Beyond
- Managing Relationships with Business Associates and Other Third Parties
- Patient Privacy Practices and Customer Satisfaction: Integrating HIPAA into Day-to-Day Clinical Practice
- Ensuring HIPAA Compliance for Across-Institution Research Projects Which Share PHI
- Healthcare Privacy and Security Issues in HIT, EHR and [**regional health information**] **RHIO** [boldface added] Initiatives
- The Future of Privacy and Security: From a Regulatory, Business, and Overall Health IT Perspective
- What Works and What Doesn't: Lessons from HIPAA, GLBA, and SOX
- Transaction, Code Sets, and Identifier Update
- [**National provider identifier**] **NPI** [boldface added] Implementation Update
- The Office for Civil Rights and Health Care Privacy
- At a Crossroads: Culturally Competent Care vs. HIPAA
- Advocating for Patient Privacy Rights (Fifteenth National HIPAA Summit: Special Edition).

Navigating these new waters can be confusing and the CMS has provided information to help small healthcare providers.

> On December 12, 2007 CMS announced the publication of a new HIPAA security educational paper entitled "Security Standards Implementation for the Small Provider." This document is the seventh and final in the series of HIPAA Security Educational Papers and is intended to assist small health care providers with coming into or maintaining compliance with the Security Rule. (U.S. Department of Health and Human Services, 2007b, ¶ 9).

HIPAA, with its privacy, confidentiality, and security regulations, became the first national rules for protecting the patient's health information. The security standards were designed to give the covered entities guidelines to follow while providing flexibility in their enactment. Each entity can determine the security measures that best suit their financial resources, operation, size, and capabilities.

Standardized electronic health records (EHR) using **electronic data interchange** (EDI) methods must be put into place. As information becomes more prevalent in electronic formats, it will be easier to collect, store, monitor, track, exchange, disseminate, and aggregate PHI across covered entities including healthcare networks and data repositories. The current **information technology (IT)**, **health information technology** (**HIT**), and informatics potential implementations are continuing to raise concerns over the security of data and the resulting attempts to secure our networks and data repositories. The addition of security measures such as encryption, passwords, firewalls, retinal recognition, dedicated phone lines, and the like have been used. As we accelerate the amount of data circumventing the globe, there is serious concern about the intimate healthcare data and information that is collected, stored, manipulated, disposed of, and shared from insurance claims, insurance enrollment and eligibility, provider identifiers, patient identifiers, and healthcare information in individual and aggregate formats. With the increasing technological capabilities, the types and amount of data that are transmitted will continue to increase exponentially. The nurse informaticist acting as or as well as the privacy officer must be concerned about the confidentiality, privacy, and access issues that arise as more and more data and information are moving internally and outside of the organization's facilities. Internally, all personnel must be trained and aware of their roles and responsibilities in the process. Everyone must collaborate and share their policies concerning communications and data transmission. External to your site, you might have several entities that you are communicating with and must recognize their policies and procedures. The discomforting piece occurs once the data and information leaves your facility; you lack control over the external entities and their personnel. The electronic communication among providers, physician-run offices and clinics, nurse practitioner-run offices and clinics, payers, hospitals, and HMOs has increased and has typically become a multientity exchange. Many different entities need to access many different pieces of a patient's health record, yet with this need for openness is also a need for closed, secure records. It is a fine line that we walk when we try to make personal health information that should be PHI easily accessible to those who need access or need to know and difficult to access for everyone else. This path has been bumpy and unsettling for many healthcare professionals. The HIPAA standards are designed to smooth the path and actually increase the amount of electronic transmissions.

There are other organizations that are assisting in the HIPAA implementation. "The American National Standards Institute (ANSI) X12N and **Health Level 7 (HL7)** [boldface added] Standards Organizations worked together to develop an electronic standard for claims attachments to recommend to HHS" (Spencer and Bushman, 2006, ¶ 2). The **American National Standards Institute** (ANSI, n.d.) was founded in 1918 and "has served as the coordinator of the U.S. voluntary standards and conformity assessment system (¶ 1). ANSI provides a "forum where the private and public sectors can cooperatively work together towards the development of voluntary national consensus standards and the related compliance programs" (¶ 2). HL7 (n.d.) "is one of several American National Standards Institute-accredited **Standards Developing Organizations (SDOs)** [boldface added] operating in the healthcare arena" (¶ 1). It states that its mission is that "HL7 provides standards for interoperability that improve care delivery, optimize workflow, reduce ambiguity, and enhance knowledge transfer among all of our stakeholders, including healthcare providers, government agencies, the vendor community, fellow SDOs and patients" (¶ 5). HL7 was initially associated with HIPAA in 1996 through the creation of a claims attachments special interest group charged with standardizing the supplemental information needed to support healthcare insurance and other e-commerce transactions. The initial deliverable of this group was six claim attachments. This special-interest group is currently known as the Attachment Special Interest Group. As the attachment projects continue, they are slated to include skilled nursing facilities, home health care, preauthorization, and referrals.

The Level Seven in Health Level Seven's name means the

> highest level of the **International Standards Organization's (ISO)** [boldface added] communications model for **Open Systems Interconnection (OSI)** [boldface added]—the application level. The application level addresses definition of the data to be exchanged, the timing of the interchange, and the communication of certain errors to the application. The seventh level supports such functions as security checks, participant identification, availability checks, exchange mechanism negotiations and, most importantly, data exchange structuring. (HL7, n.d., ¶ 5)

The OSI was an attempt to standardize networking by the ISO. HL7 addresses the distinct requirements of the systems in use in hospitals and other facilities, is more concerned with application than the other levels, and user authentication and privacy are considered (Webopedia, 2008). The lower levels address hardware, software, and data reformatting. The HL7 mission is supported through two separate groups, the XML special interest group and the structured documents technical committee. The XML special interest group makes "recommendations on use of **Extensible Markup Language (XML)** [boldface added] standards for all of HL7's platform- and vendor-independent healthcare specifications" (HL7, n.d., ¶ 21). XML began as a simplified subset of the **standard generalized markup language (SGML); Extensible markup language's (XML's)** major purpose is to facilitate the exchange of structured data across different information systems especially via the Internet. It is considered an extensible language since it permits its users to define their own elements allowing customization to enable purpose-specific development. The structured documents technical committee "support[s] the HL7 mission through development of structured document standards for healthcare" (HL7, ¶ 21). HL7 also organizes, maintains, and sustains a repository for the vocabulary terms used in its messages to provide a sharable, well defined, and unambiguous knowledge of the meaning of the data transferred.

ISO (2008a) is a "network of the national standards institutes of 157 countries, on the basis of one member per country, with a Central Secretariat in Geneva, Switzerland, that coordinates the system" (¶ 1). ISO is

> a non-governmental organization: its members are not, as is the case in the United Nations system, delegations of national governments. Nevertheless, ISO occupies a special position between the public and private sectors. This is because, on the one hand, many of its member institutes are part of the governmental structure of their countries, or are mandated by their government. On the other hand, other members have their roots uniquely in the private sector, having been set up by national partnerships of industry associations. (ISO, 2008a, ¶ 2)

This placement enables them to become a bridging organization where they can reach agreement on solutions that meet both the requirements of business as well as the broader needs of society, consumers, and users. These international agreements become standards that use the prefix ISO followed by the number of the standard. An example would be the health informatics, health cards, numbering system, and registration procedure for issuer identifiers, ISO 20302:2006, that "is designed to confirm, via a numbering system and registration procedure, the identities of both the healthcare application provider and the health card holder in order that information may be exchanged by using cards issued for healthcare service" (ISO, 2008b, ¶ 12). ISO provides standards for interoperability that improve care delivery, optimize workflow, reduce ambiguity, and enhance knowledge transfer among all of their stakeholders, including healthcare providers, government agencies, the vendor community, fellow SDOs, and patients. The standards are used on a voluntary basis since ISO has no power to force enactment.

It is evident that all of these organizations have guidelines, standards, and rules to help healthcare entities collect, store, manipulate, dispose of, and exchange secure PHI. Many SDOs are working to help develop standards. HIPAA guarantees the security and privacy of health information and curtails healthcare fraud and abuse while enforcing standards for health information.

UNITED STATES AND BEYOND

Health care was not the only focus of U.S. legislative acts. You will often see GLBA and SOX when you search for information on HIPAA. The **Gramm-Leach-Bliley**

Act (GLBA) is federal legislation in the United States to control how financial institutions handle the private information they collect from individuals. The **Sarbanes-Oxley (SOX) Act** was legislation that was put in place to protect shareholders as well as the public from deceptive accounting practices in organizations.

There are privacy and data regulations being established around the world, such as the Data Protection Act 1998 in the United Kingdom (Ministry of Justice, 2008); the Dutch Data Protection Authority (2007), which released privacy legislation guidelines on publishing personal data on the Internet; and Finland's Personal Data File Act 1988 and Personal Data Act 1999 (Data Protection Board, n.d.). New Zealand's Health Information Privacy Code 1994 had amendment number six coming into effect in November of 2007; this amendment covered such things as definitions of ethics committee, hospital, health, or disability services, health professional body, registered health professional, and health practitioner (Privacy Commissioner, 2007). Argentina's Privacy and Data Protection (2007) states that it "is the first Latin American country to be awarded the status of 'adequate country' from the point of view of European Data Protection authorities, and this breakthrough is expected to encourage other countries in the region to work towards improving data protection rights for individuals" (Privacy and Data Protection, 2007, ¶ 7). In Canada, the Personal Information Protection and Electronic Documents Act received royal assent in 2000 (Office of the Privacy Commissioner of Canada, 2004). Safe Harbor deals with "The transfer of personal data from the European Union to the USA, the regulations in Article 25 and 26 of the European Data Protection Directive serve as basis. According to these regulations, transferring data to third countries is in principle only possible if these countries guarantee an adequate level of protection as required by the Directive" (Federal Commissioner for Data Protection and Freedom of Information, n.d., ¶ 1). It is quite evident that privacy and security have become global concerns.

SUMMARY

What we would like to leave you with is that the HIPAA privacy rule is intended to enhance the rights of individuals. This rule provides them with greater access and control over their PHI. They can control its uses, dissemination, and disclosures. Covered entities must not only establish a required level of security for PHI but also sanctions for employees who violate their privacy policies and administrative processes for responding to patient requests regarding their information. Therefore, they must be able to track the PHI and note access from both a perspective of what information was accessed but also by whom and any disclosures. Finally, readers should recognize that there is global awareness of the need for pri-

THOUGHT-PROVOKING Questions

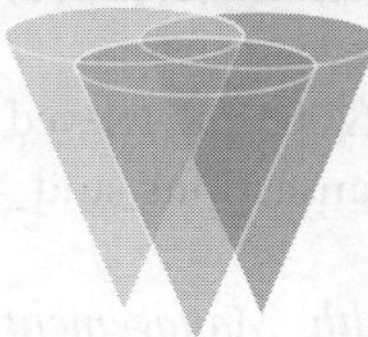

1. Why is it important to establish patient ownership of the healthcare record?
2. What are the potential negative consequences of the proposed right of amendment and correction of healthcare records by patients?
3. One of the largest problems with healthcare information security has always been inappropriate use by authorized users. How will the proposed regulations help to curb this problem?
4. How do you envision HL7 and HIPAA evolving in the next decade?
5. Imagine that you are the designated privacy officer in a healthcare institution. What types of monitoring procedures would you develop?
6. If you were the privacy officer, what would you include in your sanctions for violations policy?
7. As privacy officer, how would you address the following?
   a. Tracking each point of access of the patient's database including who entered the data.
   b. Nurses in your hospital have an access code that only gives them access to their unit's patients. A visitor accidently comes to the wrong unit looking for a patient and asks the nurse to find out what unit the patient is on.

vacy protections for personal information or PHI. Over the next years, international efforts will accelerate, enhancing international data exchange.

References

American National Standards Institute (ANSI). (n.d.). *ANSI: A historical overview.* Retrieved January 17, 2008, from http://ansi.org/about_ansi/introduction/history.aspx?menuid=1

Data Protection Board. (n.d.). *Legislation for the protection of privacy.* Retrieved January 20, 2008, from http://www.tietosuoja.fi/27305.htm

Dutch Data Protection Authority (DPA). (2007, December). *Dutch DPA publication of personal data on the Internet.* Retrieved January 20, 2008, from http://www.dutchdpa.nl/downloads_overig/en_20071108_richtsnoeren_internet.pdf?refer=true&theme=purple

Egger, E. (2000). HIPAA offers hospitals the good, the bad, and the ugly. *Health Care Strategic Management, 18*(4), 1, 21–23.

Federal Commissioner for Data Protection and Freedom of Information. (n.d.). *Safe harbor.* Retrieved January 20, 2008, from http://www.bfdi.bund.de/cln_007/nn_671558/EN/EuropeanInternationalAffaires/Artikel/SafeHarbor.html

Fifteenth National HIPAA Summit: Special Edition. (2007). *Healthcare privacy and security training and professional certification.* Retrieved January 17, 2008, from http://www.hipaasummit.com/past15/index.html

Guidance on compliance with HIPAA transactions and code sets. (2003). Retrieved January 17, 2008, from http://www.dmh.ca.gov/hipaa/Transactions_and_Code_Sets.asp

Hagland, M. (1998). The gap: HIPAA and secure IT. *Health Management Technology, 19*(6), 24–26, 28, 30.

Health Level Seven (HL7). (n.d.). *What is HL7?* Retrieved January 17, 2008, from http://www.hl7.org/

Hellerstein, D. (1999). HIPAA's impact on healthcare. *Health Management Technology.* Retrieved January 24, 2008, from http://findarticles.com/p/articles/mi_m0DUD/is_3_20/ai_54396227

Hellerstein, D. (2000). HIPAA and health information privacy rules: Almost there. *Health Management Technology.* Retrieved January 24, 2008, from http://findarticles.com/p/articles/mi_m0DUD/is_4_21/ai_61523494

International Standards Organization (ISO). (2008a). *About ISO.* Retrieved on January 17, 2008, from http://www.iso.org/iso/about.htm

International Standards Organization (ISO). (2008b). *Health informatics.* Retrieved January 17, 2008, from http://www.iso.org/iso/iso_catalogue/catalogue_tc/catalogue_detail.htm?csnumber=35376

Ministry of Justice. (2008). *Data sharing and protection.* Retrieved January 20, 2008, from http://www.justice.gov.uk/whatwedo/datasharingandprotection.htm

Office of the Privacy Commissioner of Canada. (2004). *Privacy legislation.* Retrieved January 20, 2008, from http://www.privcom.gc.ca/legislation/02_06_07_e.asp

Pretzer, M. (1999). The clock is ticking on patient privacy. *Medical Economics, 76*(2), 29–30, 32.

Privacy Commissioner. (2007). *Health information privacy code.* Retrieved January 20, 2008, from http://www.privacy.org.nz/health-information-privacy-code

Privacy and Data Protection (PDP). (2007). *Data protection in Argentina.* Retrieved January 20, 2008, from http://www.protecciondedatos.com.ar [Click on the English option to access this article in English]

Savage, M. (2006). *Security news: Perfect HIPAA security impossible, experts say.* Retrieved January 17, 2008, from http://searchsecurity.techtarget.com/originalContent/0,289142,sid14_gci1268986,00.html

Spencer, J., & Bushman, M. (2006). *HIPAAdvisory: The next HIPAA frontier: Claims attachments.* Retrieved January 17, 2008, from http://www.hipaadvisory.com/action/tcs/nextfrontier.htm

U.S. Department of Health and Human Services. (2002). *Federal Register, Part V, Department of Health and Human Services: Standards for privacy of individually identifiable health information; Final rule.* Retrieved January 17, 2008, from http://www.hhs.gov/ocr/hipaa/privrulepd.pdf

U.S. Department of Health and Human Services. (2006). *Medical privacy—National standards to protect the privacy of personal health information.* Retrieved January 15, 2008, from http://www.hhs.gov/ocr/hipaa/bkgrnd.html

U.S. Department of Health and Human Services. (2007a). *Administrative simplification in the health care industry.* Retrieved January 15, 2008, from http://aspe.os.dhhs.gov/admnsimp

U.S. Department of Health and Human Services. (2007b). *Security standard overview.* Retrieved January 15, 2008, from http://www.cms.hhs.gov/SecurityStandard

Webopedia. (2008). *The 7 layers of the OSI model.* Retrieved January 17, 2008, from http://www.webopedia.com/quick_ref/OSI_Layers.asp

Weil, S. (2004). *HIPAA security rule.* Retrieved January 17, 2008, from http://www.securityfocus.com/infocus/1764

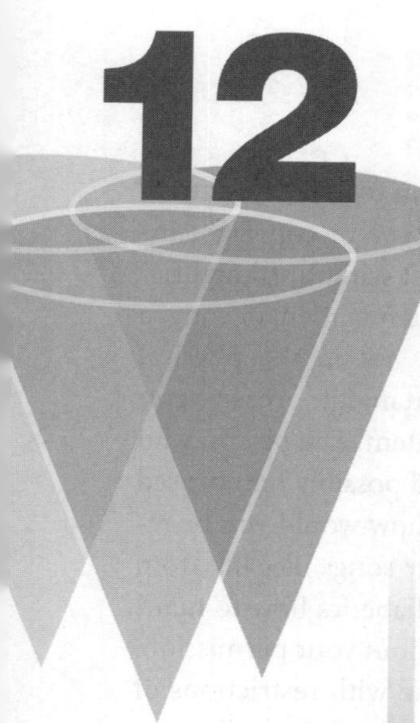

12 Securing Information in a Network

Lisa Reeves Bertin

Objectives

1. Explore information fair use and copyright restrictions.
2. Describe processes for securing information in a computer network.
3. Identify various methods of user authentication and relate authentication to security of a network.
4. Explain methods to anticipate and prevent typical threats to network security.

Key Terms

Acceptable use
Antivirus software
Authentication
Biometrics
Confidentiality
Copyright
Fair use
Firewall
Flash drive
Hacker
Integrity
Intrusion detection devices
Intrusion detection system
Jump drive
Malicious code
Malicious insider
Mask
Network
Network accessibility
Network availability
Network security
Password
Proxy server
Radio frequency identity (RFID) chip
Secure information

INTRODUCTION

In addition to complying with federal HIPAA guidelines regarding the privacy of patient information, healthcare systems also need to be vigilant in the way that they **secure information** and manage **network security**. In this chapter, we will explore some of the issues associated with managing information in a health system computer network.

FAIR USE OF INFORMATION AND SHARING

Copyright laws in the world of technology are notoriously misunderstood. The same copyright laws that cover physical books, artwork, and other creative material are still applicable in the digital world. Have you ever given a friend a CD that contains a computer game or some other type of software that you paid for and registered? Have you ever downloaded a song from the Internet without paying? Have you ever copied a section of online content from a reference site and used that content as if it was your own? Have you ever copied a picture from the Internet without asking permission from the photographer who took the picture? Have you copied and pasted information about a disease or drug

Key Terms *Continued*
Security breach
Shoulder surfing
Social engineering
Spyware
Thumb drive
Trojan horse
Virus
Worm

from a Web site and then printed out the information to give to a patient or family member? These are all examples of the type of copyright infringements enabled by technology that occur almost without thought.

The value of creative material, whether it is written content, a song, a painting, or some other type of creative work is not in the physical medium on which it is stored. The value is in the intangible areas of creativity, skills, and labor that went into creating that item. The person who created the material should be properly credited and possibly reimbursed for the use of the material. If you were a musician, how would you be reimbursed for your music if everyone just downloaded your songs illegally from the Internet? Suppose you created a game to teach type 1 diabetics how to manage their diet and other nurses copied and distributed it without your permission.

Almost all software, music CDs, and movie DVDs come with restrictions of how and why you can make copies. Most computer software developers allow for a backup copy of the software without restriction. If your hard drive fails on your computer, you are usually able to reinstall the software through the backup copy. Some software companies even allow you to transfer software to a new user. In this case, you typically are required to uninstall the software from your computer before the new owner is free to install the software on his/her computer. Most of these restrictions depend on the honesty of the user in reading and following the licensing agreement. As a result of widespread abuses, the music and film industries commonly use hardware security features that block users from making a working copy of a music CD or movie DVD.

The bottom line is to recognize that copyright laws also apply to the digital world and that you could be prosecuted for copyright violations. Technology advances have made the sharing of information easy and extremely fast. A scanner can convert any document to digital form instantly, and that document can then be shared with people anywhere in the world. Remember that the person who created that document has a right to approve of the sharing of the work. Carefully read the fine print of any software you purchase and be sure to clarify any questions regarding how you can copy the software. Avoid downloading music illegally from the Internet and do not use information from the Internet without permission to do so or citing the reference appropriately. Healthcare organizations that allow access to the Internet from a network computer should ensure that users are well aware of and compliant with copyright and **fair use** principles.

SECURING NETWORK INFORMATION

Typically, a healthcare organization will have computers linked together to facilitate communication and operations within and outside the facility. This is commonly referred to as a network. The linking of computers together and to the outside creates the possibility of a breach of network security and exposes the information to unauthorized use.

The three main areas of secure network information are **confidentiality**, availability, and **integrity**. As discussed in the ethics and HIPAA chapters (Chapters 10 and 11, respectively), an organization must follow a well-defined policy to ensure that private health information remains appropriately confidential. The confidentiality policy should clearly define what data is confidential and how the data should be handled. Employees also need to understand the procedures for releasing confidential information outside the organization or to others within the organization and what procedures to follow if confidential information is accidentally or intentionally released without authorization. In addition, the policy should contain consideration for elements as basic as the placement of monitors so that information cannot be read by passersby. **Shoulder surfing**—or watching over someone's back as that person is working—is still a major way that confidentiality is compromised.

Availability refers to network information being accessible when needed. This area of the policy tends to be much more technical in nature. An accessibility policy would cover issues associated with protecting the key hardware elements of the computer network and also cover the procedures to follow with a major electric outage or Internet outage. Food and drinks spilled onto keyboards of computer units, dropping or jarring hardware, and electrical surges or static charges are all examples of ways that the hardware elements of a computer network may be damaged. In the case of an electrical outage or a weather-related disaster, the network administrator must have clear plans for data backup, storage, and retrieval. There must also be clear procedures and alternative methods of ensuring that care delivery is largely uninterrupted.

Another way organizations protect the availability of their networks is to institute an **acceptable use** policy. Elements covered in such policy could include what types of activities are acceptable on the corporate network. For example, are employees permitted to download music at work? Restricting downloads is a very common way for organizations to avoid viruses and other malicious code from entering their networks. The policy should also clearly define what activities are not acceptable and the consequences for violations.

The last area of information security is integrity. Employees need to have confidence that the information they are reading is true. To accomplish this, organizations need clear policies to clarify how data is actually inputted, who has the authorization to change such data and to track how and when data are changed. All three of these areas use authorization and **authentication** to enforce the corporate policies. Access to networks can easily be grouped into areas of authorization; that is, users can be grouped by job title. For example, anyone with the job title of floor supervisor may be authorized to change the hours worked by an employee, but an employee with the title of patient care assistant may not make such changes.

AUTHENTICATION OF USERS

Authentication of employees is also used by organizations in their security policies. The most common ways to authenticate are by something the user knows, something the user has, or something the user is (see Figure 12-1). Something a user knows is a **password**. Most organizations today enforce a strong password policy, because free software available on the Internet can break a password from the dictionary very quickly! Strong password policies include using combinations of letters, numbers, and special characters such as plus signs (+) and ampersands (&). Policies typically include the enforcement of changing passwords every 30 or 60 days. Passwords should never be written down in an obvious place like a sticky note attached to the monitor or under the keyboard. The second area of authentication is something the user has, such as an identification (ID) card. Identification cards can be magnetic, similar to a credit card, or have a **radio frequency identity (RFID) chip** embedded into the card. The last area of authentication is **biometrics**. Devices that recognize thumb prints, retina patterns, or

FIGURE 12-1
Ways to authenticate users: (a) an ID badge; (b) examples of weak and strong passwords; (c) a finger on a biometric scanner.

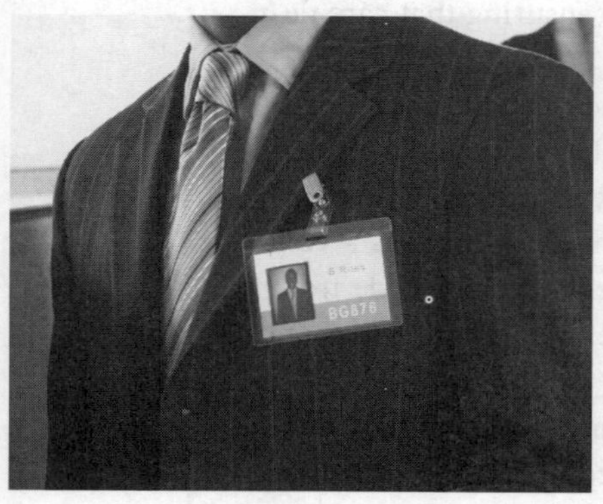

A.

Weak password: BobandSue

Strong password: M2f4#eegh/

B.

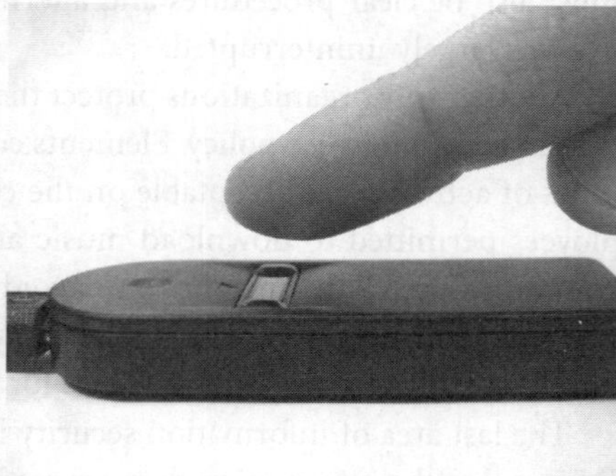

C.

SOURCES: Part A: © Photos.com. Part C: © Gary James Calder/ShutterStock, Inc.

facial patterns are available. Depending on the level of security needed, organizations will commonly use a combination of these types of authentication.

THREATS TO SECURITY

The largest benefit of a computer network is the ability to share information. However, organizations need to protect that information. A 2003 nationwide survey by the Computing Technology Industry Association (CompTIA) found that human error was the most likely cause of problems with **security breaches**. The survey indicated that only 8% were caused by purely technical errors, with more than 63% being caused by some type of human error (Gross, 2003). How do organizations approach security knowing that human beings are the most likely cause of a security breach?

The first line of defense is strictly physical. The power of a locked door, an operating system that locks down after 5 minutes of inactivity, and regular security training programs are extremely effective. Proper workspace security discipline is a critical aspect. Employees need to be properly trained to be aware of computer monitor visibility, shoulder surfing, and policy regarding the removal of computer hardware. A major issue facing organizations is removable storage devices (see Figure 12-2 as an example). CD/DVD burners, **jump drives, flash drives,** or

FIGURE 12-2
A removable storage device.

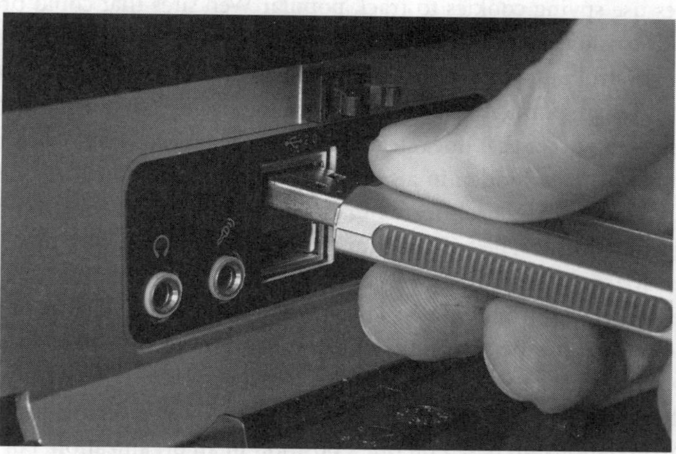

SOURCE: © Alex Kotlov/ShutterStock, Inc.

thumb drives (which use USB port access) are all potential security risks. These devices can be slipped into a pocket and thus are easily removed from the organization. One way to address this physical security risk is to limit the authorization to write files to a device. Organizations are also turning off the CD/DVD burners and USB ports on company desktops.

The most common threats a corporate network faces are **hackers, malicious code (spyware, viruses, worms, Trojan horses)**, and the **malicious insider**. Acceptable use policies help to address these problems. It is common practice for employees to be restricted from downloading files from the Internet. Downloaded files, including e-mail attachments, are the most common way viruses and other malicious code enters a computer network. Network security policies typically prohibit employees from using personal CDs/DVDs and USB drives, and thus prevent the transfer of malicious code from a personal computer to the network.

Spyware is normally controlled by limiting functions of the browser used to surf the Internet. For example, the browser privacy options can control how cookies are used. A cookie is a very small file written to the hard drive of a computer whose user is surfing the Internet. The file simply contains information about the user. For example, many shopping sites write cookies to the user's hard drive containing the user's name and preferences. When that user returns to the site, the site will greet her by name and list products she is possibly interested in. Weather Web sites send cookies to users' hard drives with their zip code so that when each user returns to that site, the local weather forecast is immediately displayed. On the negative side, cookies can also follow the user's travels on the Internet. Marketing companies use spying cookies to track popular Web sites that could provide return on advertising expenditures. Spying cookies related to marketing typically do not track keystrokes to steal user IDs and passwords. They simply exist to track what Web sites are popular, and thus are used to develop advertising and marketing strategies. Spyware that does steal user IDs and passwords contains malicious code that is normally hidden in a seemingly innocent file download. This threat to security explains why healthcare organizations typically do not allow employees to download files. The rule of thumb to protect the network and your own computer system is to only download files from a reputable site that provides complete contact information. Organizations may also use devices such as firewalls (covered in the next section) and **intrusion detection devices** to protect themselves from hackers.

Another huge threat to corporate security is **social engineering**, or the manipulation of a relationship based on one's position in an organization. For example, someone attempting to access a network might pretend to be an employee from the corporate IT office who then simply asks for an employee's digital ID and password. The outsider can then gain access to the corporate network. Once this access has been obtained, all corporate information is at risk. A second example of social engineering is a hacker impersonating a federal government agent. After literally talking an employee into revealing network information, the hacker basically has an open door to enter the corporate network.

The number one security threat to a corporate network is the malicious insider. This can be a disgruntled employee or a recently fired employee whose rights of access to the corporate network have not yet been removed. In the case of the latter, network access should be suspended immediately upon notice of termination. To avoid issues created by malicious insiders, healthcare organizations need some type of policy to monitor employee activity to ensure that employees are only carrying out duties that are part of their normal job. Separation of privileges is a common security tool; no one employee should be able to complete a task that could cause a critical event without the knowledge of another employee. For example, the employee who processes the checks and prints them should not be the same person who signs them. Another example is that the employee who alters pay rates and hours worked must submit a weekly report to a supervisor before the changes take effect. There is also software available to track and thus monitor employee activity. This software can log what files an employee accesses, if changes were made to files, and if the files were copied. Depending on the number of employees, organizations may also employ a full-time electronic auditor who does nothing but monitor activity logs.

SECURITY TOOLS

There is a wide range of tools available to an organization to protect the organizational network and information. These tools can be either a software solution such as **antivirus software** or a hardware tool such as a proxy server. These tools are only effective if used along with employee awareness training. For example, e-mail scanning is a common software tool used. All incoming e-mail messages are scanned to ensure they do not contain a virus or some other malicious code. This software can only find viruses that are currently known. Organizations can further protect themselves by training employees to never open an e-mail attachment unless they are expecting the attachment and they know the sender. This protects the organization from new viruses that are not yet included in their scanning software. E-mail scanning software and antivirus software should never be turned off and updates should be installed at least weekly, but ideally, daily. Software is also available to scan instant messages and to automatically delete spam e-mail.

Firewalls are another common tool used by organizations to protect their corporate networks when they are attached to the Internet. A firewall can be either hardware or software or a combination of both. A firewall examines all incoming messages or traffic to the network. The firewall can be set up to only allow messages from known senders into the corporate network. Firewalls can also be set up to look at outgoing information from the corporate network. If the message contains some type of corporate secret, the firewall prevents the message from leaving. Firewalls are basically electronic security guards at the gate of the corporate network.

Proxy servers also protect the organizational network. Proxy servers prevent users from directly accessing the Internet. They must first request passage from the proxy server. The server will look at the request, make sure the request is from a legitimate user, and that the destination of the request is permissible. For example, organizations can block requests to view a Web site with the word *sex* in the title. The proxy server can also lend the requesting user a **mask** to use while he or she is surfing on the World Wide Web. In this way, the corporation is protecting the identity of its employees. The proxy server keeps track of which employees are using which masks and directs the traffic appropriately.

With hacking becoming more common, healthcare organizations must have some type of protection to avoid this invasion. **Intrusion detection systems** (both hardware and software) allow an organization to monitor who is using the **network** and what files that user has accessed. Detection systems can be set up to monitor a single computer or an entire network. Corporations must diligently monitor for unauthorized access of their networks.

OFF-SITE USE OF PORTABLE DEVICES

Off-site uses of portable devices such as laptops, PDAs, home computing systems, smart phones, and portable data storage devices can help to streamline the delivery of health care. For example, home health nurses may need to access electronic protected health information (EPHI) via a wireless laptop connection during a home visit, or a physician might use a PDA to get specific patient information related to a prescription refill in response to a patient request. These mobile devices are invaluable to healthcare efficiency and responsiveness to patient need in such cases. At the very least, agencies should require data encryption when EPHI is being transmitted over unsecured networks or transported on a mobile device as a way of protecting sensitive information. Some agencies have developed a virtual private network (VPN) that the user must log in to in order to reach the network. The VPN ensures that all data transmitted via this gateway is encrypted.

Only data essential for the job should be contained on the mobile device, and other nonclinical information such as Social Security numbers should never be carried outside the secure network. Some institutions make use of thin clients, which are basic interface portals that do not keep secure information stored on them. Essentially, users must log in to the network to get the data they need. Use of thin clients may be problematic in patient care situations where the user cannot access the network easily. For example, some rural areas of the country still do not have wireless coverage. In these instances, private health information may need to be stored in a clinician's laptop or PDA.

What happens if one of these devices is lost or stolen? The agency is ultimately responsible for the integrity of the data contained on these devices and is required by HIPAA regulations (Department of Health and Human Services, 2006) to have policies in place covering such items as appropriate remote use, removal of devices from their usual physical location, and how these devices are to be protected from loss or theft. Simple rules such as covering laptops left in a car and locking car doors during transport of mobile devices containing EPHI can help to deter theft. If a device is lost or stolen, the agency must have clear procedures in place to help ensure that sensitive data does not get released or used inappropriately. The use of software packages that provide for physical tracking of the static and mobile computer inventory including laptops and PDAs are being used more widely and help in the recovery of lost or stolen devices. In addition, some software that allows for remote data deletion in the event of theft or loss of a mobile device can be invaluable to the agency in preventing the release of EPHI.

If a member of an agency is caught accessing EPHI inappropriately or steals a mobile device, the sanctions should be swift and public. Sanctions may range from a warning or suspension with retraining to termination and/or prosecution depending on the severity of the security breach. The sanctions must send a clear message to all that protecting EPHI is serious business.

The Department of Health and Human Services (2006) identifies potential risks and proposes risk management strategies for accessing, storing, and transmitting EPHI. Visit this Web site for detailed tabular information (pp. 4–6) on potential risks and risk management strategies: http://www.cms.hhs.gov/SecurityStandard/Downloads/SecurityGuidanceforRemoteUseFinal122806.pdf.

SUMMARY

The most important point I'd like to leave you with is the only completely safe network is one that is turned off! Network accessibility and network availability are necessary evils that pose security risks. The information must be available to be accessed yet secured from hackers, unauthorized users, and any other potential security breaches. It is everyone's responsibility to diligently monitor for unauthorized access of their networks, data, and/or information.

THOUGHT-PROVOKING Questions

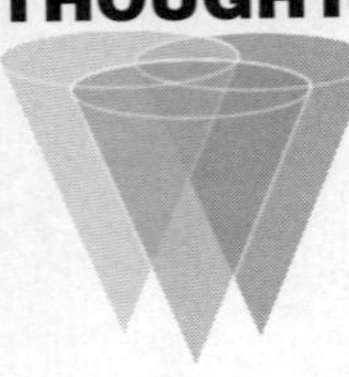

1. Jean, a diabetes nurse educator, recently read an article in an online journal that she accessed through her health agency's database subscription. The article provided a comprehensive checklist for managing diabetes in older adults that she prints and distributes to her patients in a diabetes education class. Does this constitute fair use or is this a copyright violation?
2. Sue is a chronic obstructive pulmonary disorder (COPD) clinic nurse enrolled in a master's education program. She is interested in writing a paper on the factors that are associated with poor compliance with medical regimens and associated rehospitalization of COPD patients. She downloads patient information from the clinic database to a thumb drive that she later accesses on her home computer. Sue understands rules about privacy of information and believes that since she is a nurse and needs this information for a graduate school assignment that she is entitled to the information. Is Sue correct in her thinking?

References

Department of Health and Human Services. (2006, December 28). *HIPAA security guidance.* Retrieved January 19, 2008, from Security Guidance for Remote Use Web site: http://www.cms.hhs.gov/SecurityStandard/Downloads/SecurityGuidanceforRemoteUseFinal122806.pdf

Gross, G. (2003, March 18). Human error causes most security breaches. *InfoWorld.* Retrieved January 15, 2008, from http://www.infoworld.com/article/03/03/18/HNhumanerror_1.html

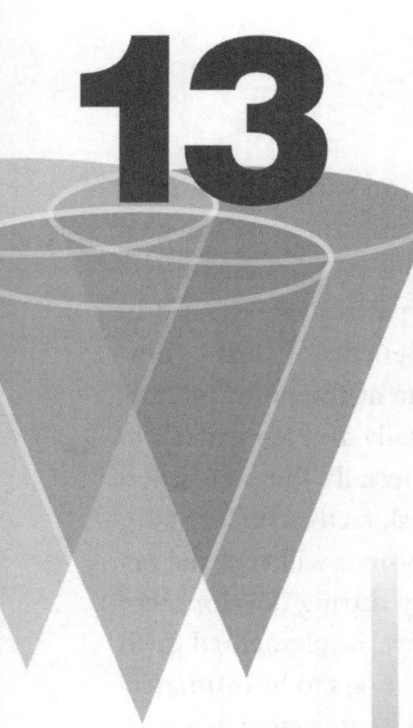

An Insider's View of the Utility of a Clinical Information System

Denise Tyler

Objectives

1. Assess an insider's description of a CIS.
2. Explore knowledge dissemination and generation tools supported by the CIS.
3. Describe quality assurance and clinical outcomes measurement supported by the CIS.
4. Explore evidence-based practice and translational research tools provided by the CIS.

Key Terms

Aggregate data
Clinical analytics
Clinical guidelines
Clinical information system (CIS)
Clinical outcomes
Clinical practice council
Coded terminology
Evidence-based practice (EBP)
Knowledge dissemination
Legacy systems
Performance improvement
Performance improvement analyst
Professional development
Quality assurance (QA)
Staff development
Translational research

INTRODUCTION

A **clinical information system (CIS)** is a technology-based system that is applied at the point of care and is designed to support the acquisition and processing of information as well as providing storage and processing capabilities. Sittig et al. provide a comprehensive definition of a CIS:

> A clinical information system is a collection of various information technology applications that provides a centralized repository of information related to patient care across distributed locations. This repository represents the patient's history of illnesses and interactions with providers by encoding knowledge capable of helping clinicians decide about the patient's condition, treatment options, and wellness activities. The repository also encodes the status of decisions, actions underway for those decisions and relevant information that could help in performing those actions. The database could also hold other information about the patient including genetic, environmental, and social contexts. (Sittig et al., 2002, ¶ 3)

Early CISs were limited in scope and provided information such as laboratory results or medication administration and drug interaction information. The goal of many organizations is to expand the scope of the CIS to a comprehensive system that provides clinical decision support, an electronic patient record, and in some instances **professional development** training tools. Benefits of such a comprehensive system could provide easy access to patient data at the point of care, structured and legible information that can be searched easily and lends itself to data mining and analysis, and improved patient safety, especially the prevention of adverse drug reactions and the identification of health risk factors such as falls. Of course, the implementation of such a comprehensive system will cost the organization both dollars and losses in clinician productivity during development and implementation. Reports from organizations that have implemented such comprehensive systems point to the critical need for the end users to be intimately involved in choosing and/or developing the CIS. Additional issues associated with implementation of a CIS include the need to interface with **legacy systems** (those already in place), privacy and security (covered in Chapters 11 and 12, which discussed HIPAA and network security, respectively), and clinician resistance to learning new technology (*Clinical Information System*, 2006).

At Kaweah Delta, staff nurses, nurse managers, support staff, and **performance improvement analysts** were all intimately involved in the design of the system used by nursing. Ancillary staff were very involved in the design of their systems as well. This has enabled a consistency in the charting done by different clinicians, while enabling their pathways to be designed according to their specific needs. As the system matures and more staff from different areas use the system both for charting and for accessing information, changes are put in place to enhance the system, and reports are created for quality assurance and reporting.

As the system evolved, views were created to incorporate an interdisciplinary display of patient education, care planning, and exchange of information for communication between providers and shift reports. These displays have greatly improved the way the information is accessed and shared. The displays and reports also allow for easier and timelier **quality assurance (QA)** of charting to provide better feedback for improvement. Reports are available online and are e-mailed out daily to clinical analysts for the review of priority assessment data to ensure accurate and timely entry of information on each new admission. These reports also help nursing administrators prioritize educational needs of staff, as well as fine tune the computerized nursing documentation to better enable staff to comply with charting requirements.

Paying attention to the human–technology interface (see Chapter 5) elements of the system is essential. Adequate testing prior to implementation can prevent problems for users. Inadequate testing can result in a negative attitude and a lack of trust in the system. This testing involves not only the system itself but the hardware used by staff (computers, printers, etc.). Getting input from both the clinicians who will be using the system and the staff who will be using the output information is critical to the success of system design and implementation.

One glitch that remains with many CISs is the quality of the printed document generated by the system. Since the systems are designed for virtual use, their display when printed can produce volumes of paper that is difficult to follow. This may be resolved one day as a result of improvements suggested by outside agencies, payers, and attorneys who may need printed reports. In the meantime, early testing of what the record will look like may not result in huge improvements, but it can at least decrease the surprise when confronted with the new printed record.

CLINICAL OUTCOMES AND QUALITY ASSURANCE SUPPORTED BY THE CIS

The ability to measure outcomes can be enhanced or impeded by the way an information system is designed and used. While many practitioners can paint a very good picture of the patient by using a narrative (free text), using this mode of expression in a clinical system without the use of a coded entry makes it difficult to analyze the care given or the patient's response. Free text reporting also leads to inconsistencies of reporting from clinician to clinician and patient information that is fragmented and/or disorganized. Obviously, this can limit the usefulness or patient data to other clinicians and interfere with the inability to run reports off of the data for QA and measurement. The other issue with using free text is that not all clinicians are skilled at this form of communication, yielding inconsistent documentation.

Integrating standardized nursing terminologies into computerized nursing documentation systems enhances the ability to use the data for reporting and further research. Saba (2007) elaborates on the benefits of using the **aggregate data** available when nursing documentation is linked to a **coded terminology** for research from practice.

The ability to refine the CIS to create different reports and displays based on the need of the user is very helpful. For example, the **performance improvement** department may want to look at charting based on safety indicators or regulatory requirements, while the clinicians caring for a patient might need to see the most recent vital signs, intake & output, results, and specific charting elements that summarize or give a picture of what is happening with that patient.

McLaughlin and Halilovic (2006) describe the use of **clinical analytics** to promote medical care outcomes research. The use of a CIS with standardized codes for patient clinical issues helps to support the rigorous analysis of clinical data. Outcomes data as a result of these analyses may include length of stay, mortality, readmissions, and complications. Future goals include the ability to compare data and outcomes across various institutions as a means of developing **clinical guidelines** or best practices guidelines. With the implementation of a comprehensive CIS, similar analyses of nursing outcomes could also be performed and shared. Such a system could also aid nurse administrators in cross-unit comparisons and staffing decisions, especially when coupled with acuity systems data. In addition, clinical analytics can support required data reporting functions, especially those required by accreditation bodies.

BOX 13-1

Clinical Outcomes Measurement

Julie A. Kenney and Ida Androwich

Currently all hospitals are required to gather data in regards to four core measures: acute myocardial infarction (MI), heart failure, pneumonia, and surgical care improvement/surgical infection prevention. Each of these four core measures is composed of evidence-based care that should be received by patients who fall into these categories. This data is required to be published on the institution's or corporation's Web site as well as be available as a hard copy on site. The data is also published on the United States Department of Health and Human Services Web site, called Hospital Compare. Hospital Compare can be found at http://www.hospitalcompare.hhs.gov/Hospital/Search/SelectConditionsAndMeasures.asp. This Web site lists each hospital's compliance with the four core measure bundles. The public can compare hospitals based on these four **clinical outcomes** measures. Each hospital supplies the information quarterly (United States Department of Health and Human Services, 2007).

With the worldwide emphasis on measuring and evaluating the quality of health care, the American Nurses Association decided that nursing should begin a program that would build a database for nursing-sensitive quality indicators and use the collected data to educate practicing nurses on quality activities and educate the public about nursing (Gallagher & Rowell, 2003). This was the beginning of the national database of nursing quality indicators (NDNQI). Facilities were recruited to gather data and return it to NDNQI, which would then store the data to begin developing facility indicator profiling and the eventual data comparison of hospitals that share similar characteristics (Gallagher & Rowell). Each facility is given a unique number in order that no identifying information is released unintentionally. Each facility decides if it wants to publicize its participation in the NDNQI project (Gallagher & Rowell).

This project has resulted in numerous studies that have used the data within the database. One study is looking at the relationship between nursing staffing and pa-

BOX Continued
13-1

tient outcomes. Currently there is little quantifiable evidence to show nursing's impact on patient outcomes, especially when looking at nursing staff ratios to patient outcomes. The database provides the ability to differentiate areas of concern down to the unit level due to the type of data that is collected (Gallagher, 2001; Gallagher & Rowell, 2003). The information is more useful when differentiated by nursing unit type than when grouped together as a whole. The separated information allows for a more accurate picture of unit level activity as compared to the institution as a whole. If the information is viewed together, a weaker unit will be balanced out by a stronger unit, which will sway the way the picture is painted by the data. In addition, the erroneous conclusions drawn by lumping unit data together will hamper the ability to provide administrative support to the unit that is struggling and provide positive reinforcement to the unit that is performing above average (Gallagher & Rowell). If an institution owns an electronic health record (EHR), a significant portion of this data can be pulled from the system, which saves the institution from employing a person to manually pull data from the paper chart. The following is the current list of data that is being collected by NDNQI (American Nurses Association [ANA], 2007):

- Patient falls
- Patient falls with injury, including level of injury
- Pressure ulcer rate
- Hospital-acquired pressure ulcer rate
- RN satisfaction
- Nursing hours per patient day
  - Registered nurse (RN) hours per patient day
  - Licensed practical/vocational nurses (LPN/LVN) hours per patient day
  - Unlicensed assistive personnel hours per patient day
- Staff mix
  - RN
  - LPN/LVNs
  - Unlicensed assistive personnel
  - Percent agency staff
- RN education/certification
- Pediatric pain assessment, intervention, reassessment cycle
- Pediatric peripheral intravenous infiltration
- Psychiatric physical/sexual abuse

Additional data collected includes the following:

- Patient population—adult or pediatric
- Hospital category (teaching, nonteaching, etc.)
- Type of unit (critical care, step-down, medical, surgical, combined medical/surgical, rehabilitation, and psychiatric)
- Number of staffed beds designated by the hospital

BOX Continued
13-1

New indicators undergoing development include the following:

- Restraints
- Practice environment scale
- Nursing turnover
- Nursing musculoskeletal injuries

The introduction of the EHR has changed the way data is collected. There is an abundance of data available for study, but due to the large number of systems and the lack of a universal medical language, transferring the data to the databases has proven difficult (Lu, Park, Ucharattana, Konicek, & Delaney, 2007). This is where nursing informatics plays a significant role. The nurse informatics specialist (NIS) works with the program developers to ensure that EHR systems are using a universal language, which will allow researchers to extract data from the EHR and import it into the database without having to translate the data into a different nomenclature. Developing and using a universal language will aid in allowing different systems to move toward interoperability.

References

American Nurses Association. (2007). *Nursing sensitive indicators.* Retrieved on September 29, 2007, from http://nursingworld.org/MainMenuCategories/ThePracticeofProfessionalNursing/PatientSafetyQuality/NDNQI/NDNQI_1/NursingSensitiveIndicators.aspx

Gallagher, R. M. (2001). Nursing quality indicators: Research proves nursing's impact on patient care. *Arkansas Nursing News, 18*(4), 23–25.

Gallagher, R. M., & Rowell, P. A. (2003). Claiming the future of nursing through nursing-sensitive quality indicators. *Nursing Administration Quarterly, 27*(4), 273–284.

Lu, D.-F., Park, H.-T., Ucharattana, P., Konicek, D., & Delaney, C. (2007). Nursing outcomes classification in the systematized nomenclature of medicine clinical terms: A cross-mapping validation. *CIN: Computers, Informatics, Nursing, 25*(3), 159–170.

United States Department of Health and Human Services. (2007). *Hospital compare Web site.* Retrieved September 29, 2007, from http://www.hospitalcompare.hhs.gov/Hospital/Search/SelectConditionsAndMeasures.asp

Quality assurance in the electronic world deals not only with quality indicators in regards to the care provided, but it also applies to the way the information is captured, displayed, and reported. Making sure that the system design and linking are done so that the discrete data elements are easy to identify whether the data is reviewed online or being used for research measurement is now important.

Reviewing the way staff are charting using the system is still necessary but should be less time consuming than it was in the paper era due to the ability to access the information from anywhere in real time as well as in the reporting functions based on the needs of the user.

EVIDENCE-BASED PRACTICE AND THE CIS

Evidence-based practice (EBP) can be thought of as the integration of clinical expertise and best practices based on systematic research to enhance decision making and improve patient care. EBP does not take away from the critical-thinking skills utilized by the expert nurse; it enhances their informed decision making. According to Simpson (2004), "Evidence-based nursing is the process by which nurses make clinical decisions using the best available research evidence, their clinical expertise, and patient preferences. Three areas of research competence are: interpreting and using research, evaluating practice, and conducting research" (p. 10).

EBP should be embedded in computerized documentation of a CIS, providing both prompts for interventions and/or different questions based on the charted assessment. These prompts can be done by required fields that display only when the criterion is met, by pop-up boxes, or even by printed reminders. How the prompts are delivered is best determined by the workflow during that process, but system capabilities and organizational policies must also be considered.

References supporting EBP should be available for review at the click of a mouse or by a few keystrokes. This ease of access to more detailed information will establish a trust among clinicians in the prompts built into the documentation system as well as increase the user's understanding of the information provided. As clinical knowledge is acquired, it can be applied to situations where the CIS prompting is not present to improve clinical decision making. The CIS prompting capabilities can also reinforce the practice of looking for evidence to support nursing interventions rather than relying on how things have been done historically. This enhances the processing and understanding of the information, as well as allowing the nurse to apply the information to other areas, increasing the knowledge obtained about why certain conditions or responses result in prompts for additional questions or actions.

For example, a healthcare agency accrediting body, the Joint Commission, has added core measures for quality as part of its reporting and inspection process. When parts of the nursing process such as problem identification and care planning are embedded in the documentation, they may become such an integral part of the workflow that staff at the bedside no longer consciously separate them out as unique actions. This reflects well on the system design but can make it difficult for care providers to explain to regulatory agencies such as the Joint Commission what they are doing. Preparing staff involved in bedside care to effectively communicate what they are doing can be a challenge. Some institutions rely on standardized clinical practice guidelines that can be modified for application to individual patients. In this way, there is a clear illustration for the application of the nursing process to clinical care.

In order to incorporate EBP into the practice of clinical nursing, the information needs to be embedded in the computerized documentation system so that it is part of the workflow. The most typical way of embedding this timely information is through clinical practice guidelines. The resulting interventions and clinical outcomes need to be measurable and reportable for further research. The supporting documentation for the EBP needs to be easily retrievable and meaningful. Links, reminders, and prompts can all be used as vehicles for transmission of this information. The format needs to allow for rapid scanning, with the ability to expand the amount of information when more detail is required or desired. Balancing a consistency in formatting with creativity can be difficult but worth the effort to stimulate an atmosphere for learning.

EBP is supported by **translational research**. Translational research is a "dynamic and fluid exchange of scientific and clinical knowledge" (Clements & Crane, 2006, p. 42). This is an exciting movement that has enormous potential for the sharing and use of EBP. By creating a fluid sharing of research and application between research experts (those who know) and clinical experts (those who do) at the bedside, more meaningful research and improved clinical outcomes should result. The use of translational research to support EBP may help to close the gap between what we know (research) and what we do (practice).

THE CIS AS A STAFF DEVELOPMENT TOOL

Joy Hilty, RN from Kaweah Delta, came up with a creative way to provide **staff development** or education without taking staff away from the bedside to a classroom setting. She created pop-up boxes on the opening charting screens for all staff who chart on the computer. These pop-ups vary in color and content and include a short piece of clinical information, along with a question. Staff can earn "vacations" from these pop-ups for up to 14 days by e-mailing the correct answer to the question. This media has provided information, stimulation, and a definite benefit: the vacation from the pop-up boxes. The pop-up box education format has encouraged staff to share the answers, thus creating interaction, **knowledge dissemination**, and reinforcement of the education provided.

This same logic can be utilized to reinforce new standards of care based on current evidence. By adding interaction to embedded practices, the information is reinforced. As this information is repeatedly utilized and reinforced, an awareness of the way the information can be used to improve patient care is developed. When the information is applied to other similar situations, knowledge has been achieved.

Embedding EBP into nursing documentation can also increase the compliance with Joint Commission core measures, such as providing information on influenza and pneumovac vaccinations to at-risk patients. In my experience at Kaweah Delta, educating staff via classes, flyers, and storyboards was not successful in improving compliance with the documentation of immunization status or offering education on the vaccinations to at-risk patients. Embedding the prompts, information, and related questions in the nursing documentation with a link to the protocol as well as educational material has improved the compliance to 96% for pneumococcal vaccinations and to 95% for the influenza vaccination (Hettinger, 2007).

Creating an environment that encourages and expects professional development and learning needs to be a consistent expectation across all levels of an organization. The volume of information available makes it extremely difficult to find information that is current, valid, and applicable to the problem or question at hand. Relying on memory or past knowledge may not be the best way of providing care based on current evidence. Further, maintaining knowledge on best practices based on current research is almost impossible due to the sheer volume of information. In an attempt to provide the medical community with a way to manage this volume of information, several companies have developed strategies for reviewing research and have developed software applications where this information can be easily retrieved. These knowledge vendors are now working with clinical systems to embed this knowledge and provide links to timely and continuously updated information.

By embedding a standard language into the computerized documentation, the data can be used for instruction as well as facilitating the sharing of information for research. This sharing of information will improve the ability to track the effects of nursing interventions. Many institutions have implemented **clinical practice councils** that use the information generated by the CIS to design clinical education programs. Councils may also update policies or procedures or clinical practice guidelines according to changes based on the analysis of institutional strengths, weaknesses, and goals.

SUMMARY

The CIS is a technology-based system that is applied at the point of care and is designed to support the acquisition and processing of information as well as providing storage and processing capabilities. Early CISs were limited in scope.

Today, the goal of many organizations is to expand the scope of the CIS to a comprehensive system that provides clinical decision support, an electronic patient record, and in some instances professional development training tools. Benefits of such a comprehensive system could provide easy access to patient data at the point of care, structured and legible information that can be searched easily and lends itself to data mining and analysis, and improved patient safety, especially the prevention of adverse drug reactions and the identification of health risk factors such as falls. Quality assurance is a positive outcome from CISs and the clinical analytics promote medical care outcomes research. The incorporation of EBP and the integration of clinical expertise and best practices based on systematic research to enhance decision making and improve patient care will further enhance the system. The use of translational research to support EBP may help to close the gap between what we know (research) and what we do (practice). As a staff development medium, embedding the prompts, information, and related questions in the nursing documentation with a link to the protocol as well as educational material has improved the compliance. CISs are becoming more robust and are assuming increasing roles in the healthcare delivery system.

The most important thought I'd like to leave you with is that I believe the clinicians of the future will be linked to a national database where evidence is documented. With minimal effort, the research can be analyzed, and when appropriate, it will be linked to the CIS in a way that is intuitive and informative. Alerts will be patient and provider specific. The steps required of the clinician to find current, reliable information will be almost transparent, and the information will be presented in a personalized manner based on user preferences stored in the CIS.

THOUGHT-PROVOKING Questions

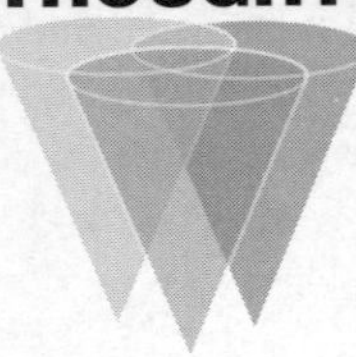

1. You have been asked to prioritize the requirements of a clinical documentation system. It has already been determined that ease, usability, and dependability are priorities. What else would you include in the system requirements?
2. You have been asked to design a test scenario for a new CIS. What are some of the details you would test? Who would you involve?
3. You are asked about a diagnosis with which you are unfamiliar. Where would you start looking for information? How would you determine how valid the information is?

References

Clements, P. T., & Crane, P. A. (2006, spring). Building bridges: The importance of translational forensic nursing research. *Journal of Forensic Nursing, 2*(1), 42–44.

Clinical information system. (2006, August 10). Retrieved January 26, 2008, from Biohealthmatics.com Web site: http://www.biohealthmatics.com/technologies/his/cis.aspx

Hettinger, M. (2007, March). *Core measure reporting: Performance improvement.* Kaweah Delta Health Care District publication.

McLaughlin, T., & Halilovic, M. (2006). Clinical analytics, rigorous coding bring objectivity to quality assertions. *Medical Staff Update Online, 30*(6). Retrieved January 20, 2008, from http://med.stanford.edu/shs/update/archives/JUNE2006/analytics.htm

Saba, V. K. (2007). *Clinical care classification (CCC) system manual: A guide to nursing documentation* (2nd ed.). New York: Springer.

Simpson, R. L. (2004). Evidence-based nursing offers certainty in the uncertain world of health care. *Nursing Management, 35*(10), 10–12.

Sittig, D., Hazlehurst, B., Palen, T., Hsu, J., Jimison, H., & Hornbrook, M. (2002, spring). A clinical information system research landscape. *The Permanente Journal, 6*(2). Retrieved January 26, 2008, from http://xnet.kp.org/permanentejournal/spring02/landscape.html

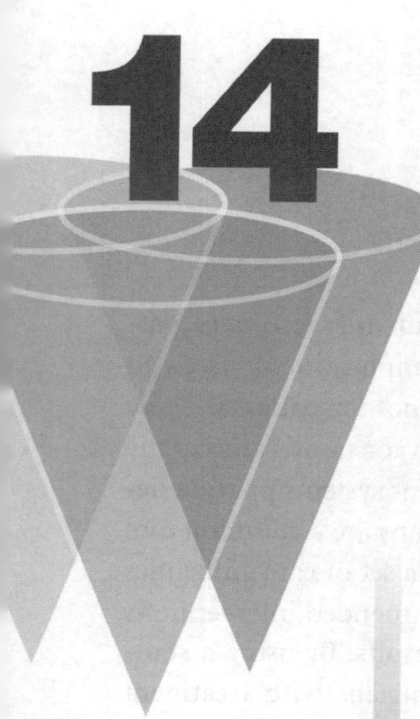

Administrative and Clinical Health Information Systems

Marianela Zytkowski and Susan M. Paschke

Objectives

1. Explore agency-based health information systems.
2. Evaluate how administrators use core business systems in their practice.
3. Assess the function and clinical information output from selected information systems used in healthcare organizations.

Key Terms

Acuity system
Admission, discharge, and transfer (ADT) system
Attribute
Care plan
Case management information system (CMIS)
Clinical documentation system
Clinical information system (CIS)
Collaboration
Column
Communication system
Computerized physician order entry system (CPOE)
Core business systems
Data dictionary
Data file
Data mart
Data mining
Data warehouse (DW)
Database

INTRODUCTION

In order to compete in the ever-changing healthcare arena, organizations require quick and immediate access to a variety of types of information, data, and bodies of knowledge for daily clinical, operational, financial, and human resource activities. Information is continuously shared between units and departments within organizations and healthcare systems and is also required or requested from other healthcare organizations, regulatory and government agencies, educational and philanthropic institutions, and consumers.

Healthcare organizations integrate a variety of clinical and administrative types of **information systems.** These systems collect, process, and distribute patient-centered data to aid in managing and providing care. Together they create a comprehensive record of the patient's medical history. Each of these systems is unique in the way they function and provide information to clinicians. An understanding of how each of these types of systems works within healthcare organizations is fundamental in the study of informatics.

Key Terms *Continued*

Database management system (DBMS)
Decision support
Drill-down
Electronic medical record (EMR)
Entity
Entity relationship diagram (ERD)
Field
Financial system
Information system (IS)
Information technology (IT)
Key field
Knowledge exchange
Laboratory information system
Managed care information systems (MCIS)
Master patient index (MPI)
Order entry system
Patient care information system (PCIS)
Patient care support system
Patient centered
Pharmacy information system
Picture and archiving communication system (PACS)
Primary key
Query
Radiology information system (RIS)
Record
Relational database management system (RDBMS)
Repository
Row
Scheduling system
Stakeholder
Standardized plan of care
Table

TYPES OF INFORMATION SYSTEMS IN HEALTHCARE ORGANIZATIONS

Case Management Information Systems

Case management information systems (CMISs) identify resources, patterns, and variances in care to prevent costly complications related to chronic conditions and enhance the overall outcomes for patients. These systems span past episodes of treatment and search for trends among the records. Once a trend is identified, case management systems provide **decision support** promoting preventive care. Care plans are a common tool found in case management systems. A **care plan** is a set of care guidelines that outline the course of treatment and the recommended interventions that should be implemented to achieve optimal results. By using a **standardized plan of care**, these systems present clinicians with treatment protocols to maximize their outcomes and support best practices. Case management information systems are especially beneficial for patient populations with a high cost of care and complex health needs such as the elderly or patients with chronic disease conditions. One example of case management systems at work is in treating patients with acquired immune deficiency syndrome (AIDS). The case management system applies a care plan to treat the patient in order to better manage care from outpatient to inpatient visits where opportunistic infections such as *Pneumocystis carinii* pneumonia (PCP) are common complications (Dijerome, 1992). Avoiding these types of complications requires identifying the right resources for care and implementing preventive treatments across all medical visits. Ultimately this preventive care will decrease the costs of care for these patients and support a better quality of life. These systems increase the value of individual care while controlling the costs and risks associated with long-term health care. Case management systems assimilate massive amounts of information obtained over a patient's lifetime by reaching far beyond the walls of the hospital and track care from one medical visit to the next (Simpson & Falk, 1996). Information collected by case management systems is processed in a way that helps to reduce risks, ensure quality, and decrease costs.

Communication Systems

Communication systems promote the interaction between healthcare providers and patients. Communication systems have historically been separate from other types of health information systems and from one another. Healthcare professionals overwhelmingly recognize the value of these systems so they are more commonly integrated into the design of other types of systems as a newly developing standard within the industry. Examples of communication systems include call light systems, wireless phones, pagers, e-mail, and instant messaging, which have traditionally been forms of communication targeted at the clinicians. However, communication systems are more frequently beginning to target patients and their families. Patients are now able to access their electronic chart from home via Internet connections. They can update their own medical record to inform their physician of changes to their health or personal practices, which impact their physical condition. Inpatients in hospital settings also receive communication directly to their room. Patients and their families review individualized messages with scheduled tests and procedures for the day and confirmation of menu choices for their meals. These types of systems may also communicate educational messages such as smoking cessation advice.

As health care begins to introduce more of this technology into practice, the value of having communication tools integrated with other types of systems is recognized. Integrating communication systems with clinical applications provides a real-time approach that will facilitate care among the entire healthcare team, patients, and their families. These systems enhance the flow of communication within an organization and promote an exchange of information to better care for patients. The next generation of communication systems will be integrated with other types of healthcare systems and are guaranteed to integrate with one another.

Core Business Systems

Core business systems enhance administrative tasks within healthcare organizations. Unlike clinical information systems whose aim is to provide direct patient care, these systems support the management of health care within an organization. Core business systems provide the framework for reimbursement, support of best practices, quality control, and resource allocation. There are four common core business systems: (1) **admission, discharge, and transfer (ADT) systems**, (2) **financial systems**, (3) **acuity systems**, and (4) **scheduling systems.**

ADT systems provide the backbone structure for the other types of clinical and business systems (Hassett & Thede, 2003). Admitting, billing, and bed management departments most commonly use ADT systems. These systems contain key information upon which all other systems interface. A few examples of information that ADT systems provide include the patient name, medical record number, visit or account number, and demographic information such as age, sex, home address, and contact information. ADT systems are considered the central source for collecting this type of patient information and communicating it to other types of healthcare information systems.

Financial systems manage the expenses and revenue for providing health care. The finance, auditing, and accounting departments within an organization most commonly use financial systems. These systems determine the direction for maintenance and growth for a given facility. Financial systems often interface to share information with materials management, staffing, and billing systems to balance the financial impact of these resources within an organization. These systems report the fiscal outcomes in order to track them against the organizational goals of an institution. Financial systems are one of the major decision-making factors as healthcare institutions prepare their fiscal budgets. These systems often play a pivotal role in determining the strategic direction for an organization.

Acuity systems monitor the range of patient types within a healthcare organization using specific indicators. Acuity systems track these indicators based on the current patient population within a facility. By monitoring the patient acuity, these systems provide feedback about how intensive the care requirement is for an individual patient or group of patients. Identifying and classifying a patient's acuity can promote better organizational management of expenses and resources necessary to provide care. Acuity systems help predict the ability and capacity of an organization to care for its current population. These types of systems also forecast future trends to allow an organization to successfully strategize on how to meet upcoming market demands.

Scheduling systems coordinate staff, services, equipment, and allocation of patient beds. These systems frequently integrate with the other types of core business systems. By closely monitoring staff and physical resources, these systems provide data to the financial systems. For example, resource-scheduling systems provide information about operating room utilization or availability of intensive care unit beds and regular nursing unit beds. These systems also serve as a great asset to the financial systems when they are used to track medical equipment within a facility. Procedures and care are planned when the tools and resources are available. Scheduling systems help to track resources within a facility while managing the frequency and distribution of those resources.

Order Entry Systems

Order entry systems are one of the most important systems in use today. These systems automate the way that orders have traditionally been initiated for patients. Clinicians place orders within these systems instead of placing them with traditional handwritten transcription onto paper. Order entry systems provide major safeguards by ensuring that physician orders are legible and complete, thereby providing a level of patient safety that was historically missing with paper-based orders. These systems, **computerized physician order entry systems**

(CPOE), provide decision support and automated alert functionality that was unavailable with paper-based orders. The Institute of Medicine estimates that medical errors cost the nation approximately $37.6 billion each year; about $17 billion of those costs are associated with preventable errors. In addition, this report recommends eliminating reliance on handwriting for ordering medications and other treatment needs (Agency for Healthcare Research and Quality, 2000). Because of this global concern for patient safety due to incorrect and misinterpreted orders, healthcare organizations are incorporating these types of systems as a standard tool for practice. Order entry systems allow for clear and legible orders promoting patient safety and streamlining care.

Patient Care Support Systems

Most specialty disciplines within health care have an associated **patient care information system (PCIS)**. These patient-centered systems focus on collecting data and disseminating information related to direct care. Several of these systems have become mainstream types of systems used in health care. The four systems most commonly found include (1) clinical documentation systems, (2) pharmacy information systems, (3) laboratory information systems, and (4) radiology information systems.

Clinical documentation systems, also known as **clinical information systems (CISs)**, are the most commonly used type of patient care support system within healthcare organizations. Clinical information systems are designed to collect patient data in real time. They enhance care by providing data at the clinician's fingertips and enabling decision making where it needs to occur, at the bedside. For that reason, these systems oftentimes are easily accessible at the point of care for caregivers interacting with the patient. CIS systems are **patient centered**, meaning they contain the observations, interventions, and outcomes noted by the care team. Team members enter information such as the plan of care, hemodynamic data, lab results, clinical notes, allergies, and medications. All members of the treatment team use clinical documentation systems—pharmacists, allied health workers, nurses, physicians, support staff, and many others access the clinical record for the patient using these systems. Frequently these types of systems are also referred to as the electronic patient record or the **electronic medical record (EMR)**.

Pharmacy information systems have also become a mainstream patient care support system. These systems typically allow pharmacists to order, manage, and dispense medications for a facility. They also commonly incorporate allergies and height and weight information for effective medication management. Pharmacy information systems streamline the order entry, dispensing, verification, and authorization process for medication administration. These systems often interface with clinical documentation and order entry systems so that clinicians can order and document the administration of medications and prescriptions to patients while having the benefits of decision support alerting and interaction checking.

Laboratory information systems were perhaps some of the first systems ever used in health care. Because of this strong history within medicine, laboratory systems have been models for the design and implementation of other types of **patient care support systems.** Laboratory information systems report on blood, body fluid, and tissue samples along with biological specimens that are collected at the bedside and received in a central laboratory. These systems provide clinicians with reference ranges for tests indicating high, low, or normal values in order to make care decisions. Often the laboratory system provides result information directing clinicians towards the next course of action within a treatment regime.

The final type of patient care support system commonly found within health care is the **radiology information system (RIS)** in radiology departments. These systems schedule, result, and store information as it relates to diagnostic radiology procedures. One common feature found in most radiology systems is a **picture archiving and communication system (PACS)**. These systems may also be stand-alone systems, separate from the main radiology system, or they can be integrated with RIS and CIS. These systems collect, store, and distribute medical images such as computed tomography (CT) scans, magnetic resonance imaging (MRI), and X-rays. PACS replace traditional hard copy films with digital media that is easy to store, retrieve, and present to clinicians. The benefit of RIS and PACS systems is their ability to assist in diagnosing and storing vital patient care support data.

As technologies evolve, so will our databases and information systems (see Box 14-1 for more information on databases). The mobility of our patients geographically as well as within one healthcare delivery system challenges information systems since data must be captured wherever and whenever the patient receives care. In the past, **managed care information systems (MCIS)** began to address these issues. Ciotti and Zodda (1996) stated that the MCIS "can nimbly cross organizational boundaries, includes an enterprise-wide **master patient index (MPI)**, and offers access across provider, geographic, and departmental lines" (¶ 10). This means that data can be obtained at any and all of the patient areas. The patient tracking mechanisms continue to be honed while the financial impact of health care has been changing our systems as well. The information systems that we currently use make it possible for nurses and physicians to make clinical decisions while being mindful of their financial ramifications. We will continue to see vast improvements in our information systems.

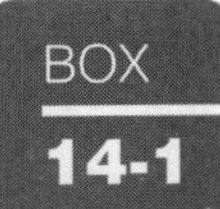

Databases, Data Warehousing, Data Mining, and Data

Dee McGonigle and Kathleen Mastrian

The most basic element of a database system is the data. Data refers to raw facts that can consist of unorganized text, graphics, sound or video. As you remember from Chapter 2, information is data that has been processed—it has meaning; information is organized in a way that people find meaningful and useful. Even useful information can be lost if one is mired in tons of unorganized information. Computers can come to the rescue by helping to create order out of chaos. Computer science and information science are designed to help us cut down the amount of information to a more manageable size and organize it so that we can cope with it more efficiently through the use of databases and database programs technology. Learning about basic databases and database management programs is paramount so that we can apply data and information management principles in health care.

Databases are structured or organized collections of data that are typically the main component of an information system. Databases and database management software allow the user to input, sort, arrange, structure, organize, and store data and turn it into useful information. One can set up a personal database to organize recipes, music, names and addresses, notes, bills, and other data. In health care, the databases and information systems make key information available to healthcare providers and ancillary personnel in order to promote the provision of quality patient care.

Databases are comprised of **fields** or **columns** and **records** or **rows**. Within each record, one of the fields is identified as the **primary key** or **key field**. This primary key contains a code, name, number, or other bit of information that acts as a unique identifier for that record. In your healthcare system, for example, your patient is assigned a patient number or ID that is unique for that patient. As you compile related records, you create data files or tables. A **data file** is a collection of related records. Therefore, **databases** consist of one or more related data files or **tables**. The term **entity** represents a table and each field within the table becomes an **attribute** of that entity. The database developer must critically think about the attributes for each specific entity. For example, the entity disease might have the attributes of chronic disease, acute disease, or communicable disease. The name of the entity, disease, would imply that the entity is about diseases. The fields or attributes would be chronic, acute, or communicable. The **entity relationship diagram (ERD)** specifies the relationship among the entities in the database. Sometimes the implied relationships are apparent based on the entities' definitions; however all relationships should be specified as to how they relate to one another. There are typically three relationships—one to one, one to many, and many to many. A one-to-one relationship would exist between the entities of the table about a patient and the table about the patient's birth. The one-to-many relationship could exist when one entity is repeatedly used by another entity. The one-to-many relationship could then be a table **query** for age that

BOX Continued
14-1

could be used numerous times for one patient entity. The many-to-many relationship would reflect entities that are all used repeatedly by other entities. This is easily explained by the entities of patient and nurse. The patient could have several nurses caring for her/him and the nurse could have many patients assigned to her/him (see Figure 14-1). When describing and discussing databases, depending on the context, the terms **entity** and **attribute** are used or **table** and **field** are used.

The relational model is a database model that describes data in which all data elements are placed in relation in two-dimensional tables; the relations or tables are analogous to files. Relational databases follow or conform to the relational model. A

FIGURE 14-1
Example of an entity relationship diagram (ERD).

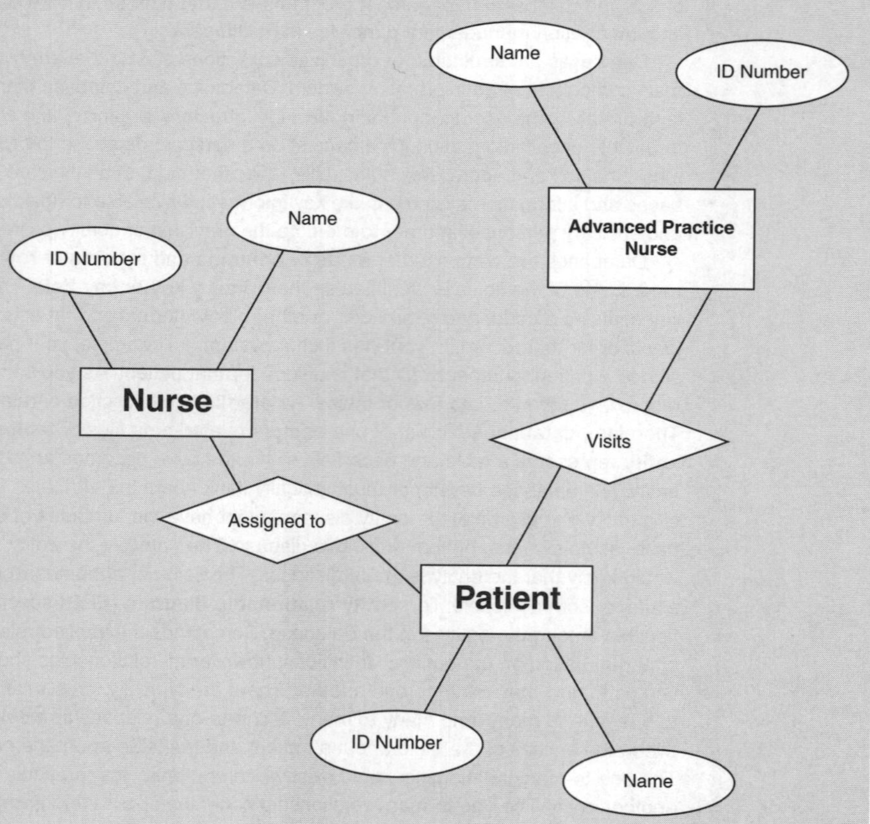

BOX *Continued*
14-1

relational database management system (RDBMS) is a system that manages data using the relational model. A relational database could link a patient's table to a treatment table, for example, by a common field such as the patient ID number. In order to keep track of the tables that comprise a database, the **database management system (DBMS)** uses software called a **data dictionary**. The data dictionary contains a listing of the tables and their details including field names, validation settings, and data types. The data type refers to the type of information such as a name, a date, or a time. The DBMS is such an important program because before it was available, many health systems and businesses had dozens of database files with incompatible formats. Because patient data comes from a variety of sources, these separated, isolated data files required duplicate entry of the same information, thereby increasing the risk of data entry error. The design of the relational databases eliminates data duplication. Some examples of popular database management system software includes Microsoft's Access or Visual FoxPro, Corel's Paradox, Oracle's Oracle Database 10g, or IBM's DB2.

On a large scale, a **data warehouse (DW)** is an extremely large database or **repository** that stores all of an organization's or institution's data and makes this data available for **data mining**. The DW can combine an institution's many different databases in order to provide management personnel flexible access to the data. On the smaller scale, a **data mart** represents a large database where the data used by one of the units or a division of a healthcare system is stored and maintained. For example, a university hospital system might store clinical information from its many affiliate hospitals in a data warehouse, and each separate hospital might have a data mart housing its data.

There are many ways to access and retrieve information in databases. Searching information in databases can be done through the use of a query as is used in Microsoft's Access database. A query asks questions of the database to retrieve specific data and information. Data mining software sorts thorough data in order to discover patterns and ascertain or establish relationships. This software discovers or uncovers previously unidentified relationships among the data in a database by conducting an exploratory analysis looking for hidden patterns in data. Using this software, the user searches for previously undiscovered or undiagnosed patterns by analyzing the data stored in a DW. **Drill-down** is a term that means the user can view DW information by drilling down to lower levels of the database to focus on information that is pertinent to her/his needs at the moment. As users move through databases within the healthcare system, they can move from enterprise-wide data warehouses to data marts. For example, an infection control nurse might notice a pattern of methicillin-resistant *Staphylococcus aureus* (MRSA) infections in the local data mart (a single hospital within a larger system). The nurse may want to find out if the outbreak is local (data mart) or more widespread in the system (data warehouse). The nurse might also query the database to determine if there are certain patient attributes (such as age or medical diagnosis) that are associated with the incidence of

BOX Continued

10-1

infection. These data mining capabilities are also quite useful for those who wish to conduct clinical research studies. For example, one might query a database to tease out attributes (patient characteristics) associated with asthma-related hospitalizations.

There are five typical clinical applications for databases: hospitals, clinical research, clinical trials, ambulatory care, and public health. Some healthcare systems are connecting their hospitals together since they have chosen a single clinical information system (CIS) to capture data systemwide. In this case, healthcare organizations are modeling after businesses where multiple application programs share a pool of related data.

What we would like you to think about is how potent databases can be in health care. Databases are organized collections of data that can transform data into information by allowing you to access only the data and information you need for a specific task. The terms *data file* and *entity* both represent a table within a database. A field is commonly also called an attribute. Depending on the context, the terms *entity* and *attribute* are used for table and field.

DEPARTMENT COLLABORATION AND KNOWLEDGE/INFORMATION EXCHANGE

The implementation of systems within health care is the responsibility of many people and departments. All systems require a partnership of collaboration and knowledge sharing in order to successfully implement and maintain successful standards of care. **Collaboration** is the sharing of ideas and experiences for the purposes of mutual understanding and learning. **Knowledge exchange** is the product of collaboration when sharing an understanding of information promotes learning from past experiences to make better decisions in the future.

Depending on the type of project, collaboration occurs at many different levels within an organization. At an administrative level, collaboration among key **stakeholders** is critical to the success of any project. Stakeholders have the most responsibility for completing the project. They have the greatest influence in the overall design of the system, and ultimately, stakeholders are the ones who are most impacted by a system implementation. Together with the organizational executive team, stakeholders collaborate on the overall budget and time frame for a system implementation.

Collaboration also occurs among the various departments impacted by the system. These groups are frequently comprised of representatives from **information technology**, clinical specialty areas, support services, and software vendors.

Once a team is assembled, it defines the objectives and goals of the system. The members work to strategically align their goals with the goals of the organization where the system is to be used. The focus for these groups is on planning, resource management, transitioning, and ongoing support of the system. This collaboration determines how the project will be managed, what the deliverables for the project are, who will be accountable for the project, what time frame the project will occur in, opportunities for process improvement using the system, and how resources will be allocated to support the system.

From collaboration comes the exchange of information and ideas through knowledge sharing. Specialists exchange knowledge within their respective areas of expertise to assure that the system will work for an entire organization. From one another, they learn requirements that will make the system successful. This exchange of ideas is what makes healthcare information systems so valuable. A multidisciplinary approach assures that systems will work in the complex environment of healthcare organizations with diverse and complex patient populations.

What the Future Holds

The integration of technology within healthcare organizations has limitless possibilities. As new types of systems emerge, clinicians will become smarter and more adept at implementing these tools into daily practice. Success will be achieved when health care incorporates technology systems in a way that they are not viewed as separate tools to support healthcare practices, but necessary instruments to provide health care. Patients, too, will become more savvy at utilizing healthcare information systems as a means of communication and managing their personal and preventive care. In the future, these two mindsets will become expectations for health care and not simply a high-tech benefit as they are often viewed today. *The future is exciting.* See Box 14-2 for June Kaminski's views on what the future holds.

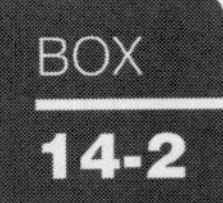

Looking to the Future

June Kaminski

The coming trends in wearable technology, smaller and faster handheld and portable computer systems, and high quality voice-activated inventions will further facilitate the utility of computers in nursing practice and professional development. The field of computer science will continue to contribute to the evolving art and science of nursing informatics. New trends promise to bring wide-sweeping and, hopefully, positive

BOX *Continued*
14-2

changes to the practice of nursing. Computers and other technologies have the potential to support a more client-oriented healthcare system where clients truly become active participants in their own healthcare planning and decisions. Mobile health technology, telenursing, sophisticated electronic health records, and next-generation technology are predicted to contribute to high quality nursing care and consultation within healthcare settings, including patients' homes and communities.

Computers will become more powerful yet more compact, which will contribute to the development of several technological initiatives that are still in their infancy. The following list includes some of these initiatives.

- **Voice-activated communicators** are already being developed in Silicon Valley by companies like Vocera Communications, Inc. This new technology will permit nurses and other healthcare professionals to use wireless, hands-free devices to communicate with each other and to record data. This hands-free communication and data recording can promote this technology, which promises to become a user-friendly and cost-effective way to increase clinical productivity.
- **Game and simulation technology** promises to offer realistic, innovative ways to teach nursing content in general, including nursing informatics concepts and skills. The same technology that powers video games can be used to create dynamic educational interfaces to help student nurses learn about pathophysiology, care guidelines, medication usage, and a host of other topics. These applications can also be very valuable for client education and health promotion materials. The serious-games industry is just beginning to develop. Video game producers are now looking beyond mere entertainment to address public and private policy, management, and leadership issues and topics, including health care-related ones. For instance, the *Games for Health Project*, initiated by the Robert Wood Johnson Foundation, is working on developing best practices to support innovation in healthcare training, messaging, and illness management.
- **Virtual reality (VR)** is another technological breakthrough that will become common in nursing education and professional development. Basically, VR is a three-dimensional computer-generated world where a person (with the right equipment) can move about and interact as if he or she were actually in the visualized location. The person's senses are immersed in this VR world using special gadgetry such as head-mounted displays, data gloves, joysticks, and other hand tools. The equipment and special technology provides a sense of presence that is lacking in multimedia and other complex programs.
- **Mobile devices** will be used more by nurses both at the point of care and in planning, documenting, interacting with the healthcare team, and in research. According to Suszka-Hildebrandt (2000),

  > There are strong indicators that nursing is ready to move quickly to adopt this new technology and utilize it to its full potential at the point-of-care. We anticipate the rate of adoption for mobile information systems within nursing to be rapid, and it will ulti-

BOX Continued

14-2

mately equal and perhaps exceed that of physicians. Mobile Nursing Informatics will be at the core of nursing in the 21st century. Ready access to data and analytical tools will fundamentally change the way practitioners of the health sciences conduct research, and approach and solve problems. (p. 3)

These predicted innovations are only some of the many computer and technological applications being developed. As nurses gain proficiency in capitalizing on the creative, time-saving, and interactive capabilities emerging from information technology research, the field of nursing informatics will grow in similar proportions.

Reference

Suszka-Hildebrandt, S. (2000). Mobile information technology at the point-of-care. *PDA Cortex.* Retrieved March 27, 2008, from http://www.rnpalm.com/mitatpoc.htm

SUMMARY

The most important thought I would like to leave you with is that when it comes to healthcare information technology, the possibilities are endless. Ultimately, it is not the type of systems that are important but the method in which they are put into practice.

THOUGHT-PROVOKING Questions

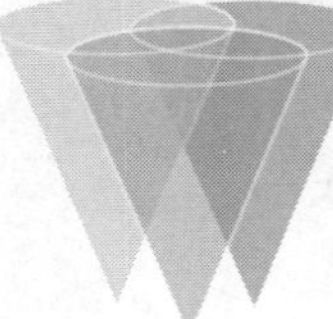

1. What type of technology exists today that could be converted into new types of information systems to be used in health care?
2. How could collaboration and knowledge sharing at a single organization be used to help individuals preparing for information technology at a different facility?
3. Discuss the administrative information systems and their applications.

References

Agency for Healthcare Research and Quality. (2000). *Medical errors: The scope of the problem. An epidemic of errors.* Retrieved August 10, 2007, from http://www.ahrq.gov/qual/errback.htm

Ciotti, V., & Zodda, F. (1996). Selecting managed care information systems. *Journal of the Healthcare Financial Management Association, 50*(6), 35–36. Retrieved March 27, 2008, from http://findarticles.com/p/articles/mi_m3257/is_n6_v50/ai_18515376

DiJerome, L. (1992). The nursing case management computerized system: Meeting the challenge of health care delivery through technology. *Computers in Nursing, 10*(6), 250–258.

Hassett, M., & Thede, L. (2003). Information in practice: Clinical information systems. In B. Cunningham (Ed.), *Informatics and nursing opportunities and challenges* (2nd ed., rev., pp. 222–239). Philadelphia: Lippincott Williams & Wilkins.

Simpson, R. L., & Falk, C. (1996). Technology and case management. In J. Hodgson (Ed.), *Information management in nursing and healthcare* (pp. 144–152). Springhouse, PA: Springhouse Corporation.

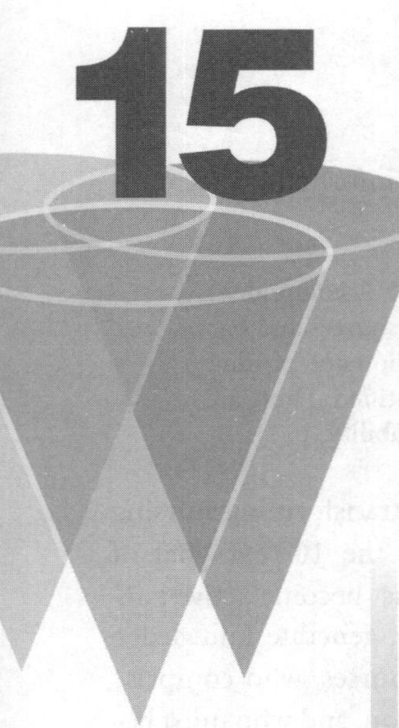

The Electronic Health Record and Clinical Informatics

Emily B. Barey

Objectives

1. Describe the common components of an electronic health record (EHR).
2. Assess the benefits of implementing an EHR.
3. Explore the ownership of an EHR.
4. Evaluate the flexibility of the EHR in meeting the needs of clinicians and patients.

Key Terms

Administrative processes
Connectivity
Decision support
Electronic communication
Electronic health record (EHR)
Healthcare information
Medicaid management information systems (MMIS)
Order entry management
Patient support
Personal health records (PHR)
Population health management
Reporting
Results management

INTRODUCTION

The United States healthcare system faces the enormous challenge to improve the quality of care and simultaneously control costs. **Electronic health records (EHRs)** have been proposed as one possible solution to achieve this goal (Institute of Medicine [IOM], 2001). In January 2004, President George W. Bush raised the profile of electronic health records in his State of the Union address by outlining a plan to ensure that most Americans would have an electronic health record by 2014. He stated that "by computerizing health records we can avoid dangerous medical mistakes, reduce costs, and improve care" (Bush, 2004). This proclamation generated an increased demand for understanding what electronic health records are and how to promote their adoption.

There are four aims of this chapter. The first is to describe the common components of an EHR. The second and third aims are to review the benefits of implementing an EHR and to provide an overview of successful ownership of an EHR. The fourth aim is to discuss the flexibility of an electronic record in meeting the needs of both clinicians and patients. Finally, as "The Future" section reveals, this is an exciting time for health care and information technology. According to Arnold et al. (2007),

> the HIMSS Global Task Force investigated a battery of EHR components within each country, including security, quality, financing sources and barriers. Four common threads that hinder EHR implementation and produce a kinship between every effort around the globe were identified. These are: Communication, Standardization, Funding, and Interoperability (p. 1).

The TIGER (2006) summit on evidence and informatics transforming nursing stated that, "the nation is working full-speed to realize the 10-year goal of Electronic Health Records for its citizens" (p. 1). Nurses must become active participants in this effort to capture **healthcare information**, generate knowledge and enhance patient care. "This is a critical juncture for nurses, who comprise 55% of the health care workforce, number more than 3 million, and who must become more aware and involved at every level of the Informatics Revolution" (TIGER, p. 1). Although EHR standards are evolving and barriers to adoption remain, the collective work has a positive momentum that can only benefit clinician and patient alike.

COMPONENTS

Overview

The definition of an EHR is evolving. A survey of the literature reveals that there are many different definitions, each with its own terminology and developed with a different audience in mind. The sources range from the federal government (CCHIT, 2007), the Institute of Medicine (2003), the Healthcare Information and Management Systems Society (HIMSS, 2007), and the National Institutes of Health (2006), among others (Robert Wood Johnson [RWJ], 2006). See Box 15-1 to review the many terms and definitions used.

BOX 15-1

What's in a Name?

Julie A. Kenney and Ida Androwich

With the advent of the EHR came a myriad of terms and definitions. The HIMSS (2006) defines an EHR as "a longitudinal electronic record of patient health information produced by encounters in one or more care settings" (p. 123). According to the HIMSS, the EHR should include items such as past medical history, patient demo-

BOX Continued
15-1

graphics, immunizations, medication history, and many additional items. The EHR has the ability to automate and streamline the caregivers' workflow as well as support patient care activities and in addition may be used for decision support, quality management, and outcomes reporting (HIMSS, 2006).

An EHR may be referred to as an electronic medical record (EMR) or a computer-based patient record (CPR) (Waegemann, 2003). These three terms are often used interchangeably, but there are subtle differences. Waegemann (2003) calls the EHR the generic term for all electronic patient care systems. A slight difference exists between the CPR and the EMR, with the CPR being an all-inclusive lifetime patient record that would include information from all medical specialties, including dentists and psychiatrists. The CPR would be the medical record that President Bush (White House, 2004) was referring to in his call for a nationwide interoperable EHR. The EMR would be an all-inclusive record as well, but it would be institution or corporation specific and would not interact with EHRs that were outside of the institution or corporation (Waegemann).

References

Healthcare Information and Management Systems Society (HIMSS). (2006). *HIMSS dictionary of healthcare information technology terms, acronyms and organizations.* Chicago: Healthcare Information and Management Systems Society.

Waegemann, C. P. (2003, May). EHR vs. CPR vs. EMR: Whatever you call it, the vision is of superior care through uniform, accessible health records. *Healthcare Informatics Online.* Retrieved on July 10, 2007, from http://www.providersedge.com/Ehdocs/ehr_articles/EHR_vs_CPR_vs_EMR.pdf

White House. (2004). *Incentives for the use of health information technology and establishing the position of the national health information technology coordinator.* Executive order dated April 27, 2004. Retrieved on July 16, 2005, from http://www.whitehouse.gov/news/releases/2004/04/print/20040427-4.html

The IOM definition is the most widely referenced, however, and provides a good starting point. The definition is useful because it has distilled all the possible features of an EHR into eight essential components with an emphasis on functions that promote patient safety, a more universal denominator that everyone in health care can accept. The eight components include health information and data, results management, order entry management, decision support, electronic communication and **connectivity**, patient support, administrative processes, and reporting and population health management (IOM, 2003). Each is described in more detail here.

Health Information and Data

Health information and data is the patient data required to make sound clinical decisions including demographics, medical and nursing diagnoses, medication lists, allergies, and test results (IOM, 2003).

Results Management

Results management is the ability to manage results of all types electronically, including laboratory and radiology procedure reports, both current and historical (IOM, 2003).

Order Entry Management

Order entry management is the ability of a clinician to enter medication and other care orders, including laboratory, microbiology, pathology, radiology, nursing, supply orders, ancillary services, and consultations directly into a computer (IOM, 2003).

Decision Support

Decision support is the computer reminders and alerts to improve the diagnosis and care of a patient including screening for correct drug selection and dosing, medication interactions with other medications, preventive health reminders in areas such as vaccinations, health risk screening and detection, and clinical guidelines for patient disease treatment (IOM, 2003).

Electronic Communication and Connectivity

Electronic communication and connectivity is the online communication among healthcare team members, their care partners, and patients including e-mail, Web messaging, and an integrated health record within and across settings, institutions, and telemedicine (IOM, 2003).

Patient Support

Patient support is the patient education and self-monitoring tools, including interactive computer-based patient education, home telemonitoring, and telehealth systems (IOM, 2003).

Administrative Processes

Administrative processes are the electronic scheduling, billing, and claims management systems including electronic scheduling for inpatient and outpatient visits and procedures, electronic insurance eligibility validation, claim authorization and prior approval, identification of possible research study participants, and drug recall support (IOM, 2003).

Reporting and Population Health Management

Reporting and **population health management** are the data collection tools to support public and private reporting requirements including data represented in a standardized terminology and machine-readable format (IOM, 2003).

Different vendor EHR systems will combine different components in their offerings, and often a single set of EHR components will not meet the needs of all clinicians and patient populations. For example, a pediatric setting may demand functions for immunization management, growth tracking, and more robust order entry features to include weight-based dosing (Spooner, 2007). These may not be provided by all EHR systems. In addition, the IOM (2003) definition focuses on care delivery functions and deliberately avoids addressing EHR infrastructure functions such as security and privacy management, controlled medical vocabularies, and interoperability standards. These additional capabilities are often required in the practical setting and to achieve further goals, such as the ability to share patient health information between different healthcare provider organizations.

After President Bush's State of the Union address in 2004, the Office of the National Coordinator for Health Information Technology (ONCHIT) was established to address these nuances and gaps in defining an EHR. The primary mission of ONCHIT is to assure users of health information technology systems that those systems "provide needed capabilities, securely manage information and protect confidentiality and work with other systems without reprogramming" (Department of Health and Human Services, 2007, ¶ 1). In order to accomplish this, ONCHIT contracted the Certification Commission for Healthcare Information Technology (CCHIT) to develop specific functionality, security, and interoperability criteria to evaluate EHR systems. These criteria will provide the needed detail to further refine the definition of an EHR and to promote the ability to share patient information across healthcare settings. Criteria for the ambulatory setting were released in 2006, and inpatient criteria were released in 2007 with an initial emphasis on order entry and medication management. CCHIT plans to release updated ambulatory and inpatient criteria in 2008, along with new criteria for child health, cardiology, and emergency department areas (CCHIT, 2007).

ADVANTAGES

There are mixed reviews of the advantages of an EHR. Much has been written about the potential promise of reduced cost, improved quality, and outcomes, but very little of it has been substantiated except anecdotally (Sidorov, 2006). Possible methods to estimate EHR benefits include using vendor-supplied data that has been retrieved from their customer systems, synthesizing and applying studies of overall EHR value, creating logical engineering models of EHR value, summarizing focused studies of elements of EHR value and conducting and applying information from site visits (Thompson, Osheroff, Classen, & Sittig, 2007). However, the time and effort involved completing this work is further burdened by the fact that there is no standard by which to measure adoption or expected benefits (RWJ, 2006; Thompson et al.). This makes it difficult to benchmark and generalize results across the industry.

What we do know is that the four most common benefits are an increased delivery of guideline-based care, an enhanced capacity to perform surveillance and monitoring for disease conditions, a reduction in medication errors, and a decreased utilization of care (Chaudhry et al., 2006). These findings were echoed by two similar literature reviews. The first focused on the use of informatics systems for chronic illness and found that the processes of care most positively impacted were guideline adherence, visit frequency (i.e., a decrease in emergency department visits), provider documentation, patient treatment adherence, and screening and testing (Dorr et al., 2007).

The second review was a costs and benefits analysis of health information technology completed by the Agency for Healthcare Research and Quality (AHRQ) that studied the value of an EHR in the ambulatory care and pediatric settings, including its overall economic value. The AHRQ highlighted the common findings already described and also noted that most of the data available for review is from six leading healthcare organizations in the United States, underscoring the challenge of generalizing these results to the broader healthcare industry (Shekelle, Morton, & Keeler, 2006). Finally, all three literature reviews cited indicated that there are a limited number of hypothesis-testing studies and even fewer that reported cost data. It is important to consider the financial aspect of the EHR (see Box 15-2).

The descriptive studies, however, do have value and should not be hastily dismissed. While not as rigorous in their design, they do describe advantages to an EHR well and often also include useful implementation recommendations learned from practical experience. Among these types of reviews, EHR advantages include simple benefits such as no longer having to interpret poor handwriting and handwritten orders to reduced turnaround time for lab results in an emergency department and to administration of the first dose of antibiotics in an inpatient nursing unit (Husk & Waxman, 2004; Smith et al., 2004).

In the ambulatory care setting, evidence of improved management of cardiac-related risk factors in patients with diabetes and effective patient notification of

BOX 15-2

Costs of Implementing an EHR

Julie A. Kenney and Ida Androwich

The electronic health record (EHR) has been touted as the tool that will change health care. In April 2004, President Bush issued an executive order to develop a nationwide interoperable EHR within 10 years, as well as to establish a new position, the national health information technology coordinator (White House, 2004). This executive order provided momentum to the IOM recommendations that the EHR will assist in providing safer patient care (Tang, 2005, Slide 13). With this rush to implement the nationwide EHR, it is estimated that "annual spending on Health Care IT will reach $10.8 billion by 2012—led by growth in the market for **Medicaid management information systems (MMIS)**" (INPUT, 2008a, ¶ 1). The tremendous cost and complexity of implementing a nationwide electronic health record has been compared to sending men to the moon in Apollo 11 (Larkin, 2005). As the government moves forward, it is estimated that the "federal health information technology (IT) spending will grow from $3.2 billion in 2008 to over $4.5 billion in 2013" (INPUT, 2008b, ¶ 1).

Implementing a nationwide EHR has the ability to make individuals' medical records available to all healthcare providers. In order for this to happen, a few things will need to take place first. According to Larkin (2005), the underlying infrastructure will require major changes in the following:

- A healthcare financing system with built-in economic initiatives
- Cooperation and information sharing between competing healthcare organizations
- Workflow changes in both the clinical area and the physician's offices

Placing this infrastructure will result in healthcare workers reassessing how they work and how they think about their work (McLane, 2005). Healthcare currently works in silos, with little interaction between the silos. In order to improve patient safety and increase communication between healthcare workers, a complete redesign of the healthcare system must take place (Cobb, 2004; Larkin, 2005). Larkin points out that health care should not rush the process because automating bad processes will result in bad results being obtained faster. The processes must be reassessed and redesigned where necessary before implementing a new initiative. The healthcare field needs to come to the realization that while the EHR may initially be an economic drain, it has the potential to boost revenue by making informed medical decisions possible, reducing medical errors, and reducing unnecessary procedures (Brown, 2005; Larkin, 2005). Health care is on the verge of realizing the tremendous benefit the EHR will bring to it.

References

Brown, N. (2005). Driving EMR adoption: Making EMRs a sustainable profitable investment. *Health Management Technology, 26*(5), 47–48.

continues

BOX Continued
15-2

Cobb, D. (2004). Improving patient safety—How can information technology help? *AORN Journal, 80*(2), 295–302.

INPUT. (2008a). *State & local health care technology spending to reach $10.8 billion by 2012.* Retrieved March 28, 2008, from http://www.input.com/corp/press/detail.cfm?news=1353

INPUT. (2008b). *Federal health IT market to reach $4.5 billion by 2013.* Retrieved March 28, 2008 from http://www.input.com/corp/press/detail.cfm?news=1361

Larkin, H. (2005). Uncle Sam wants your EHR. *H & HN: Hospitals and Health Networks, 79*(2), 38–40, 42, 44.

McLane, S. (2005). Designing an EMR planning process based on staff attitudes toward and opinions about computers in healthcare. *CIN: Computers, Informatics, Nursing, 23*(2), 85–92.

Tang, P. (2005). *Going digital with patients: IT's about patient safety.* Retrieved on March 27, 2008 from http://hi.uwaterloo.ca/hitalks/Futures-2005/Tang.pdf

White House. (2004, April 27). *Incentives for the use of health information technology and establishing the position of the national health information technology coordinator* [Executive order]. Retrieved on July 16, 2005, from http://www.whitehouse.gov/news/releases/2004/04/print/20040427-4.html

medication recalls have been demonstrated (Jain et al., 2005; Reed & Bernard, 2005). Two other unique advantages that have great potential are the ability to use the EHR and decision support functions to identify patients who qualify for research studies or who qualify for prescription drug benefits offered by pharmaceutical companies at safety-net clinics and hospitals (Embi et al., 2005; Poprock, 2005). Without an EHR system, these are very difficult and costly to accomplish. Despite limited standards and published studies, there is enough evidence to warrant pursuing widespread implementation of the EHR (Halamka, 2006) and certainly enough to warrant further study of the EHR's use and benefit.

OWNERSHIP

The implementation of an EHR has the potential to affect every member of a healthcare organization. The process of becoming a successful owner of an EHR has multiple steps and requires integrating the EHR into both the organization's day-to-day operations and long-term vision, and the clinician's day-to-day practice. All members of the healthcare organization, from the executive level to the clinician at the point of care, must feel a sense of ownership in order to make the implementation successful for themselves, their colleagues, and their patients. Successful ownership of an EHR may be defined in part by the level of clinician adoption of the tool, and this section will review key steps and strategies for the selection, implementation and evaluation, and optimization of an EHR in pursuit of that goal.

Historically, many systems were developed locally by the information technology department of a healthcare organization. It was not unusual for software developers to be employed by the organization to write needed systems and interfaces between them. As commercial offerings were introduced and matured, it became less and less common to see homegrown or locally developed systems. As a result, the first step of ownership is typically a vendor selection process. During this step, it is important to survey the organization's level of interest, identify possible barriers to participation, document desired functions of an EHR, and assess the willingness to fund the implementation (Holbrook, Keshavjee, Troyan, Pray, & Ford, 2003). Although clinicians should drive the project, the assessment should also include the need and readiness of the executive leadership, information technology, and project management teams. It is essential that leadership understands that this type of project is as much about redesigning clinical work as it is about technically automating it, and that they agree to hold accountability for its success (Goddard, 2000). In addition, this preacquisition phase should also concentrate on understanding the current state of the health information technology industry in order to identify appropriate questions and the next steps in the selection process (American Organization of Nurse Executives, 2006). These first steps will begin to identify any organizational risks toward a successful implementation and will pave the way for initiating a change management process to educate the organization about the future state of delivering health care with an EHR system.

The second step of the selection process is to select a system based on the organization's current and predicted needs. It is common during this phase to see a demonstration of several vendors' EHR products. Based on the completed needs assessment, the organization should establish key evaluation criteria to compare the different vendors and products. The criteria should include both subjective and objective items that cover topics such as common clinical workflows, decision support, reporting, usability, technical build, and maintenance of the system. Providing the vendor with these guidelines will ensure the process meets the organization's needs; however, it is also essential to let the vendor demonstrate a proposed future state from its own perspective. This is critical to ensuring that its vision and the organization's vision are well aligned. It also helps spark additional dialogue about the possible future state of clinical work at the organization and the change required in obtaining it. The demonstrations will provide not only the ability to compare and contrast the features and functions of different systems, but also a good way to engage the organization's members in being a part of this strategic decision.

Implementation planning should occur concurrently with the selection process, particularly the assessment of the scope of the work, initial sequencing of the EHR components to be implemented, and resources required. However, it begins in earnest once a vendor and product have been selected. In addition to further refining the implementation plan, this is also the time to identify key metrics by which to measure its success. As described earlier, there are numerous benefits an organization may realize from implementing an EHR. The organization should choose metrics that match its overall strategy and goals in the coming years and may include expected improvements in financial, quality, and clinical outcomes. Common metrics include reducing the number of duplicate lab tests through duplicate orders alerting and reducing the number of adverse drug events through the use of barcode medication administration. To be sure benefits are realized, it is important to avoid choosing so many that they become meaningless or unobtainable, to carefully and practically define those that are chosen, to measure before and after the implementation, and to assign accountability to a member of the organization to ensure the work is completed.

The implementation plan should also account for the long-term optimization of the EHR. This step is commonly overlooked and often results in benefits falling short of expectations because the resources are not available to realize them permanently. It also often means the difference between end users of EHRs merely surviving the change as opposed to becoming savvy about how to adopt the EHR as another powerful clinical tool like the stethoscope. Optimization activities of the EHR should be considered a routine part of the organization's operations, should be resourced accordingly, and should emphasize the continued involvement of clinician users to identify ways that the EHR can enable meeting the overall mission of the organization. Many organizations start an implementation of an EHR with the goal of transforming their care delivery and operations. Different than simply automating a previously manual process, transformation often includes improving the process to realize improved patient care outcomes or added efficiency. Although some transformation will be experienced with the initial use of the system, the majority of this work is done postimplementation and is reliant on widespread clinician adoption of the EHR. As such, it thus makes optimization a critical component to successful ownership of an EHR. Review Box 15-3 for the barriers as well as methods for successful acceptance.

FLEXIBILITY AND EXPANDABILITY

Health care is as unique as patients themselves. It is delivered in a variety of settings, for a variety of reasons over the course of a patient's lifetime. In addition, patients rarely receive all their care from one healthcare organization, and choice

BOX
15-3

Resistance to Implementation

Julie A. Kenney and Ida Androwich

For an implementation to be successful, a few things need to happen. The nurse informatics specialist (NIS) will need to understand and use change management theory to ensure that the implementation of the new EHR system will be successful. It is a well-known fact that nurses can make or break a system implementation. A nursing staff that is involved early in the implementation process has been found to be a major determinant in a successful implementation. Assessing nursing attitudes and concerns early in the process can aid the NIS in determining the best way to proceed with staff education and implementation rollout. Nurses may feel that the implementation that should be making their job easier may actually make it more challenging (Trossman, 2005). Nurses who feel that the system has been forced onto them will very likely be highly resistant to the change. This is why it is imperative that nurses be involved in the design, development, and implementation of the EHR. Nurses who have been involved in the implementation process will ensure that the product meets the needs of the staff, which will result in high end user satisfaction (McLane, 2005).

Another challenge facing those wishing to implement an EHR is that writing is nearly automatic for most but using a computer is not. This can be overcome by ensuring that data entry and system navigation make for a system that is user friendly (Walsh, 2004). Voice data entry is an easy way to enter data into the system and may be a way for those who are not comfortable with computers to still use the system effectively (Walsh). An additional way for staff to accept the new EHR is to ensure that they have had adequate training prior to the implementation as well as ensure continued support and education after the implementation. The implementation of a new EHR system entails the staff to make significant changes to how they work and how they handle patient information. The NIS who is familiar with change management and the NI process should have an integral role in the redesign of workflow processes in order to ensure a smooth transition from a paper record to an electronic record. Many excellent EHR systems that have been installed fail due to poor implementation planning. It is imperative that nurses are employed in the information systems (IS) department (Trossman, 2005).

References

McLane, S. (2005). Designing an EMR planning process based on staff attitudes toward and opinions about computers in healthcare. *CIN: Computers, Informatics, Nursing, 23*(2), 85–92.

Trossman, S. (2005). Bold new world: Technology should ease nurses' jobs, not create a greater work load. *American Journal of Nursing, 105*(5), 75–77.

Walsh, S. (2004). The clinician's perspective on electronic health records and how they can affect patient care. *BMJ: British Medical Journal, 328*(7449), 1184–1187.

is a cornerstone of the American healthcare system. An electronic health record must be flexible and expandable to meet the needs of patients and caregivers in all these settings. However, challenges remain for doing so.

At a very basic level, there is as yet no electronic health record system available that can provide all functions for all specialties to a degree that all clinicians would successfully adopt. A good example is oncology. Most systems do not yet provide the advanced ordering features required for complex treatment planning. An oncologist could utilize a general system, but he or she would not find as many benefits without additional features for chemotherapy ordering, lifetime cumulative dose tracking, or the ability to adjust a treatment day schedule and have the remaining days of the plan recalculate a new schedule.

Further, most healthcare organizations do not yet have the capacity to implement and maintain systems in all care areas. As one physician stated, "implementing an EMR is a complex and difficult multidisciplinary effort that will stretch an organization's skills and capacity for change" (Chin, 2004, p. 47). This insight suggests that no matter how flexible the electronic health record systems become, there will always be a human flexibility factor that must be overcome. These two conditions are improving every day, particularly at larger or academic organizations, but will remain persistent for the majority of the healthcare community for some time to come.

A second challenge is the lack of standards for electronic health records. Recognizing that no single vendor or organization will develop adequate systems for all settings in the near future, the government has initiated work to accelerate the development of the standards required for individual systems to communicate effectively. This interoperability already exists for many data types such as patient demographics and laboratory results, but is still being conceived and validated for the wide variety of clinical information that is required to support all patient care settings.

In addition, financial and patient privacy hurdles must also be overcome to achieve an expansive EHR. The majority of health care is delivered by small community practices and hospitals, many of which do not have the financial or technical resources to implement an EHR. The Department of Health and Human Services recently loosened regulations so that physicians may now be able to receive healthcare IT software, hardware, and implementation services from hospitals in an effort to alleviate the cost burden on individual providers and foster adoption of the EHR.

Finally, patient privacy is a pivotal issue to determining how far and how easy it will be to share data across healthcare organizations. In addition to the Health Insurance Portability and Accountability Act (HIPAA) privacy rules, many states have regulations in place related to patient confidentiality. The recent experience of the state of Minnesota foreshadows what all states will soon be facing. In 2007, Governor Tim Pawlenty announced the creation of the Minnesota Health Information Exchange (State of Minnesota, 2007). Although the intentions of the exchange are to promote patient safety and increase healthcare efficiency across the state, it raised significant concerns about security and privacy. New questions arose about the definition of when and how patient consent is required to exchange data electronically, and older paper-based processes needed to be updated to support real-time electronic exchange (Minnesota Department of Health, 2007). For health exchanges such as these to reach their full potential, the public must be able to trust that their privacy will be protected; or else the healthcare industry risks that patients may not share a full medical history, or worse yet, may not seek care, effectively making the exchange useless.

THE FUTURE

Despite the challenges, the future of EHRs is an exciting one for patient and clinician alike. Benefits may be realized by stand-alone EHRs as described here, but the most significant transformation will come as interoperability is realized between systems. As the former national information technology coordinator in the Department of Health and Human Services, David Brailer notes the potential of interoperability:

> For the first time, clinicians everywhere can have a longitudinal medical record with full information about each patient. Consumers will have better information about their health status since personal health records and similar access strategies can be feasible in an interoperable world. Consumers can move more easily between and among clinicians without fear of their information being lost. Payers can benefit from the economic efficiencies, fewer errors, and reduced duplication that arises from interoperability. Healthcare information exchange and interoperability (HIEI) also underlies meaningful public health reporting, bioterrorism surveillance, quality monitoring, and advances in clinical trials. In short, there is little that most people want from healthcare for which HIEI isn't a prerequisite (Brailer, 2005, p. W 5-20).

SUMMARY

It is an important time for health care and technology. Electronic health records have come to the forefront and will remain central to shaping the future of health care. Along with EHRs, comes another development, **personal health records (PHR)**. See Box 15-4 to learn more about this trend. As healthcare information is

BOX 15-4

Personal Health Records (PHRs)

Julie A. Kenney and Ida Androwich

A new trend that is beginning to gain momentum is the use of personal health records (PHRs). A PHR is defined by HIMSS (2006) as "a version of the health/medical record owned by the consumer/patient" (p. 67). A PHR that is combined with an EHR would result in an interoperable system that would fulfill President Bush's request for an interoperable EHR. The PHR should be a lifelong and comprehensive view of the patient's medical history as well as be accessible from anywhere at any time (Tang & Lansky, 2005). Health management tools that are built into the PHR would allow individuals with chronic conditions to manage the disease proactively along with their healthcare providers. Individuals who utilize PHRs are concerned about how their privacy and security will be protected as well as who will have access to the records (Tang & Lansky).

Currently, there are three types of PHRs available. The first is the freestanding PHR software. This may be offered by an insurance company, a local hospital, a freestanding application on the Internet, or on a personal storage device. The greatest drawback to this type of PHR is that the information must be entered by the patient, which may result in erroneous information (Tang & Lansky, 2005; Tang, 2006; Endsley, Kibbe, Linares, & Colorafi, 2006). An example of a freestanding PHR, provided by the American Health Information Management Association (AHIMA), can be seen at http://www.myphr.com/your_record/index.asp. The second type is a PHR that is linked to a hospital's EHR. This allows the individual to access not only the information that he placed into the PHR, but information in his EHR as well. This allows patients with chronic conditions to comanage their conditions with their physicians. This setup allows the physician and individual to communicate electronically, which becomes beneficial to both parties. When the physician communicates electronically with a patient, the physician and his office staff do not have to return multiple phone calls or schedule a face-to-face meeting. The individual is able to set up appointments electronically as well as receive answers to nonemergent questions without having to schedule an appointment or make repeated phone calls to gather the needed information. This becomes a win-win situation for everyone (Tang & Lansky; Tang; Endsley et al.). The third option is one that links the individual's PHR to multiple EHRs, which allows all of the individual's caregivers to access the information. This allows for accurate and up-to-date information to be available for the caregiver to make decisions regarding the individual's care. This is what President Bush would like to see implemented. Unfortunately, the medical system and technology are not quite ready for this step (Tang & Lansky; Tang; Endsley et al.).

Ideally the PHRs should be set up using a language that is compatible with the languages the EHRs use. This would allow for interoperability to take place between the

BOX Continued
15-4

two systems. If the PHR and the EHR were to use distinct languages that were not compatible, this would set up two distinct bodies of information that would be stored in noncommunicating silos. This fragmentation needs to be prevented, as it is a waste of time and resources (Tang & Lansky, 2005). One way to prevent this is to ensure that the PHRs are capturing essential data that could be used in an EHR. Tang (2006) and Endsley and colleagues (2006) identified the following items that this could include:

- Personal and identification information
- Emergency contact information
- Past medical history
- Medication lists
- Allergies
- Home-monitoring data
- Laboratory test results
- Problem list
- Major illnesses/procedures
- Provider list
- Advance directives
- Family history

The benefits of the use of PHRs include improved communication between healthcare providers and individuals. Individuals become more involved in their care, which results in better compliance with treatment regimens. Physicians are able to communicate with individuals via e-mail for nonemergent issues or questions, which frees up appointment times that can be used by other individuals. This results in physicians being able to provide more efficient and cost-effective care, especially for individuals with chronic conditions. The use of PHRs along with EHRs results in increased patient safety as well as individual and physician satisfaction (Endsley et al., 2006).

Weak computer skills and lack of access to a computer mean that some individuals will not be able to able to access a PHR. There is similarly a lack of knowledge of individual and physician workflow that would help us to imagine just how the PHR would be used. Having this information would allow the developers of PHR software to adjust it to meet the needs of the individuals and physicians who use the software. Some physicians may feel threatened by the PHR as they believe that they will lose control, autonomy, and authority in the relationship with the individual patients (Tang, 2006). There is still much work to be done in this area, but use of the PHR does encourage providers and individuals to begin working together as a team, which will result in improved patient care and safety.

References

Endsley, S., Kibbe, D. C., Linares, A., & Colorafi, K. (2006). An introduction to personal health records. Retrieved on September 22, 2007, from http://www.aafp.org/fpm/20060500/57anin.html

BOX *Continued*

15-4

Healthcare Information and Management Systems Society (HIMSS). (2006). *HIMSS dictionary of healthcare information technology terms, acronyms and organizations*. Chicago: Healthcare Information and Management Systems Society.

Tang, P. C. (2006). *The missing link: Bridging the patient-provider health information gap*. Retrieved March 28, 2008 from http://www.hhs.gov/healthit/ahic/materials/meeting10/cc/Paul_Tang.pdf

Tang, P.C., & Lansky, D. (2005). The missing link: Bridging the patient–provider health information gap. *Health Affairs, 24*(5), 1290–1295.

captured at various points throughout one's life, the PHR and EHR will become vital patient information repositories.

The most important thought I would like to leave you with is that the capabilities of EHRs and the standards related to them are rapidly evolving, fueled by a national interest in improving health care while reducing cost. There is a wealth of descriptive data available pointing to the benefits of an EHR; however there is a dearth of quantitative research related to the EHR. Nursing must stay engaged in this evolution and help shape its direction, as it has already proven to have a significant impact on our practice and our patients.

THOUGHT-PROVOKING Questions

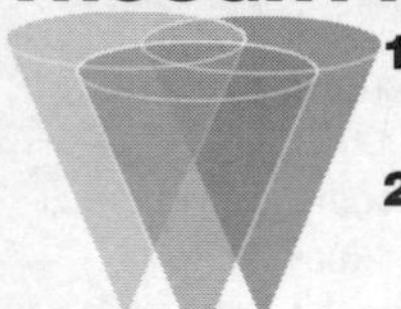

1. What are the implications for nursing education as the EHR becomes the standard for caring for patients?
2. What are the ethical considerations related to interoperability and a shared electronic health record?

References

American Organization of Nurse Executives. (2006, September). *Defining the role of the nurse executive in technology acquisition and implementation.* Washington, DC: Author. Retrieved October 12, 2007, from http://www.aone.org/aone/pdf/Guiding%20Principles%20for%20Acquisition%20and%20Implementation%20of%20Information%20Technology.pdf

Arnold, S., Wagner, J., Hyatt, S. J., & Klein, G. M., and the Global EHR Task Force Members. (2007). *Electronic health records: A global perspective overview.*

Retrieved July 30, 2007, from http://www.himss.org/content/files/DrArnold20011207EISPresentationWhitePaper.pdf

Brailer, D. J. (2005, January 19). Interoperability: The key to the future healthcare system. *Health Affairs—Web Exclusive*, W 5-19–W 5-21. Available from http://content.healthaffairs.org/cgi/reprint/hlthaff.w5.19v1

Bush, G. W. (2004). *State of the Union address.* Retrieved July 30, 2007, from http://www.whitehouse.gov/news/releases/2004/01/20040120-7.html

Certification Commission for Healthcare Information Technology (CCHIT). (2007). *Certification commission announces new work group members.* Retrieved July 30, 2007, from http://www.cchit.org/about/news/releases/Certification-Commission-Announces-New-Work-Group-Members.asp

Chaudhry, B., Wang, J., Wu, S., Maglione, M., Mojica, W., Roth, E., et al. (2006). Systematic review: Impact of health information technology on quality, efficiency, and costs of medical care. *Annals of Internal Medicine, 144*(10), E-12–E-22.

Chin, H. L. (2004). The reality of EMR implementation: Lessons from the field. *The Permanente Journal, 8*(4), 43–48.

Department of Health and Human Services. (2007). *HIT Certification: Background.* Retrieved March 28, 2008, from http://www.dhhs.gov/healthit/certification/background

Dorr, D., Bonner, L. M., Cohen, A. N., Shoai, R. S., Perrin, R., Chaney, E., et al. (2007). Informatics systems to promote improved care for chronic illness: A literature review. *Journal of the American Medical Informatics Association, 14*(2), 156–163.

Embi, P. J., Jain, A., Clark, J., Bizjack, S., Hornung, R., & Harris, C. M. (2005). Effect of a clinical trial alert system on physician participation in trial recruitment. *Archives of Internal Medicine, 165*, 2272–2277.

Goddard, B. L. (2000). Termination of a contract to implement an enterprise electronic medical record system. *Journal of American Medical Informatics Association, 7*, 564–568.

Halamka, J. D. (2006, May). Health information technology: Shall we wait for the evidence? [Letter to the editor]. *Annals of Internal Medicine, 144*(10), 775–776.

Healthcare Information and Management Systems Society (HIMSS). (2007). *Electronic health record.* Retrieved July 30, 2007, from http://www.himss.org/ASP/topics_ehr.asp

Holbrook, A., Keshavjee, K., Troyan, S., Pray, M., & Ford, P. T. (2003). Applying methodology to electronic medical record selection. *International Journal of Medical Informatics, 71*, 43–50.

Husk, G., & Waxman, D. A. (2004). Using data from hospital information systems to improve emergency care. *Academic Emergency Medicine, 11*(11), 1237–1244.

Institute of Medicine. (2001). *Crossing the quality chasm: A new health system for the 21st century.* Washington, DC: National Academies Press.

Institute of Medicine. (2003). *Key capabilities of an electronic health record system: Letter report.* Washington, DC: National Academies Press.

Jain, A., Atreja, A., Harris, C. M., Lehmann, M., Burns, J., & Young, J. (2005). Responding to the rofecoxib withdrawal crisis: A new model for notifying patients at risk and their healthcare providers. *Annals of Internal Medicine, 142*(3), 182–186.

Minnesota Department of Health. (2007, June). *Minnesota Health Records Act—HF 1078 fact sheet.* Minneapolis, MN: Author. Retrieved October 12, 2007, from http://www.health.state.mn.us/e-health/mpsp/hrafactsheet2007.pdf

National Institutes of Health. (April, 2006). *Electronic health records overview.* McLean, Virginia: The MITRE Corporation.

Poprock, B. (2005, September). *Using Epic's alternative medications reminder to reduce prescription costs and encourage assistance programs for indigent patients.* Presented at the Epic Systems Corporation user group meeting, Madison, WI.

Reed, H. L., & Bernard, E. (2005). Reductions in diabetic cardiovascular risk by community primary care providers. *International Journal of Circumpolar Health, 64*(1), 26–37.

Robert Wood Johnson Foundation (RWJ). (2006). Health information technology in the United States: The information base for progress. Retrieved July 30, 2007, from http://www.rwjf.org/programareas/resources/product.jsp?id=15895&pid=1142&gsa=1

Shekelle, P. G., Morton, S. C., & Keeler, E. B. (2006). *Costs and benefits of health information technology. Evidence report/technology assessment, No. 132* [Prepared by the Southern California Evidence-based Practice Center under Contract No. 290-02-0003]. Agency for Healthcare Research and Quality Publication No. 06-E006. Rockville, MD: Agency for Healthcare Research and Quality.

Sidorov, J. (2006). It ain't necessarily so: The electronic health record and the unlikely prospect of reducing healthcare costs. *Health Affairs, 25*(4), 1079–1085.

Smith, T., Semerdjian, N., King, P., DeMartin, B., Levi, S., Reynolds, K., et al. (2004). *Nicolas E. Davies Award of Excellence: Transforming healthcare with a patient-centric electronic health record system.* Evanston, IL: Evanston Northwestern Healthcare. Retrieved July 30, 2007, from http://www.himss.org/content/files/davies2004_evanston.pdf

Spooner, S. A., & The Council on Clinical Information Technology. (2007). Special requirements of electronic health record systems in pediatrics. *Pediatrics, 119,* 631–637.

State of Minnesota, Office of the Governor. (2007). *New public-private partnership to improve patient care, safety and efficiency.* Retrieved October 12, 2007, from http://www.governor.state.mn.us/mediacenter/pressreleases/2007/PROD008303.html

Technology Informatics Guiding Education Reform (TIGER). (2006). *Evidence and informatics transforming nursing.* Retrieved March 28, 2008, from http://www.amia.org/inside/releases/2006/tiger_press%20release_amia.pdf

Thompson, D. I., Osheroff, J., Classen, D., Sittig, D. F. (2007). A review of methods to estimate the benefits of electronic medical records in hospitals and the need for a national database. *Journal of Healthcare Information Management, 21*(1), 62–68.

Supporting Consumer Information and Education Needs

Kathleen Mastrian and Dee McGonigle

Objectives

1. Define health literacy and e-health.
2. Explore various technology-based approaches to consumer health education.
3. Identify barriers to use of technology and issues associated with health-related consumer information.
4. Imagine future approaches to technology-supported consumer health information.

Key Terms

Blog
Digital divide
Domain name
e-brochure
e-health
eHealth Initiative
Empowerment
Grey gap
Health literacy
HONcode
Interactive media
Know-do gap
Static medium
Trust-e
Voice recognition
Web quest
Weblog

INTRODUCTION

Imagine that you have decided to take up running as your preferred form of exercise in a quest to get in shape. You start slowly by running a half mile and walking a half mile. You gradually build up your endurance and find yourself running nearly every day for longer distances and longer periods of time. You first notice a nagging pain in the right hip that over a few weeks gradually spreads to the center of the right buttocks and then down the right leg. You try rest and heat, but nothing seems to help. You visit your doctor, and she suggests that you have developed piriformis syndrome and prescribes a series of stretching exercises, ice to the involved area, and rest. You are intrigued by the diagnosis and upon your return home you log on to the Internet and begin a search for information about piriformis syndrome. When you type the words into your favorite search engine, you get 60,500 results for your query. Your use of the Internet to seek health information mirrors the behavior of many consumers who increasingly rely on the Internet for health-related information. The challenge for consumers and healthcare professionals alike is the proliferation of information on the Internet and the need to learn how to recognize when information is accurate and useful for the situation at hand.

In this chapter, we will explore consumer information and education needs and how technology may help to meet those needs, and at the same time create ever-increasing demands for health-related information. We will begin with a discussion of health literacy, e-health, and health education and information needs, and we will explore various approaches by healthcare providers to using technology to promote health literacy. We will also examine the use of games, **Web quests**, and simulations as means of increasing health literacy among the school-age population. Issues associated with the credibility of Web-based information and barriers to access and use will also be discussed. Finally, we will explore future trends related to technology-supported consumer information.

CONSUMER DEMAND FOR INFORMATION

This is the Information Age; many people want to be in the know. We demand news and information and we want immediate results and unlimited access. This is increasingly true with health information. More and more people, in a trend known as consumer **empowerment**, are interested in taking control of their health and are not satisfied being dependent on a healthcare provider to supply them with information. The Pew Internet and American Life Project survey report of 2006 (Fox, 2006) indicates that 8 in 10 Americans who are online have searched for health information. The most frequent health topic searches (64%) are related to a specific disease or medical problem that the searcher or a member of the family is experiencing. Other frequent topics of health-related searches are medical treatments or procedures (51%), nutrition and diet (49%), exercise or fitness (44%), and drug information (37%). The survey tracked 8 million searches for health information by American adults in a single day and suggests that most begin their searches with a search engine. The impacts of the searches were reported as both positive and negative. The impacts ranged from affecting decisions about their care (58%), changes in the approaches to overall health maintenance (55%), providing material for asking questions of healthcare providers (54%), to feeling overwhelmed (25%) or confused (18%) by materials they found online about their health (Fox, 2006).

It is important to note that this survey is limited to those who are online and does not reflect the health information needs or demands of those who are not online. The **digital divide** is the term used to describe the gap between those who have and those who do not have access to online information. Fox (2007b) reports that the current estimate of connectivity among Americans is 71%. She also identifies a **grey gap** in that only 32% of persons over the age of 65 have ever gone online or lived in a connected household. Similarly, in another report from the Pew Internet group, Fox (2007a) describes connectivity disparities among various races and ethnicities, including Latinos, non-Hispanic Whites, and non-Hispanic Blacks, and analyzes the influences of English-speaking ability and level of education on connectivity. Nurses and healthcare providers need to be aware of the various components of the digital divide to ensure that our patients/clients are receiving the health information they need in a format that they are interested in and can comprehend.

Missen and Cook (2007), discuss the potential impact that technology-based health information dissemination can have on the **know-do gap** in developing countries. The know-do gap reflects the fact that solutions to global health problems exist but are not implemented in a timely fashion because of the lack of access to important health information. The Internet connections in developing countries are widely scattered and may not be efficient/sufficient for viewing healthcare information. Missen and Cook describe the use of a freestanding hard drive that has been loaded with hundreds of CDs of health-related information in a Web page format that responds to a search command. This is a great example of providing technologies that work with the constraints of the situation. Another example of addressing the digital divide is the growing number of health-related Web sites that support a Spanish language format.

HEALTH LITERACY AND HEALTH INITIATIVES

The goal of **health literacy** for all is one that is widely embraced in many sectors of health care, and a major goal of Healthy People 2010. Those of us who have been practicing for some time recognize that informed patients have better outcomes and pay more attention to their overall health and changes in their health than those who are poorly informed. Some of the earliest formally developed patient education programs that included post-op teaching, diabetes education, cardiac rehabilitation, and diet education were implemented in response to research that suggested the positive impact of patient education on health outcomes and satisfaction with care. Glassman (2008) recently updated the National Network Libraries of Medicine Web page on health literacy (http://nnlm.gov/outreach/consumer/hlthlit.html). She concludes from the research on the economic impact of health literacy that those with low health literacy have less ability to properly manage a chronic illness and tend to use more healthcare services than those who are more literate. In addition, she uses results of health research to demonstrate the impact of low health literacy and the incidence of disease.

Glassman (2008) updated the National Network of Libraries of Medicine health literacy site that states, "Health literacy is defined in *Healthy People 2010* as: 'The degree to which individuals have the capacity to obtain, process, and understand basic health information and services needed to make appropriate health decisions'" (¶ 2). For example, healthcare providers depend on a patient's ability to understand and follow directions associated with preparation for surgery or taking medications. We also assume, sometimes erroneously, that people will correctly interpret symptoms of a serious illness and act appropriately. The ability to locate and evaluate health information for credibility and quality, to analyze the various risks and benefits of treatments, and to calculate dosages and interpret test results are among the tasks Glassman (2008) identifies as essential for health literacy. Other important and less easily learned health literacy skills are the ability to negotiate complex healthcare environments and understanding the economics of payment for services. Parker, Ratzan, and Lurie (2003) estimate that at least one third of all Americans have health literacy problems and lament that in a time-is-money economic climate, healthcare practitioners are not always reimbursed for patient education activities.

The **eHealth Initiative** (eHI) was developed to address the growing need for managing health information and to promote technology as a means of improving health information exchange, health literacy, and healthcare delivery. See the eHealth Initiative Web site for more information (http://www.ehealthinitiative.org/default.mspx). While the scope of the eHealth Initiative goes beyond health literacy, a major goal continues to be empowering consumers to better understand their health needs and to take action appropriate to those needs. Poor interoperability among healthcare systems and failure to completely embrace national data standards for health care continue to be identified as barriers to the eHealth Initiative. Further, concerns about privacy and security of information and the failure to invest appropriately in technology have slowed the development of this important initiative. Several states developed viable health information networks as part of the eHI: see Utah Health Information Network (http://www.uhin.com/) and the Vermont Cooperative Consumer Health Information Project (http://library.uvm.edu/dana/vthealth/) as examples of attempts to implement e-health initiatives.

HEALTHCARE ORGANIZATION APPROACHES TO EDUCATION

Healthcare organizations (HCOs) use a wide variety of approaches and tools to promote patient education and health literacy. While the old standby for disseminating information was and sometimes still is the paper-based flyer, some HCOs are recognizing that today's consumers are more attracted to a dynamic rather than **static medium**. In addition, the cost of designing and of printing pamphlets and flyers becomes prohibitive when one considers the rapidity of change of information. That is, the brochure may be outdated almost as soon as it is printed. One approach is to have patient education information stored electronically so that changes can be made as needed or information can be better tailored to the specific patient situation and then printed out and reviewed with the patient. Another old standby approach that is still widely used is the group education class. These classes initially were developed in response to helping people manage chronic health problems (e.g., diabetes) and were typically scheduled while people were hospitalized. Now, many HCOs also sponsor health promotion education classes as a way of marketing their facilities and showcasing some of their expert practitioners.

The movement from static to dynamic presentations began in many HCOs as DVDs and videotapes that were shown in groups or broadcast on demand over dedicated channels via the televisions in a patient's room. HCOs are now also taking advantage of the fact that patients and families are captive audiences in waiting rooms and promote education via pamphlet distribution, health promotion programs broadcast on TV, and health information kiosks. The kiosks are typically a computer station and often contain a variety of self-assessment tools—especially those related to risks for diabetes, heart disease, or cancer—as well as searchable pages of information about specific health conditions. The self-assessment tools represent yet another step forward in technological support for education in that in addition to being dynamic, the kiosk is also interactive. That is, on the assessment pages, the user is asked to respond to a series of questions and then the health risk is calculated by the computer program. One caution, however, is that just because the information is made available does not mean that people will participate or that they will understand what they have experienced. The level of health literacy, the digital divide, and the grey gap will still exist in these situations.

Many HCOs have invested time and money in developing interactive Web sites and believe that Web presence is a critical marketing strategy. Sternberg (2002) suggests that many Web sites begin as an **e-brochure** and progress through various stages to reach a true e-care status. Most offer physician search capabilities, e-newsletters, and call-center tie-ins. As with all patient education materials, there must be a sincere commitment to keeping information current and easily accessible. Web designers must pay particular attention to the aesthetics of the site, the ease of use, and the literacy level of those in the intended audience.

PROMOTING HEALTH LITERACY IN SCHOOL-AGED CHILDREN

Promoting health literacy in school-aged children presents special challenges to health educators. There is wide agreement that childhood obesity is a serious and growing issue and is related not only to poor choice of foods, but also to the sedentary lifestyles promoted by video games and television. In addition, the time devoted to health and physical education programs in schools has given way to the core subjects like math and science.

The Children's Nutrition Research Center has responded to these challenges by supporting the development of nutrition education programs as interactive computer games, video games, and cartoons referred to as *edutainment* (Flores, 2006). These **e-health** programs are developed specifically to appeal to the generational (highly connected and computer literate) and cultural needs of this group. Flores (2006) describes the Family Web project that uses comic strips to impart nutrition information; and Squires Quest, where the students earn points by choosing fruits and vegetables to fight the snakes and moles who are trying to destroy the healthy foods in the Kingdom of SALot. These are great examples of health education programs that are designed to appeal to this connected generation of learners and their intuitive ability to use interactive technologies.

Donovan (2005) describes an interdisciplinary Web quest designed to appeal to older school-aged children. The quest is interdisciplinary in that it requires reading comprehension, critical thinking, presentation, and writing so that core skills and health literacy skills are learned in a single assignment. Students are directed to the Web to search for information on the pros and cons of low-carbohydrate diets and obesity prevention. Students learn along the way as they search for information, collect and interpret it, and then develop a presentation and final paper.

SUPPORTING USE OF THE INTERNET FOR HEALTH EDUCATION

Nurses and other healthcare providers need to embrace the Internet as a source of health information for patient education and health literacy. Patients are increasingly turning there for instant information about their health maladies. Health-related **blogs** (short for **Weblog**, an online journal) and electronic patient and parent support groups are also proliferating at an astounding rate. We need to be prepared to arm our patients with skills to identify credible Web sites. We also need to participate in the development of well-designed, easy-to-use health education tools. Finally, we need to convince payers of the necessity of health education and the powerful impact it has on promoting and maintaining health. See Box 16-1 to read more about health education.

The Health on the Net (HON) Foundation (2005) survey describes the certifications and accreditation symbols that identify trusted health sites. The **HONcode** and **Trust-e** were identified as the two most common symbols that power users look for. The survey also indicates that Internet users look at the

BOX 16-1

Considerations for Patient Education

Julie A. Kenney and Ida Androwich

Nurses need to take many things into account when teaching patients. Nurses need to assess a patient's willingness to learn, his reading ability, how he learns best, and how much he already knows about the subject. Nurses also need to take cultural differences and language differences into account when teaching a patient. If the nurse chooses to use an electronic method to educate the patient, digital natives—patients who have grown up with technology—will need to be taught differently than digital immigrants—those who have been forced to learn technology (Educational Strategies, 2006). Digital natives are typically born after 1982 and may also be referred to as Generation Y. This generation will prefer to learn using technology. The younger group will learn quite well if information is presented in a format they are accustomed to such as an interactive video game to introduce them to a topic. This group would also be comfortable using information that they could access via their iPods and MP3 players (Maag, 2006). Those born before 1982 will have learning styles that range from preferring to learn in a classroom setting to reading a book about the topic to learning using a hands-on, interactive approach (Educational Strategies).

References

Educational strategies in generational designs. (2006). *Progress in Transplantation, 16*(1), 8–9.

Maag, M. (2006). Pod casting and MP3 players: Emerging education technologies. *CIN: Computers, Informatics, Nursing, 24*(1), 9–13.

Patient Education Web Sites

American Academy of Family Physicians
http://www.familydoctor.org

American Cancer Society
http://www.cancer.org

American Heart Association
http://www.americanheart.org

CDC
http://www.cdc.gov

Krames (products to purchase)
http://www.krames.com

Merck (products to purchase as well as free information for patients)
http://www.merckservices.com/portal/site/merckservices/&tcode=K09FA

Thomson—Educational products for nurses (requires a subscription)
http://www.micromedex.com/products/nurses
http://www.micromedex.com/products/carenotes/cn_brochure.pdf

domain name and will frequently gravitate toward university sites (.edu), government sites (.gov), and HCO sites (.org). Half of the survey respondents were in favor of the use of a **domain name** called .health to identify quality health information Web sites. In contrast, Pew/Internet (2006) indicates that nearly 75% of online searchers do not check the date or the source of information they are accessing on the Web and 3% of online health seekers report knowing someone who was harmed by following health information found on the Web.

The U.S. National Library of Medicine and the National Institutes of Health sponsor MedlinePlus, a Web site that has a tutorial for learning how to evaluate health information as well as an electronic guide to Web surfing that is available in both English and Spanish. The site is found at http://nccam.nih.gov/health/webresources. This guide explains the major things you should evaluate when you access health related resources on the Web (NCCAM, 2008). Suggest that your patients visit this site to become better at identifying whether or not a Web site is credible before they adopt the recommendations provided. The clinician is very important in patient education. Refer to Box 16-2 to review effective education methods used in teaching patients and their families.

BOX 16-2

A Clinician's View on Patient Education

Denise D. Tyler

Knowledge dissemination in nursing practice includes sharing information with patients and families so that they understand their healthcare needs well enough to participate in developing the plan of care, make informed decisions about their health, and ultimately comply with the plan of care, both during hospitalization and as outpatients.

There are several effective methods for educating patients and their families. Providing one-on-one as well as classroom instruction are traditional and valuable forms of education. One-on-one education is interactive and can be adjusted anytime during the process based on the needs of the individual patient or family, and can be supplemented by written material, videos, and Web-based learning applications. Classroom education can be beneficial since patients and families with similar needs or problems can network, thus enhancing the individual experience. However, the ability to interact with each member of the group and to tailor the educational experience based on individual needs may be limited by the size and dissimilarities of the group. Individual follow-up should be available when possible.

Paper-based education that is created, printed, and distributed by individual institutions and/or providers can be very effective since they can be distributed at any time and reviewed when the patient feels like learning. Many agencies, such as the Centers for Disease Control and Prevention (CDC), have education for patients avail-

BOX Continued
16-2

able on their Web sites. These can be reviewed online, or they can be printed by healthcare providers or patients. Organizations can also develop and distribute information and instructions specific to their policies and procedures. Printed educational material can also be purchased from companies who employ experts in the subject matter as well as instructional design.

One of the newer sources of patient education information is the Internet. Many hospitals and healthcare organizations provide proprietary information such as directions, information on procedures, and instructions on what to expect during hospitalization in this manner. Other health organizations such as the National Institutes of Health provide detailed information on their Web sites. Clinicians should be cautious when recommending Web sites to patients and families, as not all sites are reliable or valid.

Many companies who provide clinical information systems (CISs) also include patient education materials linked to the clinical system via an intranet. Thus, standardized instructions that are specific to a procedure or disease process can be printed from this computer-based application. Discharge instructions that are interdisciplinary and patient specific can often be modified via drop-down lists or selectable items that can be deleted or changed by the clinician. This ability to modify prior to printing provides more consistent and individualized instruction. The computer-based generation of instruction is preferable to free text and verbal instruction modification because it also allows the information to be linked to a coded nursing language and thus easily used for measurement and quality assurance reporting. Relevant triggers may be embedded in the CIS as well. For example, when a patient answers "yes" to smoking, smoking cessation information should automatically print, or a trigger should remind the nurse to explore this with the patient and then provide the patient with preprinted information on smoking cessation.

Integration of standardized discharge instructions and patient education into the clinical system is another way to improve the compliance and documentation of education along with streamlining the workflow of clinicians. Printing the information to give to the patient should be seamless to the clinician who is charting. The format should be logical and easy to read. The more transparent the process, the more efficient the system and the easier it is to use for the clinician. What I envision for the future is a system that will "remember" the style of learning preferred by patients and their families, prompt the provider to print handouts, and program the bedside computer/video education system based on their previous selections and surveys. This interactive patient and family education will be integrated into the clinical system and the patient's personal health record.

Some providers have developed a list of credible Web sites that is shared with patients or family members. Recommendations might include the U.S. Department of Health and Human Services sponsored healthfinder site (http://www.healthfinder.gov), a Web site dedicated to helping consumers find credible information on the Internet. Other excellent sources of reliable information are the National Institutes of Health (http://www.nih.gov), the Centers for Disease Control and Prevention (http://www.cdc.gov) and the National Health Information Center (http://www.health.gov/nhic).

FUTURE DIRECTIONS

Predicting future directions for technology-based health education is somewhat difficult, because we may not be able to completely envision the technology of the future. We can predict, however, that some current technologies will be used increasingly to support health literacy. For example, audio and video podcasts may become more commonplace in health education and be provided as free downloads from the Web sites of HCOs. **Voice recognition** software used to navigate the Web may reduce the frustration and confusion associated with attempting to spell complex medical terms. On the other hand, the confusion and frustration may increase if the patient/client is unable to pronounce the terms. Voice interactivity should help to reduce the disparity associated with those who have limited keyboard or mousing skills.

Those who are frequent e-mail users may be interested in being able to communicate with physicians and other healthcare personnel via e-mail, rather than the telephone. This idea may meet some resistance by physicians who perceive the e-mail correspondence as bothersome and time consuming. However, it is possible that work efficiency might also increase if patients and their needs were screened via e-mail prior to an office visit. For example, as a result of an e-mail correspondence in lieu of an initial office visit, medications could be changed or diagnostic tests could be performed prior to the office visit. In addition, patients could be directed to an interactive screening form housed on a Web site where they would answer a series of questions that would help them make a decision about whether they should call for an appointment, head for the emergency room, or self-manage the issue. If self-management is the outcome of the screening tool, then the patient or caregiver could be directed to a credible Web site for more information. The idea is not to interfere with or replace the face-to-face visit, but to supplement the physician–patient relationship and perhaps streamline the efficiency of healthcare delivery. McCray (2005) suggests that physicians may be resistant to providing e-mail consultations and recommending health-related Web sites because of the potential for malpractice liability.

Piette (2007) describes the use of interactive behavior change technology (IBCT) to improve the effectiveness of diabetes management. The goal of the IBCT is to improve communication between patients and healthcare providers and provide educational interventions to promote better disease management between visits. The combination of electronic medication reminders, meters that track glycemic control longitudinally, and PDA-based calculators all supported the behavioral interventions necessary to better manage the diabetes.

SUMMARY

One thought we would like to leave you with is that the consumer empowerment movement will continue to drive the need for access to quality health education and support programs. We must be willing to meet our patients where they are and design materials that are both user friendly and meet the skills and interests of the user.

THOUGHT-PROVOKING Questions

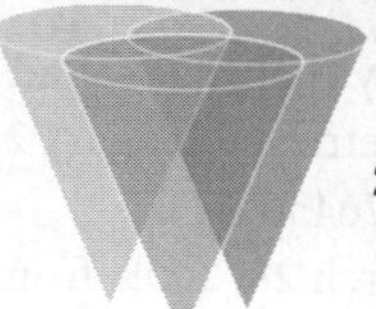

1. How do you envision technology enhancing patient or consumer education in your setting?
2. Formulate a plan evidencing a potent patient education episode on MRSA. Provide a rationale for each approach and describe a tool you would use to educate the patient and his or her family.

References

Donovan, O. (2005). The carbohydrate quandary: Achieving health literacy through an interdisciplinary WebQuest. *The Journal of School Health, 75*(9), 359–362. Retrieved January 2, 2008, from Health Module database (Document ID: 924409661).

Flores, A. (2006). Using computer games and other media to decrease child obesity. *Agricultural Research, 54*(3), 8–9. Retrieved January 2, 2008, from Research Library Core database (Document ID: 1005199991).

Fox, S. (2006, October 29). *Online health search 2006.* Retrieved January 15, 2008, from http://pewinternet.org/pdfs/PIP_Online_Health_2006.pdf

Fox, S. (2007a, March 14). *Latinos online.* Retrieved January 15, 2008, from http://pewinternet.org/pdfs/Latinos_Online_March_14_2007.pdf

Fox, S. (2007b, June 22). *Broadband, cell phones, and the continuing reality of the grey cap.* Retrieved January 15, 2008, from http://pewinternet.org/PPF/r/101/presentation_display.asp

Glassman, P. (2008). *Health literacy.* Retrieved March 28, 2008, from http://nnlm.gov/outreach/consumer/hlthlit.html

Health on the Net (HON) Foundation. (2005). *Analysis of 9th HON survey of health and medical Internet users.* Retrieved January 17, 2008, from http://www.hon.ch/Survey/Survey2005/res.html

McCray, A. (2005). Promoting health literacy. *Journal of the American Medical Informatics Association, 12*(2), 152–163. Retrieved January 2, 2008, from ProQuest Nursing & Allied Health Source database (Document ID: 810410751).

Missen, C., & Cook, T. (2007). *Appropriate information-communications technologies for developing countries.* Retrieved March 28, 2008, from http://www.who.int/bulletin/volumes/85/4/07-041475/en/index.html

National Center for Complementary and Alternative Medicine (NCCAM)/National Institutes of Health. (2008). *10 things to know about evaluating medical resources on the Web.* Retrieved March 28, 2008, from http://nccam.nih.gov/health/webresources

Parker, R., Ratzan, C., & Lurie, N. (2003). Health literacy: A policy challenge for advancing high-quality health care. *Health Affairs, 22*(4), 147. Retrieved January 2, 2008, from ABI/INFORM Global database (Document ID: 376436551).

Pew/Internet (2006). *The future of the internet II.* Retrieved March 28, 2008, from http://news.bbc.co.uk/1/shared/bsp/hi/pdfs/22_09_2006pewsummary.pdf

Piette, J. (2007). Interactive behavior change technology to support diabetes self-management: Where do we stand? *Diabetes Care, 30*(10), 2425–2432. Retrieved January 2, 2008, from Health Module database (Document ID: 1360494771).

Sternberg, D. (2002). Building on your quick wins. *Marketing Health Services, 22*(3), 41–43. Retrieved January 2, 2008, from ABI/INFORM Global database (Document ID: 155769441).

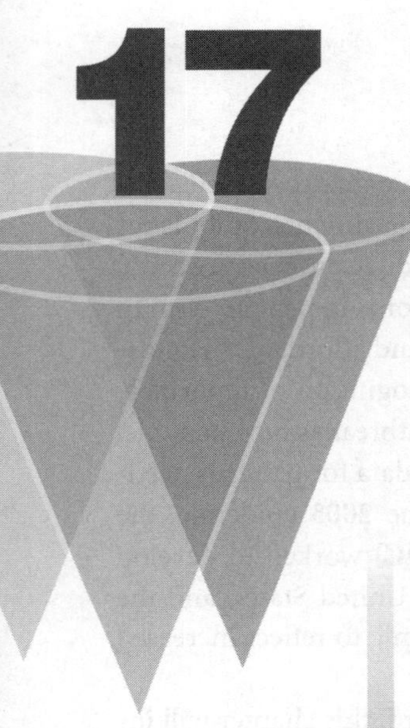

17 Using Informatics to Promote Community/Population Health

Margaret Ross Kraft and Ida Androwich

Objectives

1. Provide an overview of community and population health informatics.
2. Describe informatics tools for promoting community and population health.
3. Define the roles of federal, state, and local public health agencies in the development of public health informatics.

Key Terms

Behavioral Risk Factor Surveillance System (BRFSS)
Bioterrorism
Centers for Disease Control and Prevention (CDC)
Community risk assessment (CRA)
Epidemiology
National Center for Public Health Informatics (NCPHI)
National health information network (NHIN)
National Health and Nutrition Examination Survey (NHANES)
Public health (PH)
Public health informatics (PHI)
Public health interventions
Regional health information organization (RHIO)

INTRODUCTION

In late fall of 2002, severe acute respiratory syndrome (SARS) appeared in China. By March of 2003, SARS became recognized as a global threat. According to World Health Organization (WHO) data, more than 8,000 persons from 29 countries became infected with this previously unknown virus, and more than 700 persons died. The last SARS cases in 2004 were due to laboratory acquired infections. In addition to isolation and quarantine for diagnosed cases, computerized global **surveillance** and data collection helped to avert the potentially negative impact of a widespread global epidemic. Many surveillance systems, loosely termed **syndromic surveillance** systems, use data that are not diagnostic of a disease but that might indicate the early stages of an outbreak. Outbreak detection is the overriding purpose of syndromic surveillance for terrorism preparedness. Enhanced case-finding and monitoring the course and population characteristics of a recognized outbreak also are potential benefits of syndromic surveillance. New

Key Terms *Continued*
Risk assessment
Suicide Prevention Community Assessment Tool
Surveillance
Surveillance data systems
Syndromic surveillance
Youth Risk Behavior Surveillance System (YRBSS)

data have been used by **public health** personnel to enhance surveillance, such as patients' chief complaints in emergency departments, ambulance log sheets, prescriptions filled, retail drug and product purchases, school or work absenteeism, and medical signs and symptoms in persons seen in various clinical settings. With faster, more specific, and affordable diagnostic methods and decision-support tools, timely recognition of reportable diseases with the potential to create a substantial outbreak is now possible. Tools for pattern recognition can be used to screen data for patterns needing further public health investigation. During the 2003 epidemic, the **Centers for Disease Control and Prevention** (CDC) worked to develop surveillance criteria to identify persons with SARS in the United States, and the surveillance case definition changed throughout the epidemic to reflect increased understanding of SARS (CDC, 2007).

Utilizing the SARS outbreak description as a springboard, this chapter will introduce the reader to community and population health informatics. We will describe informatics tools for promoting community and population health and define the roles of federal, state, and local public health agencies in the development of **public health informatics (PHI)**.

USING THE FOUNDATION OF KNOWLEDGE MODEL

The collection and processing of population health data creates the information that becomes the basis for knowledge in the field of public health. There is an ever-increasing need for timely information about the health of communities, states, and countries. Knowledge about disease trends and other threats to community health can improve program planning, decision making and care delivery. Patients seen from the perspective of major health threats within their communities can benefit from opportunities for early intervention. Information technology now allows for the integration and analysis of diverse data sources in a spatial-temporal context that supports the development of predictive models and the development of timely interventions (Kopp et al., 2002).

The core public health functions are: "The assessment and monitoring of the health of communities and populations at risk to identify health problems and priorities; The formulation of public policies designed to solve identified local and national health problems and priorities; To assure that all populations have access to appropriate and cost-effective care, including health promotion and disease prevention services, and evaluation of the effectiveness of that care" (MedTerms, 2007). "Public health is a field that encompasses an amalgam of science, action, research, policy, advocacy and government" (Yasnoff, Overhage, Humphreys, & LaVenture, 2001, p. 536).

Historically, Dr. John Snow might be designated the father of public health, because in 1854, he plotted information about cholera deaths and was able to determine that the deaths were all around the same water pump in London. He convinced authorities that the cholera deaths were associated with that water pump, and when the pump handle was removed, cholera disappeared. It was Dr. Snow's focus on the cholera population rather than on a single patient that led to his discovery of the cholera outbreak (Vachon, 2005).

Florence Nightingale should also be recognized as an early public health informaticist. Her recommendations about medical reform and the need for improved sanitary conditions were based on data about morbidity and mortality that she compiled from her experiences in the Crimea and in England. Her efforts led to a total reorganization of how and which healthcare statistics should be collected (Dossey, 2000).

Just as information has been recognized as an asset in the business world, health care is now recognized as information intensive requiring timely, accurate information from many different sources. Health information systems address the collection, storage, analysis, interpretation, and communication of health data and information. Many health disciplines such as medicine and nursing have developed their own concepts of informatics integrating computer, information, and cognitive science with the science of the professional domain. That trend has reached the field of public and community health, and public health informatics (PHI) represents "a systematic application of information and computer science and technology to public health (PH) practice, research and learning" (Yasnoff, O'Carroll, Koo, Linkins, & Kilbourne, 2000, p. 67). This area of informatics differs from others because it is focused on the promotion of health and disease prevention in populations and communities. PHI efficiently and effectively organizes and manages data, information, and knowledge generated and used by public health professionals to fulfill the core functions of public health: assessment, policy, and assurance (ATSDR, 2003). Public health changes the social conditions and systems that affect everyone within a given community. It is because of public health that we understand the importance of clean water, the danger of secondhand smoke, and the fact that seat belts really do save lives (Public Health Institute, 2008).

The scope of PHI practice includes knowledge from a variety of additional disciplines including management, organization theory, psychology, political science, and law, as well as fields related to PH such as **epidemiology**, microbiology, toxicology, and statistics (O'Carroll, Yasnoff, Ward, Ripp, & Martin, 2003). Public health informatics focuses on applications of information technology (IT) that "promote the health of populations rather than individuals, focus on disease prevention rather than treatment, focus on preventive intervention at all vulnerable points" (O'Carrroll et al., 2003, pp. 3–4). PHI addresses the data, information, and knowledge that public health professionals generate and use to meet the core functions of public health (PHDSC, 2007b). Yasnoff and others (2000) have defined four principles that define and guide the activities of PHI. These principles are (1) applications promote the health of populations, (2) applications focus on disease and injury prevention, (3) applications should explore prevention at "all vulnerable points in the causal changes" (p. 69) and (4) PHI must reflect the "governmental context in which public health is practiced" (p. 69).

The Institute of Medicine (IOM) defines the role of public health as "fulfilling society's interest in assuring conditions in which people can be healthy" (as cited in Khoury, 1997, p. 176). Functions of public health include prevention of epidemics and the spread of disease, protection against environmental hazards, promotion of health, disaster response and recovery, and providing access to health care (PHDSC, 2007).

COMMUNITY HEALTH RISK ASSESSMENT (TOOLS FOR ACQUIRING KNOWLEDGE)

As the public has become more aware of harmful elements in the environment, **risk assessment** tools have been developed. Such tools allow assessment of pesticide use, exposure to harmful chemicals, contaminants in food and water, and toxic pollutants in the air to determine if potential hazards need to be addressed. A risk assessment may also be called a threat and risk assessment. "A 'threat' is a harmful act such as the deployment of a virus or illegal network penetration. A 'risk' is the expectation that a threat may succeed and the potential damage that can occur" (PCMag.com Encyclopedia, 2007).

"Risk factor assessments complement vital statistics data systems and morbidity data systems by providing information on factors earlier in the causal chain leading to illness, injury or death" (O'Carroll, Powell-Griner, Holtzman, & Williamson, 2003, p. 316).

"Health risk assessments are used to estimate whether current or future exposures will pose health risks to broad populations" (CEPA, 1998, p. 4) and are used to weigh the benefits and costs of various program alternatives for reducing exposure to potential hazards. They may impact public policy and regulatory decisions. Health risk assessment is a constantly developing process based in sound science and professional judgments. There are usually four basic steps ascribed to risk assessment. They include hazard identification, exposure assessment, dose-response assessment, and risk characterization. Hazard identification seeks to determine the types of health problems that could be caused by exposure to a potentially hazardous material. All research studies related to the potentially hazardous material are reviewed to identify potential health problems. Exposure assessment is done to determine the length, amount, and pattern of exposure to the potentially hazardous material. Dose response is an estimation of how much exposure to the potential hazard would cause varying degrees of health effects. Risk characterization is an assessment of the risk of the hazardous material causing illness in the population (CEPA, 1998). The question the risk assessment has to answer is how much risk is acceptable?

Risk factor systems are used throughout the country and may be local, regional, or national in scope. Risk assessment tools exist for specific health issues such as the **Suicide Prevention Community Assessment Tool**, which addresses general community information, prevention networks, and the demographics of the target population as well as community assets and risk factors. Other risk assessment tools include the **Youth Risk Behavior Surveillance System (YRBSS)**, the **Behavorial Risk Factor Surveillance System (BRFSS)**, and the **National Health and Nutrition Examination Survey (NHANES)**. Pennsylvania's Office of Mental Retardation began an assessment initiative in 1998 to collect information on the movement of this specific population from state-operated facilities into community settings. The goal of this assessment process was to ensure that this population had access to necessary health care and that their needs were being met (PHRAP, 1998).

Determining the presence of risk factors in a community is a key part of a **community risk assessment (CRA)**. Communities may be concerned about what in the environment affects or may affect the community's health, the level of environmental risk, and other factors that should be included in public health planning. Ball (2003) defines value as "a function of cost, service, and outcome" (p. 41). The value of a community risk assessment is in providing information crucial to planning, building consensus of how to mobilize community resources, and allowing for comparison of risks with those of other communities. The goal of a CRA is risk reduction and improved health. A CRA may identify unmet needs and opportunities for action that may help set new priorities for local public health units. A CRA may also be used to monitor the impact of prevention programs.

AGENCY SUPPORT OF EPIDEMIOLOGY AND THE MONITORING OF DISEASE OUTBREAKS

There is a need to define the role of federal, state, and local PH agencies in the development of PHI and IT applications. The availability of IT today challenges all stakeholders in the health of the public to adopt new systems to provide adequate disease surveillance and challenges us to improve outmoded processes.

Preparedness in public health means more timely detection of potential health threats, situational awareness, surveillance, outbreak management, countermeasures, response, and communications. These needs are advancing the scope of epidemiologic surveillance, which includes data on disease incidence and prevalence and physical environment profiles. Surveillance uses health-related data that signal a sufficient probability of a case or an outbreak that warrants further public health response. Although historically syndromic surveillance has been utilized to target investigations of potential infectious cases, its utility to detect possible outbreaks associated with **bioterrorism** is increasingly being explored by public health officials (CDC, 2007). Early detection of possible outbreaks can be achieved through timely and complete receipt, review, and investigation of disease case reports, by improving the ability to recognize patterns in data that may be indicative of a possible outbreak early in its course and through receipt of new types of data that can signify an outbreak earlier in its course. New types of data might include identification of absences from work or school, increased purchases of healthcare products, including specific types of over-the-counter medications, presenting symptoms to healthcare providers, and laboratory test orders (CDC, 2007). A comprehensive surveillance effort supports timely investigation and identifies data needs for managing the public health response to an outbreak or terrorist event.

Geographic information systems are now being used to look at the geographic prevalence and incidence of disease, identification of at-risk populations, differentiation of risk factors, intervention planning in anticipation of epidemics, and local and global monitoring of disease in a real-time perspective (Kopp et al., 2002).

In order to appropriately process public health data, PHI has a need for a standardized vocabulary and coding structure. This is especially important as national public health data is collected so that data variables can be understood across systems and between agencies. A standardized vocabulary must address local language use vs. universal language usage for public health.

In the early 1990s, the CDC launched a plan for an integrated surveillance system that moved from stand-alone systems to networked data exchange built with specific standards. Early initiatives were the National Electronic Telecommunications System for Surveillance (NETSS) and the Wide-ranging Online Data for Epidemiologic Research (WONDER). Six current initiatives reflect this early vision:

- PulseNet USA: A surveillance network for food-borne infections
- The National Electronic Disease Surveillance System (NEDSS): Facilitates reporting on approximately 100 diseases with data feeding directly from clinical laboratories allowing for early detection

- Epidemic Information Exchange (Epi-X): A secure communication system for practitioners to access and share preliminary health surveillance information
- Health Alert Network (HAN): A state and nationwide alert system
- Biosense: Provides improved real-time biosurveillance and situational awareness in support of early detection
- Public Health Information Network (PHIN): Promotes standards and software solutions for the rapid flow of public health information.

Certainly the events of September 2001 have created an acceleration in the need for informatics in public health practice. Today response requirements include fast detection, science, communication, integration, and action (Kukafka, 2006). In 2005, the CDC created the **National Center for Public Health Informatics (NCPHI)** to provide leadership in the field. This center aims to protect and improve health through PHI (McNabb, Koo, Pinner, & Seligman, 2006).

Information is vital to public health programming. The data processed into public health information can be from administrative, financial, and facility sources. Encounter, screening, registry, clinical, and laboratory data as well as surveillance data may be included. It has been recommended that the functions of population health beyond surveillance need to be integrated into the electronic health record and the personal health record. Such an initiative might allow for population level alerts to be sent to clinicians through these electronic record systems. Data on vital statistics from state and local governments are also used for public health purposes. It should be noted that databases created with public funds are public databases that are available for authorized public representatives for public purposes (Freedman & Weed, 2003).

APPLYING KNOWLEDGE TO HEALTH DISASTER PLANNING AND PREPARATION

The availability of data and speed of data exchange can have a significant impact on critical PH functions like disease monitoring and syndromic surveillance. Currently surveillance data are limited and historical in nature. Special data collections are needed to address specific public health issues, and investigations and emergencies are addressed and managed with paper. The future of PHI will offer real-time surveillance data available electronically, and investigations and emergences will be managed with the tools of informatics. "**Surveillance data systems** [boldface added], e.g., systems for infectious diseases, store information on exposure or trends in adverse health effects over a specified period of time that can be used by public health officials for planning, evaluation, or implementation of **public health interventions** [boldface added]"(ATSDR, 2003). "Syndromic surveillance for early outbreak detection is an investigational approach where health department staff, assisted by automated data acquisition and generation of statistical signals, monitor disease indicators continually (real time) or at least daily (near real time) to detect outbreaks of diseases earlier and more completely than might otherwise be possible with traditional public health methods" (Buehler, Hopkins, Overhage, Sosin, & Tong, 2004, ¶ 7)

INFORMATICS TOOLS TO SUPPORT COMMUNICATION AND DISSEMINATION

The revolution in IT has made the capture and analysis of health data and the distribution of healthcare information more achievable and less costly. Since the early 1960s, CDC has used IT in its practice and PHI emerged as a specialty in the 1990s. PHI has become more important with improvements in information technology, changes in our care delivery system, and the challenges related to emerging infections, resistance to antibiotics, and the threat of chemical and biological terrorism. Two-way communication between public health agencies, community clinicians, and clinical laboratories can identify clusters of reportable and unusual diseases. As a result, health departments can consult on case diagnosis and management, alerts, surveillance summaries, and clinical and public health recommendations. Ongoing healthcare provider outreach, education, and 24-hour access to public health professionals leads to the discovery of urgent health threats. The automated transfer of specified data from a laboratory database to a public health data repository improves the timeliness and completeness of reporting notifiable conditions.

PH information systems represent a partnership of federal, state, and local public health professionals. Such systems allow the capture of large amounts of data, rapid exchange of information, and strengthened links between these three system levels. Dissemination of prevention guidelines and communication among PH officials, clinicians, and patients has become a major benefit of PHI. IT solutions can be used to provide accurate and timely information that will guide public health actions. In addition, the Internet has become a universal communications pathway and allows individuals as well as population groups to be more involved and responsible for management of their own health status.

Few PH professionals have received formal informatics training and may not be aware of the potential impact of IT on their practice. A working group formed at the University of Washington Center for public health informatics has published a draft of PHI competencies needed (Karras, 2007). These competencies include:

- Supporting development of strategic direction for PHI within the enterprise.
- Participating in development of knowledge management tools for the enterprise.

- Utilizing standards.
- Assuring that knowledge, information, and data needs of project or program users and stakeholders are met.
- Managing information system development, procurement, and implementation.
- Managing IT operations related to project or program (for public health agencies with internal IT operations).
- Monitoring IT operations managed by external organizations.
- Communicating with cross-disciplinary leaders and team members.
- Participating in applied public health informatics research.
- Developing public health information systems that are interoperable with other relevant information systems.
- Supporting use of informatics to integrate clinical health, environmental risk, and population health.
- Implementing solutions that assure confidentiality, security, and integrity, while maximizing availability of information for public health.
- Conducting education and training in PHI (CPHI, 2007).

Information technology is also valuable in the promotion of individual health literacy and knowledge that may encourage individuals to accept more personal responsibility for their health status and make more informed decisions about their health. Improved health status in individuals contributes to improved population health.

USING FEEDBACK TO IMPROVE RESPONSES AND PROMOTE READINESS

Improvement of community health status and population health depends on effective public and healthcare infrastructures. In addition to information from public health agencies, there is now interest in the capture of information from hospitals, pharmacies, poison control centers, laboratories, and environmental agencies. Timely collection of such data allows early detection and analysis that can increase the rapidity of response with more effective interventions. Yasnoff and his colleagues (2000) identify the grand challenges still facing PHI as the development of national public health information systems, a closer integration of clinical care with public health, and concerns of confidentiality and privacy.

Population health data must be considered an important part of the infrastructure of all **regional health information organizations (RHIOs)**, which are the building blocks for a **national health information network (NHIN)**. "These efforts call for collaboration of various organizations and agencies interested in clinical, public health and population health information to promote and protect the public's health"(PHDSC, 2007b). The public health data includes information about surveillance, environmental health, and preparedness systems and has client information like immunization registries as well as laboratory results reporting and analysis. It can provide information about outbreaks, patterns of drug-resistant organisms, and other trends that can help improve the accuracy of diagnostic and treatment decisions (LaVenture, 2005). An RHIO/NHIN can also support public health goals through broader opportunities for participation in surveillance and prevention activities, improved case management and care coordination, and increased accuracy and timeliness of information for disease reporting (LaVenture).

Public health informatics strives to ensure that health data systems will meet the data needs of all organizations interested in population health as national and international standards are developed for healthcare data collection. This includes standardization of environmental, sociocultural, economic, and other data that are relevant to population health (PHDSC, 2007b). Table 17-1 provides the

TABLE 17-1
Important PHI Sites

Name	Address	Web Site
American Public Health Association	APHA 800 I Street, NW Washington, DC 20001	www.apha.org
Center for Public Health Informatics	CPHI University of Washington 1100 NE 45th Street, Suite 405 Seattle, WA 98105	www.cphi.washington.edu
Centers for Disease Control and Prevention	Centers for Disease Control and Prevention 1600 Clifton Road Atlanta, GA 30333	www.cdc.gov
National Center for Public Health Informatics	The National Center for Public Health Informatics (NCPHI) 1600 Clifton Road NE Mailstop E-78 Atlanta, GA 30333	www.cdc.gov/ncphi
Public Health Data Standards Consortium	Public Health Data Standards Consortium c/o Johns Hopkins Bloomberg School of Public Health 624 North Broadway, Room 325 Baltimore, MD 21205	www.phdsc.org

names, addresses, and URLs for important organizations dedicated to public health data and informatics.

SUMMARY

The two most important thoughts we'd like to leave you with are: (1) the issue is not what data to collect but how to collect and share it; and (2) there is an ever-increasing need for timely information about the health of communities, states, and countries.

THOUGHT-PROVOKING Questions

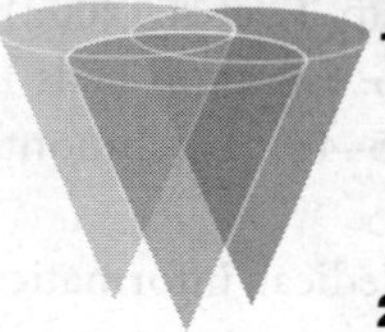

1. Imagine that you are a public health informatics specialist and you and your colleagues have determined that the threat of a new strain of influenza indicates a need for a mass inoculation program. What public health data would have been used to determine the need for such a program?
2. What data will be collected to determine the success of such a program?

References

Agency for Toxic Substances and Disease Registry (ATSDR). (2003, February 6). *ATSDR glossary of terms.* Retrieved August, 30, 2007, from http://www.atsdr.cdc.gov/glossary.html

Ball, M. (2003). Better health through informatics: Managing information to deliver value. In P. O'Carroll, W. Yasnoff, M. E. Ward, L. Ripp, & E. Martin (Eds.), *Public health informatics and information systems* (pp. 39–51). New York: Springer-Verlag.

Buehler, J. W., Hopkins, R. S., Overhage, J. M., Sosin, D. M., & Tong, V. (2004). *Framework for evaluating public health surveillance systems for early detection of outbreaks.* Retrieved September 20, 2007, from http://www.cdc.gov/MMWR/preview/mmwrhtml/rr5305a1.htm

California Environmental Protection Agency (1998). *A guide to health risk assessment.* Retrieved August 30, 2007, from http://www.oehha.ca.gov/risk/layperson/index.html

Center for Public Health Informatics (CPHI). (2007). *Draft competencies V7 for the public health informatician.* Seattle: University of Washington. Retrieved August 15, 2007, from http://www.cphi.washington.edu/projects/phi-comp/comp-phinformaticians/PHI_Competencies%20v7%2002207-3.pdf

Dossey, B. M. (2000). *Florence Nightingale: Mystic, visionary, healer*. Springhouse, PA: Springhouse Corporation.

Freedman, M. A., & Weed, J. A. (2003). National vital statistics system. In P. O'Carroll, W. Yasnoff, M. Ward, L., Ripp, & E. Martin (Eds.). (2003). *Public health informatics and information systems* (pp. 269–285). New York: Springer-Verlag.

Khoury, M. J. (1997). Genetic epidemiology and the future of disease prevention and public health. *Epidemologic Reviews, 19*(1), 175–180.

Karras, B. (2007). *Competencies for the public health informatician.* Seattle: University of Washington. Retrieved August 15, 2007, from http://www.cphi.washington.edu/projects/phi-comp/comp-phinformaticians

Kopp, S., Shuchman, R., Strecher, V., Gueye, M., Ledlow, J., Philip, T., et al. (2002). Public health applications. In R. Bashshur, S. Mandil, & G. Shannon (Eds.), *Telemedicine/telehealth: An international perspective* (pp. 35–48). Larchmont, NY: Mary Ann Liebert, Inc.

Kukafka, R. (2006, September). *Public health informatics.* Medical informatics course for health professionals. Woods Hole, MA.

LaVenture, M. (2005, May). *Role of population/public health in regional health information exchanges.* PHDSC/eHealth Initiative annual conference, Washington, DC.

McNabb, S., Koo, D., Pinner, R., & Seligman, J. (2006). *Informatics and public health at CDC.* Retrieved August 30, 2007, from http://www.cdc.gov/mmwr/preview/mmwrhtml/su5502a10

MedTerms. (2007). *Definition of public health.* Retrieved August 30, 2007, from http://www.medterms.com/script/main/art.asp?articlekey=5120

O'Carroll, P., Powell-Griner, E., Holtzman, D., & Williamson, G. D. (2003). Risk factor information systems. In P. O'Carroll, W. Yasnoff, M. Ward, L. Ripp, & E. Martin (Eds.), *Public health informatics and information systems* (pp. 316–334). New York: Springer-Verlag.

O'Carroll, P., Yasnoff, W., Ward, M., Ripp, L., & Martin, E. (Eds.). (2003). *Public health informatics and information systems.* New York: Springer-Verlag.

PCMag.com Encyclopedia. (2007). *Risk assessment.* Retrieved September 3, 2007, from http://www.pcmag.com/encyclopedia_term/0,2542,t=risk+assessment&i=50556,00.asp

Pennsylvania's Health Risk Assessment Process (PHRAP). (1998). Retrieved September 30, 2007, from http://www.hsri.org/docs/QF_HealthRiskAssessmentPA.pdf

Public Health Data Standards Consortium (PHDSC). (2007a). *Tutorial module 1: What is public health.* Retrieved August 30, 2007, from www.phdsc.org/knowresources/tutorials/module1

Public Health Data Standards Consortium (PHDSC). (2007b). *Tutorial module 8: Viewing public health data and data standards in a larger context.* Retrieved August 30, 2007, from www.phdsc.org/knowresources/tutorials/module1

Public Health Institute. (2008). *PHI—Public health 101.* Retrieved May 29, 2008, from http://www.phi.org/ph101.html

Vachon, D. (2005, May-June). Dr. John Snow blames water pollution for cholera epidemic. *Old News, 16*(8), 8–10. Retrieved September 1, 2007, from www.ph.ucla/epi/snow

Yasnoff, W. (2003). Introduction to PH informatics. In P. O'Carroll, *Public health informatics and information systems* (pp. 3–15). New York: Springer-Verlag.

Yasnoff, W., O'Carroll, P., Koo, D., Linkings, R., & Kilbourne, E. (2000). Public health informatics: Improving and transforming public health in the Information Age. *Journal of Public Health Management Practice, 6*(6), 67–75.

Yasnoff, W., Overhage, M., Humphreys, B., & LaVenture, M. (2001). A national agenda for public health informatics. *Journal of the American Medical Informatics Association, 8*(6), 535–545.

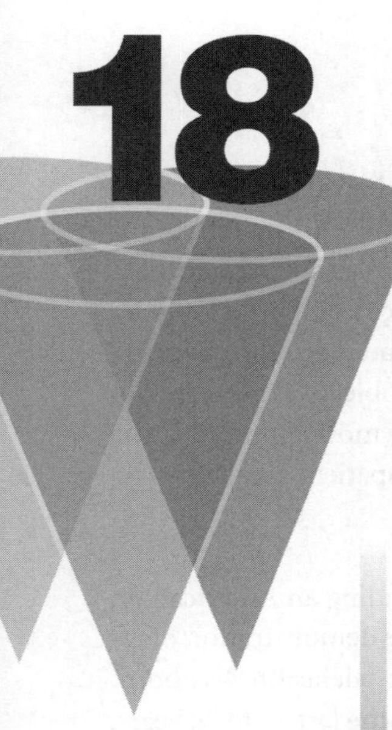

Overview of Home Telehealth[1]

Sheldon Prial and Schuyler F. Hoss

Objectives

1. Review the historical development of telehealth.
2. Identify the clinical and economic benefits of telehealth.
3. Explore the professional roles associated with telehealth.
4. Predict future uses of telehealth.

Key Terms

Communications hub
Digital health record (DHR)
Home health agency (HHA)
Long-term care facility
Payer organization
Peripheral devices
Real environment data
Telehealth
Telehealth hardware
Telehealth software
Trending
Triage
Visiting Nurse Association (VNA)

INTRODUCTION

The term *tele* means "distant, at a distance, over a distance" (Merriam-Webster's Online Dictionary, n.d.). Think about your telephone or your television and how signals are transmitted over a distance. We often take terminologies for granted without really thinking about what they mean. When *tele* is attached to health, it refers to health care that is performed or delivered over a distance. Home **telehealth** allows the caregiver to be in contact with the patient without requiring a face-to-face encounter. With the United States graying rapidly and chronic patient populations growing dramatically, the ability for this type of patient interaction has become a necessity. This capacity to supervise patients away from an office is predicted to continue to grow rapidly and may reach an $8 billion per year world-wide market value by 2012 (Health Data Management, 2007). The ability to provide better healthcare access is the number one benefit of using telehealth. By reducing the need for face-to-face interaction with the patient, the nurse, physician, or even the technician can be much more

[1]Some of the information contained in this chapter is primarily the result of private consulting done by the authors and study conclusions by the Northwest Healthcare Management client database.

productive. When information is collected in the home, it becomes much more convenient for the patient, and the quality and timeliness of the information is improved dramatically. Home telemonitoring should be viewed as an enhancement to care, for it allows more direct, physical intervention to occur only when it is actually needed. Care is not directed by prescheduled appointment or subjective perceptions of condition; it can instead be determined by objective measures of physical status. With telehealth, it can also be delivered at the most appropriate site of care, reducing reliance on emergency departments and inpatient facilities.

HISTORY OF TELEHEALTH

The late President John F. Kennedy gave NASA a goal of landing an American on the moon. The surprise benefit of the space program was the demonstration of effective remote monitoring of the astronauts, thus modern telehealth was born. While most of the advances in telehealth have taken place in the last 20 to 30 years, Craig and Patterson (2005) describe much earlier uses such as the use of bonfires to alert neighboring villages of the arrival of bubonic plague during the Middle Ages. Postal services and telegraphs were used to transmit health information in the mid-19th century; while 1910 marks the first transmission of stethoscope sounds over a telephone. Radio communications were employed to provide medical support for crews on ships; the Seaman's Church Institute of New York (1920) and the International Radio Medical Center (1938) are two examples of organizations founded to provide health support at a distance. These services were later expanded to cover air travel (Craig & Patterson). The National Institutes of Mental Health supported a program in the mid-1950s that connected seven state hospitals in four different states via a closed-circuit telephone system (Venable, 2005). As technology evolved, its use in health care continued to grow. The first reported use of television to monitor patients in a clinical facility occurred in the 1950s, which then led to the development of interactive closed-circuit applications in the mid-1960s. These early TV applications to health care occurred within the facility but still had the benefit of extending the reach of the caregivers because they did not need to be in the same room to effectively monitor their patients. Craig and Patterson suggest that ever-evolving technologies in digital transmission, the falling costs of computing in general, and the explosion of mobile phones and satellite communications will sustain the advance of telehealth. Let's shift our attention to home telehealth.

HOME TELEHEALTH HARDWARE

In the typical patient home, you will find **telehealth hardware**—equipment that captures objective vital sign data. Some systems use interactive self-reporting devices to capture subjective information on how a patient feels as well. The values obtained from the patient are then collected and transmitted by a communication hub. **Peripheral devices** used in home telehealth can include any item with a digital readout. Generally this equipment is self-administrated by the patient or is administered by a family caregiver. Examples of the most commonly used peripheral devices include:

- Weight scale
- Blood pressure monitor
- Pulse oximeter
- Thermometer
- Glucometer
- Spirometer
- Prothrombin time, international normalized ratio (PT/INR) meter
- Digital camera (to capture images of wounds)
- PDA-based or telephonic self-reporting devices

Specialty equipment used in managing cardiac, respiratory, transplant, and bariatric patients are commonly used as well. While live video has long been available, use of interactive visual technology is limited in field applications because of the need to have a dedicated clinician sitting on the receiving end. The cost and scheduling complexity associated with the use of live video has limited its application.

The **communications hub** is a device that captures and assists in the transmission of information from peripheral equipment. A processor organizes the data, appropriately encrypts it to assure confidentiality, and transmits it to appropriate decision makers. Data can be transmitted via traditional phone lines, the Internet, or over wireless networks. Typically the hub will be a small box, to which peripheral equipment is connected.

HOME TELEHEALTH SOFTWARE

As important as the gathering of data is the organizing of information to support decision making by clinical professionals. The **telehealth software** supporting home telehealth programs has become much more sophisticated, allowing for greater numbers of patients to be better managed by a single clinician. Areas of significant improvement in software include **trending**, **triage**, communications protocols, access, and sharing.

Trending

One of the advantages of home telemonitoring is the creation of a **digital health record** (DHR) that allows information to be recorded over time. If a patient takes his/her weight and blood pressure daily, most software will graphically display this data over time so that subtle trends can be observed. This type of trend data is much more useful in identifying emerging or developing conditions than snapshot data that is collected every 6–8 weeks at a physician's office. Trend information can also be developed for groups of patients or populations, allowing for population-based analyses of interventions. It is possible to gather trend information on chronic obstructive pulmonary disease (COPD) patients, patients of a particular physician, or all patients receiving a certain medication, for example.

Triage

Most home telemonitoring systems set an acceptable range of values for an individual patient when he or she is enrolled in the monitoring program. If oxygen saturation, blood pressure, or weight values, for example, go above or below predetermined amounts, then the software will alert the appropriate party. More sophisticated software will look at readings from multiple pieces of equipment on a single patient and can give higher priority to patients at risk of an acute episode. This helps clinicians better organize their work and arrange for appropriate interventions.

Communications

Advanced telemonitoring software has sophisticated electronic notification protocols. It is often predetermined when information will be communicated and to whom it is sent. Sophisticated protocols can be developed related to both routine and alert information organizing communications with physicians, nurses, and caregivers. Some systems also have the capacity to communicate back to the patient or seek additional information under predetermined circumstances.

Data Access and Information Sharing

Many telemonitoring systems house information in Web-based formats. This allows for easy access to the data from any location that has access to the Internet. Multiple parties can simultaneously share and view data. Information can also be conveniently transmitted to other clinicians and is updated almost immediately when new values are received. Web-based records are fully HIPAA compliant when appropriate protections and controls are in place.

HOME TELEHEALTH PATIENTS

Any patient who has a condition that must be monitored is a candidate for home telemonitoring. Patients with chronic illnesses have particularly benefited from ongoing monitoring in order to prevent acute episodes. Patients who are homebound or have limited access to transportation are also appropriate for monitoring.

Chronic Disease Patients

Given demographics and advances in medical practice, we have experienced unprecedented growth in patients with chronic diseases. Those patients are at significant risk of having an acute episode when subtle but significant changes in their medical condition occur. The ability to identify these changes in a timely fashion allows for changes in medication, lifestyle, or treatment to occur. Identification of a 3-pound weight gain over 5 days in a congestive heart failure (CHF) patient allows for interventions that prevent an emergency room visit and subsequent hospitalization. The most common categories of chronic patients that are currently monitored include those with CHF, COPD, diabetes, or those who require long-term wound care.

These patients, particularly those with higher acuity levels, are at significant risk of having a medical crisis that necessitates emergency or unplanned acute interventions. There are many other categories of chronic patients who are less susceptible to a health crisis, but would greatly benefit from home telemonitoring in an effort to both improve care and reduce costs.

At-Risk Populations

Telemonitoring can be used effectively on patients who are at risk for an episode of acute illness. Patients who have a predisposition to disease are at risk of medical problems associated with employment, lifestyle, or location, or those patients who have displayed early signs of potential serious health problems could be placed on preventive monitoring. Monitoring is used to ensure that interventions are timely and acute incidents avoided. Such technology could be part of a healthcare early warning system and could support preventive models of care.

Isolated Patients

Home telemonitoring obviously is effective for patients who cannot physically access healthcare services. The homebound elderly have been among the first to benefit from this technology in conjunction with the home health services they receive. With increasing limits on the ability of patients to receive services in the home due to staffing shortages and coverage limitations, telemonitoring technology will take on greater importance in managing homebound patients.

Patients in remote geographic areas have been long-time users of telemedicine interventions. With few rural healthcare facilities being built and access problems becoming more difficult, the use of technology in the home will increase. Even in suburban and rural areas, access is becoming more problematic, requiring greater use of home telemonitoring interventions. A lack of primary care and emergency resources in many urban core areas has many health systems looking at managing certain patients through telemonitoring options and better staging patient access. Telemedicine also is effective for patients in institutions such as prisons for whom it is logistically difficult to have them travel to traditional care sites.

Hospitalized Patients

Home telemonitoring has proven effective in managing the flow of patients into and out of hospitals and other inpatient facilities. Patients are monitored to determine when they are admitted, how long they are expected to stay, and to prevent unfunded readmissions. Patients undergoing semielective procedures can be better staged with scheduling options when they are monitored in the home prior to admission. If there is an observed deterioration in a condition, a procedure can be accelerated or planned interventions changed. Monitoring can also be used effectively in length of stay (LOS) reduction strategies. Physicians and surgeons are more confident to discharge early when they know that vital signs will be monitored and any decline in condition noted in a timely fashion. Use of monitoring effectively allows for an extension of step-down models of care into the patient's home. These LOS management strategies have been particularly useful in situations where there is a lack of available hospital beds. Unplanned readmissions are a serious patient care and financial management issue for hospitals. The use of monitoring in the home has consistently reduced unplanned and unfunded readmissions by being able to obtain reliable information on the patient and intervene appropriately to keep the patient at home.

Emergency Response Situations

Telemedicine will likely be a major component of effectively managing patients in a major disaster, large-scale nuclear/biochemical attack, or in the case of an outbreak of highly infectious disease. In such a situation, traditional healthcare delivery systems may be overwhelmed and patients will need to be more effectively triaged and managed by remote providers. Telemedicine applications allow for a dramatic extension of patient management and triaging options and allow off-site providers to be involved in care. If an infectious or communicable disease is involved, patient isolation could be accomplished in the home using telemedicine technology.

Concerned Patients and Families

Perhaps the largest potential market for home telemonitoring are patients and families who want to have reliable and objective information that allows for their involvement in healthcare decision making. At one extreme would be a young person who wants to monitor physiological data as part of a personal wellness or fitness program. At the other extreme might be families that want information on the status of a terminally ill loved one in another city. In between there is a wide range of opportunities for individuals and families to obtain information that promotes realistic and meaningful dialogue with healthcare professionals.

Assisted Living/Subacute Patients

In assisted living facilities or subacute care centers, a kiosk can be used to obtain vital signs for large groups of people. Vital sign reports can then be forwarded on a regularly established schedule to physicians and others involved in the patient's care. This allows for better individual care management and lends itself to developing intervention strategies and education options to benefit the entire population of a facility. Some facilities have even used access to telemonitoring systems as an inducement to attract potential residents.

BENEFITS OF TELEHEALTH

Home monitoring technology has been used successfully on tens of thousands of patients. Several consistent benefits have been observed. While many of these benefits improve the quality of patient care, there are also significant impacts on both costs and patient satisfaction.

Clinical Benefits

One of the great advantages of using home telemonitoring technology is that it provides a more realistic measure of vital signs and **real environment data**. Information gathered in a clinic or physician office setting is often within a range of accuracy but not necessarily reflective of typical values. Data collected in the home is more reflective of usual circumstances. When measures are taken at a similar time and in a set location every day, there is greater consistency in measures, allowing for the observation of subtle changes. This is important in developing interventions for conditions such as CHF, and it also can strongly influence patient compliance.

Patient information obtained by a **home health agency (HHA)** can be more than 1 week old before it is reviewed by clinical decision makers. This delay makes it very difficult to manage unstable or complex patients effectively. This may result in an underutilization of home-based interventions and greater reliance on more costly institutional models of care. Telehealth monitoring may improve the timeliness of clinical decision making and appropriate interventions.

As mentioned previously, having access to patient trend data allows for new levels of sophistication in medical management in a home setting. Appropriately displayed trend data allows for instant identification of pertinent changes in a patient's condition over time. Without trend data, some of the more subtle changes would be invisible to medical managers.

The effects of changes in a plan of care or medications can be readily observed when home telemonitoring technology is used. Vital sign response to changes in medication levels can often be observed in a matter of hours. Longer term changes such as associated activity levels, diet, or patient compliance can also be tracked. Periods of noncompliance can also be identified with certain categories of patients as a result of physiological readings.

Almost all home telemonitoring systems create some form of a DHR that can be integrated with electronic medical records. This allows for easy access to patient information, tracking and trending of data, and enhanced coordination of care. The DHR can also be used to expedite the billing functions and to simplify prior authorization and concurrent review processes.

The ability to quickly and efficiently share information allows multiple parties to better coordinate care and decision making. The use of contemporaneous information allows for meaningful collaboration among providers in different locations. Some organizations are currently using Web-based case conferences to jointly review and discuss mutual patients and to develop agreed-upon care plans. Nurse and physician care coordination has been particularly enhanced.

The continuous stream of patient data afforded by telehealth allows for the development of flexible plans of care that are driven by patient circumstances and needs. This allows for much more customization of care plans that can be modified by achieved benchmarks. Home health agencies have demonstrated the effective use of as-needed models of visits as opposed to preset frequencies. Other interventions can likewise be calibrated with patient status.

The use of telemonitoring has been demonstrated to dramatically reduce the need for hospital and other acute care services. Reductions of between 40 and 75% in the utilization of inpatient resources and emergency transport are routinely documented for chronic patients with diagnosis such as CHF and COPD. Not only does this result in a profound reduction in costs, but it also contributes to improved satisfaction and patient sense of confidence in managing their disease state.

The information developed through home telemonitoring programs dramatically increases levels of patient and family involvement in care. Objective data reduces reliance on subjective feelings in decision making. Extended family anxiety is reduced, and compliance levels tend to increase significantly.

Economic Benefits

The use of home telemonitoring is expected to dramatically reduce the costs of caring for many types of patients. Telemedicine may also make a significant economic contribution by increasing the efficiency and productivity of clinicians. As the cost for providing health care in the United States continues to rise, the importance of home telehealth will increase. Home telehealth may be a very effective way to both save money and improve the quality of care.

The ability to study a patient's vital signs and compare them to previous readings can reveal subtle changes in his or her condition. Once a trend is identified, early interventions can be implemented to prevent emergency room (ER) visits and unnecessary hospitalizations. Home telemonitoring can be particularly effective in reducing unnecessary acute care costs for CHF and COPD patients by identifying slight changes in vital signs. This allows for changes in medication, diet, or activity levels that prevent acute episodes.

If the ER visits are dramatically reduced and institutionalization is used only as the last resort, several benefits will occur. Emergency rooms will become what they are intended to be for—emergencies—not a substitute for physician visits. Emergency transportation costs are similarly reduced. Hospitals will have rooms available for those who must be admitted. Those who can be monitored and cared for at their home will not be filling a hospital bed. The amount of money that will be saved can dramatically reduce the cost of health care in the United States and greatly improve the services available. Home telemonitoring is viewed by medical economists as the most promising tool on the horizon to control and contain healthcare costs.

Objective data on a patient's condition allows patients to be treated or cared for in the most cost effective setting. In the absence of timely information, there is greater use of acute care options such as the emergency room or hospital. Assuring that a patient received care in the most clinically appropriate and cost-effective setting is particularly important for patients with chronic illness. An additional benefit to home telemonitoring is that it allows chronically ill persons to be maintained in the home for longer periods of time rather than being transferred to skilled care or long-term care settings. Patient compliance also tends to increase when monitoring is utilized, resulting in better illness management and more cost-effective care. This contributes to not only significant cost savings, but also an increase in the patient's independence and quality of life.

The productivity of caregivers can be dramatically enhanced when home telemonitoring strategies are effectively employed. In an era of serious shortages in trained professionals, this can have a significant impact on the ability of providers to accept and effectively care for patients. Clinical professionals visiting patients in their home spend a significant amount of time traveling to patient homes and recording patient data. The use of telemedicine allows for a reduction in the physical visits nurses must make, freeing up their time to accept and manage additional patients. Likewise, when automated systems are collecting and organizing information that the nurse would otherwise have to input into nursing notes or patient records, there is additional time created for hands-on care with new patients. Home health agencies that have effectively used home telehealth have enjoyed this benefit of increased nursing productivity, thus allowing nurses to carry one to two additional patients per week. Caseloads are growing as our population ages. Unfortunately, the number of clinical professionals to serve them is not growing at the same rate. Home telehealth has provided the tool to be able to increase their caseloads without reducing the quality of their work.

Home monitoring systems utilize software that creates a DHR. The information obtained from patients can thus be organized, trended, and communicated efficiently. It can also be integrated with other electronic medical record (EMR) formats. The monitoring equipment collects and transmits the data. This eliminates the need for clinicians to gather and record information in a manual file. Decision-making software based on the violation of parameters or patient norms is often integrated to allow for the immediate identification and triaging of patients with potential health issues. Timely and appropriate data management increases caregiver productivity and clinical coordination effectiveness.

Another benefit afforded by telehealth is improved scheduling options for the visiting nurse or home health agencies. Under the prospective payment system, agencies can use technology to monitor patients and reduce the need for physical visits in the home. Physical visits are made when the physiological data indicates a need and are not driven by arbitrary visit frequencies. This flexibility enhances productivity and improves the ability to better cluster visits geographically in order to reduce travel and transportation time.

ROLES OF CLINICAL PROFESSIONALS

Clinicians at several levels have an important role in making a home telemonitoring program successful. As with most aspects of health care, developing a team approach enhances the contribution of each clinician and improves the outcomes for the patient. As home telemonitoring is relatively new, the respective roles of clinicians have not been clearly defined. As the technology is more widely utilized, there will be greater clarity in function and responsibility.

Nurses

Nurses are key to making any home telemonitoring program successful. Nurses have an important role in identifying patients who are appropriate for monitoring. Visiting nurses, as well as nurses in physician's office or clinic settings, will often be among the first clinicians to recognize a patient that could benefit from home monitoring. Nurses are also generally involved in reviewing data generated by home monitoring systems. Another critical nursing role is the triaging of patients when they are found to exceed preset limits or parameters. Case management and triage models of intervention are effectively employed by nurses to identify and respond to problems in an appropriate fashion. Finally, nurses are very involved in working with other clinicians in developing follow-up or intervention strategies. The great benefit of this technology in nurses' hands is that it supports more immediate and less complex interventions.

Home telemonitoring also is an effective strategy in assuring that the nurse's time is spent on those patients who have genuine needs. The triage capability of home telemonitoring software allows nurses to direct their time and expertise to patients requiring interventions. In home health in particular, this allows for better scheduling, enhanced alignment of clinician skills with patient needs, and improved productivity.

Physicians

Physicians have traditionally been limited in their role in managing the homebound or chronic patient. While the physician is required to make decisions on necessary care, medication, and other services, they have only limited access to timely information on the client. As a result, they may be basing care decisions on physiological data that can be several days old, lab values that are dated, and observations that may have been made in an office or other artificial setting. Home telemedicine allows the physician to have virtually real-time, objective information that is obtained in the patient's home environment.

As with the nurse, the physician's time can be appropriately focused on patients with more pressing needs as a result of home telemonitoring software's triage capability. Telemonitoring also makes information sharing with nurses, therapy clinicians, and specialty physicians more timely and practical. Web-based team conferences can be facilitated using the data obtained from telemonitoring systems. Treatments and interventions can be effectively adjusted based on changing patient circumstances. Physicians have used the technology to monitor the effects of emergency medical technicians (EMTs) and nurse interventions in the home, adjust medication dosages, change recommended diet or activity levels, and alter therapy protocols. The physician, however distant from the patient's home, can be actively involved with patients in their home through reports and other information provided. This has the double benefit of keeping the physician fully informed and providing the patient peace of mind in knowing that his or her health is being adequately monitored. It is likely that in the future specialty physicians will be designated to monitor and respond to telehealth patients, much as hospitalists currently attend to patients in acute care facilities.

Case Managers

One of the greatest frustrations for care managers is obtaining accurate and appropriately organized information that allows them to make reasonable decisions on care alternatives. This lack of information results in the use of higher-cost care than is necessary and in interventions that may not be optimal to patients' real needs and circumstances. Sending a nurse to visit the patient at home simply to gather vital signs is generally impractical and too expensive. With the use of home telehealth, that problem is resolved. Technology allows case managers to effectively collaborate with the patient's physician and nurse in developing optimal care plans that are more cost effective due to reduced reliance on hospital and emergency response resources. Access to this information significantly reduces tensions and mistrust by clinicians in working with case managers by basing decision making on objective data.

Technical Support Personnel

Because of the sophistication and reliability of the equipment used in the home to collect patient information, technician-level personnel play a key role in delivering, setting up, maintaining, and recovering equipment. Support personnel can also be involved in educating patients on the use of technology, troubleshooting problems associated with the hardware and software, and recalibrating equipment. This reduces the need for nurses being involved in the logistical aspects of home telemonitoring.

Tech-level personnel can also perform some of the information management tasks associated with getting data to clinical decision makers. Base station monitoring personnel are used by many telemonitoring providers with preset communications protocols followed for transmitting clinically relevant data. The use of technicians allows nurses and physicians to be involved in analyzing the patient data and in developing appropriate clinical responses. Effective use of tech-level personnel frees up nurses and physicians to focus on patient needs, maintain care at the highest level, and show tremendous monetary savings.

WHO IS USING HOME TELEMONITORING?

Home telemonitoring is currently in its infancy, with relatively few patients actually being monitored. This will change very dramatically over the next several years as the benefits of using the technology are better understood and there is more widespread acceptance of the equipment. Many analysts believe that home telemonitoring will ultimately become a multibillion-dollar a year business. It is estimated that as many as 25 million Americans could have the cost of their health care reduced and their clinical outcomes improved by using the technology that is currently available. A discussion of some of the emerging markets for the use of home telemonitoring follows.

Home Health Agencies

Home health agencies and the **Visiting Nurse Association (VNA)** have embraced home telehealth and have become the largest category of provider deploying the technology. Under the home health prospective payment system (PPS), agencies receive a fixed amount for each episode of care provided to a patient. There is a strong financial incentive to lower costs by reducing the number of visits made by caregivers. As mentioned before, caregiver productivity can be significantly increased by utilizing the technology as well. Several HHAs have also been able to improve patient outcomes by using monitoring technology. With the Centers for Medicare and Medicaid Services (CMS) creating incentives for agencies based on improved outcomes, it is expected that utilization of home monitoring will increase among home health providers.

Hospital and Health System

Hospitals and health systems have utilized home telemonitoring to achieve a number of strategic and financial objectives. Several health systems use technology to reduce rates of unfunded readmission to the hospitals. Many payors do not pay for unplanned readmissions for the same diagnosis within 30 days of a discharge. With certain chronic patients, there is a high rate of unfunded readmissions that can be significantly reduced when patients are monitored at home. Other systems use technology to better manage unfunded "frequent fliers" who routinely access emergency room or hospital services.

In recent years, hospitals have used home telemonitoring technology to better manage patient flow, particularly when there is a shortage of available inpatient beds. Admission can be delayed, LOS reduced, and planned accelerated discharge protocols (PADS) supported with technology. The result of employing the technology enhances the management of admissions, discharges, and overall LOS. The financial implication for hospitals and health systems can be very significant.

Payor Organizations

An increasing number of **payor organizations** provide coverage for home telemonitoring. Payors have the greatest incentive to use this technology as the cost savings associated with home telemonitoring accrue to their benefit. Tens of thousands of dollars can be saved for patients with long-term, chronic illnesses. The reductions in emergency room utilization and subsequent hospitalizations have a significant bottom line impact to payors. Most of the patients provided with home telemonitoring are complex CHF or COPD patients who have a high likelihood of accessing acute care service if their medical condition is not carefully managed.

Government-sponsored payors such as Medicare, Medicaid, and the Department of Veterans Affairs all have limited-scale telemonitoring programs in place. Blue Cross/Blue Shield plans, health maintenance organizations (HMOs), employer-sponsored health plans, and union benefit trust funds have also offered coverage for the technology in certain markets. It is expected that coverage will grow exponentially over the next several years as a result of greater acceptance of technology and as a result of more demonstration projects being completed. It is also anticipated that the technology will be used on an expanding range of patients. Lower monitoring costs as a result of more widespread deployment should also make monitoring appropriate for a wider range of patients. It is likely that monitoring technology will be integrated with disease state management strategies.

Long-Term Care Facilities

The ability to cost-effectively monitor residents of a nursing home, a senior citizen complex, or other **long-term care facility** is a primary concern. Kiosks have been developed for this purpose and allow for the simple and convenient collection of vital sign data and the creation of a digital health record that can be shared with other healthcare professionals. The kiosk becomes a simple means to use home telehealth in any setting where groups of people routinely congregate. The use of swipe cards or patient personal identification numbers allows one device to gather data from large numbers of individuals. Quality of care and resident satisfaction with care is likely to increase, giving peace of mind to family members.

Families and Patients

There is an ever-increasing private demand for home telemonitoring. Individuals who wish to monitor their own health status, as well as the adult children of at-risk elderly parents represent a significant potential market of private pay clients. Adult children who live great distances from their parents have a need to obtain objective information on the health status of their parents so that they can help to identify issues and participate in healthcare decision making. Likewise, patients themselves are interested in accessing accurate and timely information on their health status so that they can make proper decisions on diet, exercise, and lifestyle issues.

Employers/Wellness Programs

Health care is a vital concern for employers. They have a direct financial interest in lowering costs and are financial beneficiaries of long-term illness preventive strategies. If they can monitor their workers (offering telehealth options as a wellness program), they will see many benefits for themselves, such as reduced absenteeism and increased productivity. Effective monitoring programs can ultimately lower healthcare costs and associated insurance premiums. Some companies are now exploring the creation of financial incentives for employees who achieve healthcare objectives such as appropriate weight, reduced blood pressure, and levels of exercise. Monitoring could very well be used as a means of tracking performance in this regard.

FUTURE DIRECTIONS

The technology associated with home telehealth will become much more sophisticated and integrated over time. Clearly it is expected that monitoring equipment will become less expensive. This will most likely be a result of more widespread use of the technology lowering per unit costs and the trend toward declining prices of technology in general. Monitoring equipment will become more affordable, and this affordability will spur further demand.

Another clear future direction is that home monitoring equipment will be much more portable and likely will utilize wireless technology. This will improve flexibility and ease of use dramatically, making much of the data collection invisible to the patient.

The range of activities monitored and the sophistication of the medical devices deployed will increase significantly. Sophisticated peripherals measuring lung function and blood values are already routinely integrated with home telemonitoring systems. Diagnostic equipment will be increasingly utilized, allowing many tests currently done in outpatient labs to be done by the patient at home. Monitors will also be better integrated with other medical equipment in the home, such as infusion pumps, allowing for adjustments to be made on the basis of values received.

Home monitoring systems will be integrated with an expanded array of other equipment that monitor safety and functionality. Emergency response devices, environmental safety monitors, motion sensors, activity of daily living measures, and a host of other equipment will be integrated, providing a much more comprehensive view of the patient, his/her physical status, and ability to function. It is also likely that there will be much more interactive communication with the patient that becomes part of the DHR. Patients will be able to ask caregivers questions, receive responses and information links, and to analyze their own personal data within their DHR. This will create a true data and information hub for all health-related issues.

SUMMARY

The use of home telemonitoring represents one of our society's best opportunities to significantly reduce the cost of health care while improving outcomes. It allows the entire healthcare system to become more preventive in its orientation and allows a disease state to be much better managed. This technology will once again make the patient's home the primary site for healthcare service and intervention, reversing the trend of relying on hospitals and clinics.

All of the technology exists to support this change. Electronically embedded monitoring devices, appropriate communications protocols, and decision support software are all available today. What is required to make the use of home telemonitoring more widespread are payment systems that reward the use of the technology. It is expected that this change will occur quickly, as data on telemonitoring's efficacy becomes more widespread and available.

The most important thought we would like to leave you with is that nurses need to recognize the inevitability of the shift in patient care strategies and practices that will result from widespread use of home telemonitoring. There will be a dramatic expansion in home-based healthcare services and a requirement that nurses learn to use data and technology better in managing patient care. With the greater access to data, there will be more of a clinical focus on managing trends in an illness trajectory and less focus on responding to acute incidents.

THOUGHT-PROVOKING Questions

Consider a recent patient care scenario of yours and describe how it could have been managed at a distance.

1. What training would you need?
2. What equipment would you use?
3. How would your patient and his or her family respond to home telemonitoring?

References

Craig, J., & Patterson, V. (2005). Introduction to the practice of telemedicine. *Journal of Telemedicine and Telecare, 11*(1), 3–9. Retrieved from ProQuest Psychology Journals database (Document ID: 805776671).

Health Data Management. (2007, September 4). *Report: Home monitoring growing fast.* Retrieved April 20, 2008, from http://www.healthdatamanagement.com/news/15703-1.html

Merriam-Webster's Online Dictionary [Web]. (n.d.). *Tele-*. Retrieved May 29, 2008, from http://www.merriam-webster.com/dictionary/tele-

Venable, S. (2005). A call to action: Georgia must adopt a new standard of care, licensure, reimbursement, and privacy laws for telemedicine. *Emory Law Journal, 54*(2), 1183–1217. Retrieved from Law Module database (Document ID: 875322011).

19 Telenursing and Remote Access Telehealth

Audrey Kinsella and Kathleen Albright

Objectives

1. Explore the use of telehealth technology in nursing practice.
2. Identify the socioeconomic factors likely to increase the use of telehealth interventions.
3. Describe clinical and nonclinical uses of telehealth.
4. Specify and describe the most common telehealth tools utilized in nursing practice.
5. Explore telehealth pathways and protocols.
6. Identify legal, ethical, and regulatory issues of home telehealth practice.
7. Describe the role of the telenurse.
8. Apply the Foundation of Knowledge model to home telehealth.

Key Terms

Call centers
Central stations
Chronic disease
Home health care
Home telehealth care
Medication management devices
Patient informed consent
Peripheral biometric (medical) devices
Personal emergency response system (PERS)
Portals
Real-time telehealth
Sensor and activity monitoring systems
Store-and-forward telehealth transmission
Telehealth
Telehealth care
Telemedicine
Telemonitoring
Telenursing
Telepathology
Telephony

INTRODUCTION

Telehealth is a relatively new term in our medical/nursing vocabulary, and refers to a wide range of health services that are delivered by telecommunications-ready tools, such as the telephone, videophone, and computer. The most basic of telecommunications technology, the telephone, has been used by health professionals for many years, sometimes by nurses to counsel a patient or by doctors to change a patient's plan of care. Because of these widespread uses, we are already somewhat familiar with the value of the direct, expedient contact that telecommunications-ready tools provide for healthcare professionals. The growing field of telehealth, particularly in nursing practice, will allow us to improve care delivery services even more.

Key Terms *Continued*
Teleradiology
Web servers

In the 1970s, uses of more advanced forms of telehealth in the medical field, referred to as **telemedicine**, included **teleradiology** and **telepathology**—radiological and pathological images transmitted to specialists who were located at some distance (Allan, 2006). As additional specialties such as dermatology, ophthalmology, and others entered the telemedicine arena; telehealth use enabled even more physicians to access information about their patients regardless of distances between themselves and the patients and conventional healthcare settings.

Success in telehealth was achieved after decades were spent refining the technology, which resulted in clearer imaging, more speedy transmissions, and accurate replication of data from remote locations to a central hub. Technical advances in imaging, for example, have increased the usage of telehealth in wound care and increased specialists' satisfaction with quality of patient data received from remote sites (Kinsella, 2002b). The end results of telehealth interactions today have helped to ensure that professionals—whether working off site or directly with patients—can replicate usual clinical interactions in all specialties regardless of the distance involved in the contact.

NURSING ASPECTS OF TELEHEALTH

Understanding telehealth and the potential use of telehealth technology in nursing practice is necessary in today's changing healthcare arena. As this chapter will describe, nurses using telehealth will have much greater access to their patients' conditions and needs and be able to respond in a more timely way than would have been possible using only face-to-face visits. Patients' responses to new medications, for example, can be tracked within hours rather than several days that elapsed between face-to-face visits. The telecommunications-ready tools that can be used to achieve these results will be described, and cases that have demonstrated successful outcomes highlighted.

Today, the use of many telehealth tools by nurses *is* new. Telehealth interventions or contacts are performed off site and often require less time spent on task because of the efficiencies offered by the technology applications. Their use, however, must never be associated with less care. It is important to note that nursing activity in telehealth still follows the same best practice standards as those espoused in conventional care. We should, in fact, look at the use of telehealth tools as a means for nurses to do their work better.

The following case study indicates the capability of a **home health care** nurse's working with telehealth tools to detect and respond to a patient's condition more expediently so that needed care could be accessed.

Case Study: Early Detection of a Change in Condition

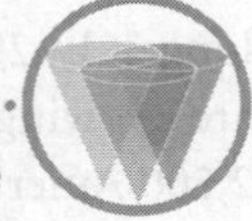

Mrs. C., an independent, 96-year-old woman, has a history of rehospitalization due to atrial fibrillation resulting from congestive heart failure (CHF) and hypertension.

After her most recent hospitalization, Mrs. C. was treated and released into home care at an agency in Washington. A home telemonitoring system that tracks and transmits patients' vital signs was placed in her home. The primary goal of placing this patient on the telemonitor was to provide daily monitoring of the patient's condition, thereby avoiding unnecessary rehospitalizations.

One morning, Mrs. C's telenurse detected an alarmingly low oxygen saturation level in the patient's transmitted data. As a result, the nurse telephoned Mrs. C. and asked her to retake her O_2 reading. The reading was confirmed and the telenurse contacted the patient's physician, who requested immediate transportation of the patient to the hospital emergency room. Medics were called and the patient was taken to the hospital, where she was diagnosed with a pulmonary embolism.

The prompt response resulted from the early detection and timely intervention enabled by the home telehealth equipment and a home health nurse's oversight. One notable fact in this case is this: although the primary goal of monitoring patients is to avoid unnecessary hospitalization, in this case, the hospitalization in fact was a necessary one for the patient as a result of her elevated blood pressure and compromised oxygen saturation levels. The patient *was still asymptomatic at the time of detection*. However, the telehealth intervention and subsequent hospitalization allowed for the embolism to be treated before any serious damage occurred.

Under the traditional home care model, this patient may only have been seen by a nurse two to three times a week. The clinician does not have knowledge of the patient's condition in between visits; however, having vital patient data tracked and transmitted daily allowed for rapid response that resulted in a positive outcome, perhaps a life-saving intervention for this patient.

DRIVING FORCES FOR TELEHEALTH

We can expect a significant increase in use of information technology tools in the coming decades in nursing venues. Its use is now and will continue to be affected by a number of factors in all of western society. We need to know these factors as drivers of the growing trend toward telehealth and technology use.

The driving factors that will influence nursing practice significantly in the next decades are demographics; nursing/healthcare worker shortages; **chronic diseases** and conditions; the new, educated consumers; and excessive costs of healthcare services that are increasing in need and kind.

Let's get even better acquainted with items on this list.

Demographics

We hear it every day: the baby boomers are getting older and people are living longer. In 2000, 13% of the American population was over 65, and the numbers are growing significantly. According to the U.S. Bureau of the Census (1993), 2,500 Americans turn 65 years old every day. Consequently, by 2040, 21% of the U.S. population—one in five Americans—will be 65 years old or older and there will be almost four times as many people over 85 as there are today, as documented by the Institute of Aging (1996). Also on the rise is the number of aged Americans living with at least one chronic disease or condition (Hoffman, Rice, & Sung, 1996), a factor alerting us to the much greater demand for planned professional care in the near future.

Nursing/Healthcare Worker Shortages

The crisis in the well-known nursing shortage is twofold: there is a greater need for nurses by more persons, particularly those living lifetimes with sometimes multiple comorbidities; and there is a significant decrease in the number of young persons entering the nursing profession. There are currently 2.9 million registered nurses (RNs) in the United States, with well over 41% of them aged 50 years old or older (U.S. Department of Health and Human Services, 2004). But nationwide, the demand for nurses is clearly exceeding supply. A recent report from the Health Resources and Services Administration (HRSA) (U.S. Department of Health and Human Services, 2002) on the shortage of RNs notes that the shortage is expected to rise from 6% today to 12% by 2010, and more than triple in size to 20% as soon as 2015.

The very serious shortage of healthcare workers in the United States must be addressed with some foresight. Although we are currently seeing more focus on training lay people such as aides and other paraprofessionals in certain nursing tasks, this venture certainly cannot replicate the clinical expertise of trained nurses skilled in nursing routines. We must, therefore, begin to look seriously at using effective adjuncts to skilled care, telehealth being one of these important adjuncts. Some have already begun to do so. For one, a recent study by the Pennsylvania Homecare Association and Penn State University (2004) looked at how telehealth can be used to address workforce issues in the home healthcare industry and determined that telehealth use may enhance nurses' job satisfaction and help to retain nurses in their current positions.

Chronic Diseases and Conditions

Chronic conditions are the leading cause of illness, disability, and death in the United States today. The aging population living with chronic diseases and conditions is expected to increase dramatically in the United States in the next decades. But many age groups are also affected by chronic diseases, not just the elderly. Currently, more than 100 million Americans are living with one or more chronic diseases or conditions. The costs of their direct medical care are excessive—as much as $539 billion a year, according to the Institute of Aging's 1996 report, *Chronic Care in America: A 21st Century Challenge.* As noted in a more recent report, from the Centers for Disease Control and Prevention (2005), medical care costs of people with chronic diseases account for more than 75% of the United States' $1.4 trillion medical care expenditures. Furthermore, by the year 2030, 148 million Americans will join these ranks, at least one third of them limited in their ability to go to school or to live independently. Securing appropriate, adequate, and affordable care services for these populations should be a national concern.

Educated Consumers

The wave of today's aging baby boomers is driving some of the usual health service practices toward a very different course. Many of these individuals are more educated than their parents and more comfortable with use of technology. They want to become more informed and involved with their care plans. These empowered consumers will be financially motivated with the introduction of consumer-directed healthcare plans that will reward healthier lifestyles and better disease management of chronic conditions. All of these circumstances will further drive the use of and the innovation of new technologies to meet consumer need. However, as Kinsella (2002a) has pointed out, this new consumer-driven trend of which the boomers are a part will not only be affected by technological innovation but will in fact affect *how* healthcare services are delivered. New plans for this new generation of consumers are very much leaning toward meeting their demands for when-needed, as-needed care—or, care services delivered on their own terms and timing.

Economics

When we connect the drivers of today's healthcare market—the demographics, nursing shortages, and increased number of persons living with chronic conditions and their extensive use of healthcare services—with excessive costs of this health care, the need for solutions is, simply, vital. The American healthcare system spends $1.4 trillion per year on conventional medical care. Much more should be expected to be spent annually in the coming decades. And so, we must ask: taking all of the driving factors of today's healthcare market into account, what do we need to do to address healthcare issues in the United States and meet the burgeoning numbers and needs of patients?

A solution is to develop a new clinical model for American health care that includes technology. And most particularly, telehealth technology should be included to fill the gap resulting from an overabundance of patients and a scarcity of healthcare providers. This concept is indicated in Figure 19-1.

Consider the use of technology that can fill current gaps in our healthcare system. Tools of telehealth can, for example, help render needed services without requiring in-person professional care at all contacts. The remote or virtual visit made by skilled clinicians is only one approach to using a range of health technologies available today. We need to learn much more about what telehealth is, how it works, and what aspects have been successful so that we can plan to incorporate its use into routine clinical care.

TELEHEALTH CARE

Let's start with a basic definition of **telehealth care**. Keep in mind, however, that telehealth is an emerging field, and definitions are subject to change and improvement as technology evolves. As recently defined by the American Telemedicine Association (2007):

> Telemedicine is the use of medical information exchanged from one site to another via electronic communications to improve patients' health status.

FIGURE 19-1
Technology fills the gap.

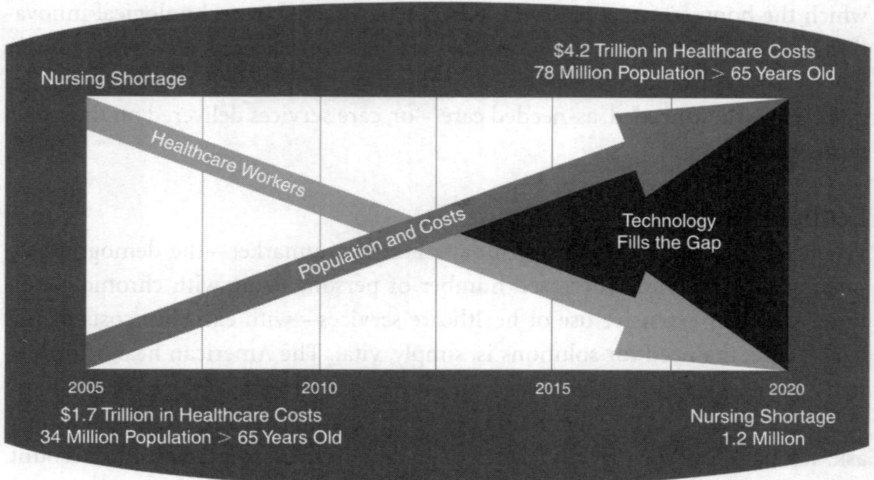

> Closely associated with telemedicine is the term "telehealth," which is often used to encompass a broader definition of remote healthcare that does not always involve clinical services. Videoconferencing, transmission of still images, e-health including patient portals, remote monitoring of vital signs, continuing medical education and nursing call centers are all considered part of telemedicine and telehealth. (¶ 1–3).

Indeed, "telehealth" is generally used as an umbrella term to describe all of the possible variations of healthcare services that use telecommunications. Telehealth can refer, as well, to clinical and nonclinical uses of health-related contacts. Delivery of patient education such as menu planning for diabetic patients or the transmission of medication reminders are examples of health-promoting aspects of telehealth.

Clinical Uses of Telehealth

Let's look at a few clinical uses for telehealth technologies and some sample clinical applications. These include:

1. Transmitting images for assessment or diagnosis. One example is transmission of digital images such as images of wounds for assessment and treatment consults.
2. Transmitting clinical data for assessment, diagnosis, or disease management. One example is remote patient monitoring and transmitting patients' objective and/or subjective clinical data such as vital signs monitoring and answers to disease management questions.
3. Providing disease prevention and promotion of good health. One example is telephonic case management and patient education provided through asthma and weight management programs conducted in schools.
4. Using telephonic health advice in emergent cases. One example is performing teletriage in call centers.
5. Using real-time video. One example is exchanging health services or education live via videoconference.

Telehealth Transmission Formats and Their Clinical Applications

Nurses must become familiar with the many and varied clinical and nonclinical transmission formats and applications of telehealth technologies so that they can make informed choices about the tools that are available for their use, as needed. Among these applications are store-and-forward telehealth, real-time telehealth, remote monitoring, and telephony.

Store-and-forward telehealth. In a **store-and-forward telehealth transmission**, digital images, video, audio, and clinical data are captured and stored on the client computer or device; then, at a convenient time, the data are transmitted securely (forwarded) to a specialist/clinician at another location where they are studied by the relevant specialist/clinician. If indicated, the opinion of the specialist/clinician is then transmitted back. Based on the requirements of the participating healthcare entities, this round-trip interaction could take from minutes to 48 hours. In many store-and-forward specialties, such as teleradiology, an immediate response is not critical. Dermatology, radiology, and pathology are common specialties that are conducive to store-and-forward technologies. Transmission of wound care images for assessment by specialty care nurses and/or other specialists has become a frequently used and important form of home telehealth nursing practice.

Real-time (or interactive) telehealth. In **real-time telehealth**, a telecommunications link between the involved parties allows a real-time or live interaction to take place. Videoconferencing equipment is one of the most common forms of technologies used in synchronous telehealth. There are also peripheral devices that can be attached to computers or to the videoconferencing equipment that can aid in an interactive examination. Use of computers for real-time two-way audio and video streaming between centers over ever-improving and cheaper communication channels is becoming common. These developments have contributed to lowering of costs in telehealth.

Examples of real-time clinical telehealth applications include:

- Telemental health—which uses videoconferencing technology to connect a psychiatric nurse with a mental health client.
- Telerehabilitation—which uses videocameras and other technologies to assess patients' progress in home rehabilitation.
- Telehomecare—which uses video technologies to observe/assess/teach patients living in rural areas.
- Teleconsultations—which use a variety of technologies to enable collaborative exchanges or consultations between individuals or among groups that are involved with a case. These teleconsults may be transmitted live using videoconferencing technology. They may, for instance, involve teaching a certain technique to a less-experienced clinician or they may provide several clinicians with an opportunity for discussing an appropriate approach to a difficult case.
- Telehospice/telepalliative care—can use real-time and/or remote monitoring to provide psychological support to patients and/or caregivers. Telehealth devices can also play a role in symptom management, in effect helping end-of-life patients to achieve an optimum quality of life.

Remote monitoring (telemonitoring or remote patient monitoring). In remote monitoring, devices are used to capture and transmit biometric data. For example, a tele-EEG device monitors the electrical activity of a patient's brain and then transmits that data to an assigned specialist. This interaction could be done in either real time or as a stored and then forwarded transmission.

Examples of **telemonitoring** include:

- Monitoring patient parameters during home-based nocturnal dialysis.
- Cardiac and multiparameter monitoring of remote ICUs.
- Home telehealth, in which examples can include daily home telemonitoring of vital signs by patients and transmitting data that enables off-site nurses to track their patients regularly and precisely and address noticeable changes through education/information suggestions about diet or exercise.
- Disease management.

***Telephony. Telephone monitoring** (telephony)* is the most basic type of telehealth. It can be described as scheduled remote care delivery or monitoring in which scheduled patient encounters via the telephone occur between a healthcare provider and a patient or caregiver (Quality Insights of Pennsylvania, 2005). More details about interaction using telephony are provided in the "Applications of Telenursing in Home Care" section.

Nonclinical Uses of Telehealth Technologies

There are also many nonclinical uses of telehealth technologies. Currently, these include:

- Distance education including continuing medical and nursing education, grand rounds, and patient education
- Administrative uses including meetings among telehealth networks, supervision, and presentations
- Research using the Internet and other online sources for information and health data management

All of these telecommunications-assisted activities overcome obstacles of distance and provide access to needed health-related information. Clearly, with telehealth, the range of patient care possibilities broadens significantly.

TELENURSING

Where do nurses using telehealth, as in telenursing, play a role in today's healthcare delivery arena? **Telenursing** refers to the use of telecommunications and information technology for providing nursing services in health care to enhance care whenever a physical distance exists between patient and nurse or between any number of nurses (Skiba, 1998). As a clinical field, telenursing is part of telehealth and has many points of contacts with other medical and nonmedical applications, such as telediagnosis, teleconsultation, and telemonitoring. Telenurses do not, in effect, work outside of the broader clinical team effort, no matter where they are located. They are indeed an integral part of the healthcare delivery team.

Applications of Telenursing in Home Care

The most developing area of telenursing today is in **home telehealth care.** An accepted definition of home telehealth care provided by Kinsella (2004) is as follows: "Home telehealth care is clinician-driven remote care delivery and education services that are delivered to the home via telecommunications-ready tools" (p. 36).

As home telehealth care evolved, the definition has expanded to include a broader arena of delivery. In fact, some have defined the home as anywhere outside of an acute inpatient setting, and so includes nursing homes, assisted living facilities, and other living situations beyond the single family home or apartment. And wherever the home setting may be, people want to be cared for there. The burgeoning senior population today, in particular, has become quite vocal about this preference. According to regular surveys by the American Association for Retired Persons (AARP) (AARP, 1996), more than 90% of seniors want to remain independent at home and age in a familiar place. Care at home is clearly a key concern and preference.

Fortuitously, today, the reach of nurses using telecommunications-ready tools in the home is now remarkably extended. Not only are the settings for home care extended beyond what was usual (the family home) in the last 4 decades of home health's formal existence, but the types of services delivered to the home are more advanced than ever before. The home care industry's newest challenge is to work with sicker patients, many of whom have been discharged from hospitals to home earlier than in the past.

This challenge to extend the range of conventional home care is why telehealth can be (and needs to be) provided to a wide range of patients, including those who:

- are immobilized
- live in remote or difficult-to-reach places
- have chronic ailments, such as chronic obstructive pulmonary disease, diabetes, and congestive heart disease
- have debilitating diseases, such as neural degenerative diseases (Parkinson's disease, Alzheimer's disease, amyotrophic lateral sclerosis)

All of these patients may stay at home and be "visited" and assisted regularly by a nurse via videoconferencing, Internet, videophone, or other telecommunications means. These telecommunications-ready tools enable home telenurses to follow through at those advanced levels of care, as needed.

Still other varied applications of home telehealth care are the care of patients in immediate postsurgical situations, those needing care of wounds and ostomies, and handicapped individuals needing physical therapy interventions or telerehabilitation. In addition to this extended range of patients who can be served with telehealth, many more patients can be seen as well when telehealth is used. For example, in conventional home health care, depending on the distances of travel involved, one nurse is able to visit up to seven patients per day. Using telenursing, however, one nurse can remotely visit or televisit 12–16 patients in the same amount of time using interactive telehealth. Over the last decade, efficiencies of telenursing have become well documented, as have the resulting improved patient care outcomes that can be expected by frequent telecontact.

Another outpatient application of telenursing is telephony-based **call centers**, which may be operated by managed care organizations, hospitals, and other health organizations. Some call centers include telemonitoring services as well, which allows the patients to stay at home and use different telehealthcare devices to transmit biometric and other medical information back to the call center. Monitoring can be intermittent or continuous. This use of the teletechnology allows the clinicians to evaluate patients' status and use the data to make decisions to better manage patients' health conditions.

Are call centers' services comparable to conventional hands-on care in the home? Many features certainly are. For instance, call centers are typically staffed by registered nurses who act as case managers or perform patient triage. These professionals can provide information and counseling to patients as part of a disease management program and as a means to educate them on their disease process. In effect, their goal is to offer appropriate access to care (from nurses at the call centers) and help patients to prevent avoidable ER visits and rehospitalizations. An example of this assistance would include a nurse calling (i.e., not waiting for a patient to contact the call center) a recently discharged diabetic patient on a regularly scheduled basis to evaluate progress at home, activity tolerance, medication compliance, foot care, and diet management. This empowering of patients towards self-management is a very significant and needed part of telenursing.

Home care telenursing can also involve other activities such as providing customized patient education in dietary or exercise needs, nursing teleconsultations, review of results of medical tests and exams, and assistance to physicians in the implementation of medical treatment protocols. The work can be wide ranging; for example, there are some home-based telecardiology programs that involve the patient, the family, the physician, and a specialized cardiac monitoring center. A multidisciplinary approach is used along with best practice-defined protocols to manage the patient, improve the patient's quality of life, and reduce healthcare costs—most particularly reduced hospitalization costs. Nurses play a key role in this network of care.

By reviewing all of these examples of telenursing practice, we can see, in effect, that nurses using telenursing can broaden their involvement in the targeted care of each of their patients. It is predicted, in fact, that home care will soon become a hub of all patient activity—the home will be where care that is begun in hospitals and other settings will be managed over the very long term and in the most cost-effective healthcare setting. Home care telenurses can well expect to play a vital and dynamic role in the changing delivery systems that are to be in place in the next decades.

TOOLS OF HOME TELEHEALTH

There is a wide and growing range of telecommunications-ready tools readily available for nurses' and patients' use in the home. Let's examine each of these tools in more detail.

Central Stations, Web Servers, and Portals

Central stations, **Web servers**, and **portals** are various terms presently used for multifunctional telehealthcare platforms and application servers. The terms indicate clinical management software programs that receive and display patients' vital signs as well as other information transmitted from a medical device, including blood pressure and glucose information. This transmission is most commonly accomplished over plain old telephone system lines (POTS); however, network access as well as wireless communication is gaining popularity as technology advances and access improves.

Central stations/Web servers are key components to telehealth that can be as minimal as a single screen display or may be more comprehensive software applications that provide various functions including triaging the data according to medical alerts, which allows clinicians to quickly identify patients requiring immediate attention. Other features found in these packages allow clinicians to build personal medical records for patients and provide trended patient data and analysis reports supporting improved patient outcomes using telehealth. In addition, some of the software packages provide remote programming capabilities that allow the clinician to remotely program the medical device in the patient's home. This application can change monitoring report times for patients, individualized alert parameters, set up reminders, and send educational content to a patient.

Peripheral Biometric (Medical) Devices

Peripheral biometric (medical) devices can consist of fully integrated systems such as a vital signs monitor, or they may be stand-alone telecommunications-ready devices such as blood pressure cuffs and blood glucose meters. Many plug directly into the household telephone jack to send data to a central server location.

There is an ever-increasing number of peripheral devices coming to market. Some examples of other peripheral devices seen in home telehealth today include pulse oximeters; prothrombin time, international normalized ratio (PT/INR) meters; spirometers; peak flow meters; ECG monitors; and card readers/writers that utilize smart card technology and enable multiple users to utilize one device.

Telephones

Telephones are already the most familiar household communications tool used in telehealth care. A telephone device can also be augmented for easier use by patients, as needed, with a lighted dial pad, an auto-dial system, and/or louder ringer.

Videocameras/Videophones

Videocameras and videophones are easily available consumer items that can be used in telehealth for show-and-tell demonstrations by nurses for patients or to capture wound healing progress, among other applications. Typically, these products can operate as a standard phone or as a video picture phone, using standard telephone lines to transmit information or interactions. It should be noted that the image quality over a POTS is limited by the bandwidth of POTS technology. It favors assessment rather than diagnostic quality images. These imaging capabilities will improve as integrated services digital network (ISDN) lines become more widely available in the home environment. Typically, medical centers and hospitals have access to larger bandwidth capabilities for image transmission and viewing, thus assuring high-quality diagnostic images and point-to-point consultations in hospital- or medical center-based settings.

Personal Emergency Response Systems

Personal emergency response systems (PERSs) are well-known signaling devices worn as a pendant or otherwise made easily accessible to patients to ensure their safety and to access emergency care when needed, usually in case of a fall. A preset telephone number is alerted by the patient's pushing a button on the pendant, and predesignated emergency help is dispatched. Many newer sensor options for tracking patients at home are being incorporated into multifunctioning PERS devices, such as alerting a central call center to water flooding or smoke in a patient's home. See the next section for details on these sensors and monitors.

Sensor and Activity-Monitoring Systems

Sensor and activity-monitoring systems can track activities of daily living of seniors and other at-risk individuals in their place of residence. The sensors/monitoring systems can provide insight into behavior changes that might signal changes or deterioration of health status. These technologies consist of wireless motion sensors that are strategically placed around the residence and can detect motion on a 24-hour basis.

One authority on these new technologies, David J. Stern, describes their operation further (Stern, 2007), noting that data from these sensors are wirelessly sent to a receiver and base station that periodically transmits the information to a centralized server through standard phone lines. Sophisticated algorithms analyze the data, compiling each individual's normal patterns of behavior including bathroom usage, sleep disturbance, meal preparation, medication interaction, and general levels of activity including fall detection. Deviations from these norms can be important warning signs of emerging health problems and can enable caregivers to intervene early.

In addition to widely used fire, security, and home gas detectors, there are other sensors that can monitor appliances to detect whether a household appliance is turned on or off and can sometimes switch the appliance on and off for the resident. Typical applications for affixing programmable sensors can include lamps, television sets, irons, and kitchen stoves. Such sensors might be very valuable for ensuring the safety of elderly, forgetful persons who live alone. One excellent example of today's sensor use for assistance with the elderly are sensors placed in or on stovetops to alert the user when he or she is standing too close to the equipment or when the kettle has overboiled. Benefits realized from these technologies include enabling people to live independently with an improved quality of life. They can also provide peace of mind for other family members living at a distance.

Medication Management Devices

Medication management devices are addressing a well-recognized major problem in health care today—medication management and compliance. According to the American Heart Association (2007), 49% of Americans use prescription drugs. In fact, 32 million people are taking three or more medications daily, with even more medications typically being taken by those 65 years of age or older.

What has become a national problem in health care today is the failure of patients to take medications as prescribed. Failing to do so can have devastating consequences, particularly for those patients living with chronic illnesses. Here are some of the facts about medication management and compliance in the United States, based on data from the National Pharmaceutical Council (2003):

- The cost of hospital admissions is an estimated $8.5 billion annually just for patients who do not take their medications as prescribed.
- About 23% of all nursing home admissions are due to failure to take medications as prescribed.
- About 10% of all hospital admissions are related to improper self-administration of medication.
- People who miss medication doses need three times as many doctor visits as others and face increased medical costs.

To address some of these very pressing problems, there are a host of telecommunications-ready medication devices available and many new ones in development. Some are as simple as a watch that reminds a person to take medications, others are pill organizers with audible reminders, and some actually can be programmed to dispense prefilled containers with medications and alert a patient or caregiver of a missed dose. Furthermore, there are medication tools that send data from the device back to a central server so that patients' medication compliance can be tracked. These telecommunications-ready devices can organize, manage, dispense, or remind, and they can play an increasingly important role in helping people live independently and manage their disease processes through medication compliance.

Special Needs Telecommunications-Ready Devices

Special needs telecommunications ready-devices can include preprogrammed, multifunctional infusion pumps for providing a range of infusion needs, including medications for pain management and other infusion delivery needs such as hydration and nutrition; peak flow meters, ECG monitors, and so on. Many such tools are in development to meet the more demanding and challenging needs of today's at-home patients. The common goal among all of these tools is that of increasing communications between the nurse and patient and providing the opportunity to effectively increase nurses' knowledge of their patients' status in a timely manner.

HOME TELEHEALTH PRACTICE AND PROTOCOLS

The tools of telehealth described above are devices that enable remote care delivery, enhance patient care, and improve outcomes. They should be incorporated into nursing practice as nurses would typically use, for example, a blood pressure cuff. It is important to note that the data received from these tools is useless without some type of clinical oversight. The tools do not replace the nurse—rather they give the nurse the ability to make more informed clinical decisions based on reliable data and a comprehensive picture of the patient's status. In home care they also direct the clinical resources to patients based on need. It becomes a patient-centered approach to care that delivers improved patient outcomes and clinical efficiencies.

Home telehealth is indeed a practice. It is a change in our current clinical model of practice for home care. We integrate the use of the telehealth tools into the practice to improve patient outcomes. But like any tool, the effectiveness is directly proportional to its application and use. Let's look more closely at how telehealth is being used to date.

Home telehealth programs will differ depending on the type of technology used and the foci of the telehealth programs. However, every program should have telehealth use criteria established. The guidelines discussed here are broad-based, generic clinical guidelines for the deployment of home telehealth developed by the Home Telehealth Special Interest Group of the American Telemedicine Association (ATA, 2002).

The first guideline focuses on ensuring that the home is suitable for home telehealth delivery; and the second example focuses on ensuring that patients sign an informed consent form *prior* to receiving telehealth services. During the initial face-to-face visit, an assessment should be conducted to determine access to utilities and safety concerns appropriate for the installation of the equipment. Informed written consent must be obtained from the client or designee before beginning the use of telehealth consultations. The consent should be part of the plan of care and stored in the clinical record. These and similar guidelines issued by other health organizations including the American Nurses Association (ANA, 2001) and the Community Health Accreditation Program (CHAP, whose guidelines are not publicly available to nonmembers) can apply to both interactive home telehealth and telemonitored activity. Patient criteria should have inclusion and exclusion guidelines established, detailing who is eligible and appropriate for each type of technology. Other criteria include establishing policies and procedures that address patient enrollment, education, and equipment setup, patient/caregiver and home assessment, **patient informed consent,** as well as privacy and confidentiality rights. In addition, a clinical plan of care that is specific to patient needs should be developed. Telehealth pathways and protocols ensure more focused work with patients and allow for targeted interventions. A sample pathway to use for a patient who is being remotely monitored is provided in Figure 19-2. Home health agencies may use such samples as templates from which to design their own in-house, customized guidelines for home telenursing practice.

In addition, in Figure 19-3, a sample protocol is provided for telemonitoring patients living with hypertension. As with use of the pathway in Figure 19-2,

FIGURE 19-2
Sample clinical pathway.

Hypertension
Daily Home Monitoring Pathway

Client Name: ______________________ **SOC:** __________

POC/Visit Frequency: 2w1, 1w8 with daily home monitoring until end of episode.
2 PRN visits to assess cardiovascular status based upon data received from daily home monitoring.
***Visits may be reduced throughout the episode based upon client assessment, daily home monitoring and the achievement of goals.**

GOALS OF DAILY HOME MONITORING & INTERMITTENT SKILLED SERVICES

1) Increase client knowledge regarding the disease process, treatment and management of hypertension utilizing the clinical data received from daily home monitoring.
2) Client will comply with treatment regimen and lifestyle changes to promote the optimum level of functioning at the time of discharge.
3) Improve clinical outcomes through the review of daily and trended data, allowing for early detection and intervention.
4) Maintain BP within parameters to avoid rehospitalization/ED visits allowing the client to remain at home with focus on self-management.

WEEK ONE: 2w1

Visit One: ______________________

- ☐ Admission SOC/OASIS
- ☐ Assess client/caregiver/home for daily home monitoring
- ☐ Initiate client/caregiver teaching as indicated
- ☐ Skilled interventions as ordered
- ☐ Evaluate appropriate parameters
- ☐ Add daily home monitoring to 485
- ☐ Installation of monitor and transmission of baseline vital signs

Visit Two: ______________________

- ☐ Installation and inservice of home monitor
- ☐ Client assessment
- ☐ Continue client/caregiver teaching as indicated
- ☐ Skilled interventions as ordered
- ☐ Discharge planning
- ☐ Assess appropriateness of parameters
- ☐ Other: ______________________

WEEK TWO: Nine: 1w8 and prn SNV based upon data from daily home monitoring

Skilled Nursing Visits:

- ☐ Client assessment
- ☐ Client/caregiver teaching as indicated
- ☐ Skilled interventions as ordered
- ☐ Confer with central station clinician as required
- ☐ Discharge planning
- ☐ Oversight and coordination of home care services and disciplines
- ☐ Assess need for continuing daily monitoring after discharge from home healthcare services
- ☐ Other: ______________________

Daily Home Monitoring:

- ☐ Daily review of clinical data
- ☐ Contact client to obtain additional subjective data if needed
- ☐ Reinforce client teaching
- ☐ Provide early detection and intervention as needed
- ☐ Confer with CM to review client status
- ☐ Weekly review of trends to evaluate client status and identify subtle changes in condition
- ☐ Fax trend reports to physician per protocol
- ☐ Assess need for continuing monitor after discharge from home care

Date	Initials	Signature

continues

FIGURE 19-2
Continued.

Client/Caregiver Teaching Client/Caregiver Demonstrates/Verbalizes:	Goal Met	Not Met	N/A	Variance
1. Goal, purpose and importance of daily home monitoring related to disease process and management of hypertension. (↓ ED visits/hospitalizations)				
2. Demonstrates correct use of Honeywell HomMed monitor and identified peripherals.				
3. Early warning signs and symptoms of hypertension and when to call 911, MD, or the agency.				
4. Measures to avoid long-term complications of hypertension.				
5. Factors affecting hypertension and preventive measures/lifestyle changes to promote or improve health.				
6. Importance of MD follow-up visits.				
7. Medications: Indications, dosage, timing, route, desired, and adverse effects.				
8. Compliance with medication regimen.				
9. Importance of diet modifications and restrictions including sodium, cholesterol, calories, and fluid balance.				
10. Compliance with diet and fluid regimen.				
11. Importance of rest, exercise, energy conservation, and pacing activities following MD guidelines.				
12. Importance of lab testing and relation of results to the continuing treatment plan.				
13. Importance of daily maintenance or improvement of VS within individually set parameters.				
14. Health-promoting behaviors at or before discharge.				

VARIANCE CODES

V1: Client physically/cognitively unable
V2: Client refuses/noncompliant
V3: Client hospitalized
V4: Client terminated services
V5: Client transferred
V6: Client moved
V7: Client expired
V8: Client other__________
V9: Caregiver none/absent
V10: Caregiver refuses
V11: Caregiver not capable
V12: Caregiver other__________
V13: Assistive aids unavailable______
V14: Assistive aid other______
V15: Environment unsafe______
V16: Environment other______
V17: New diagnosis/Comorbidity
V18: Exacerbation of disease
V19: Client no longer meets criteria for HHC
V20: Other:__________
V21: Other:__________
V22: Other:__________
V23: Other:__________
V24: Other:__________

FIGURE 19-3
Protocol for CHF.

Telemonitoring Disease Management Protocol
Chronic Heart Failure

Overview: To increase the efficiency of healthcare resouce utilization and to improve patient health status, care coordination will be enhanced with the daily collection of patient specific objective and subjective data via the HomeMed Monitor.

GOALS:

1) Improve clinical outcomes through daily collection and review of patient's objective and subjective data allowing for early detection and intervention.
2) Increase patient knowledge regarding the disease process, treatment, and management of the disease utilizing the clinical data received from daily home monitoring.
3) Improve patient compliance with treatment regimen and lifestyle changes for promotion of health and optimal daily life functioning.
4) Promote patient independence and enhance behavior modification through daily vital sign awareness and follow-up.
5) Increase patient satisfaction through avoided rehospitalizations/ED visits/inappropriate clinic utilization and promotion of self-management in home.

CARE MANAGEMENT OVERVIEW: PATIENT IDENTIFICATION AND EDUCATION

Home Monitoring Patient Identification/ Installation

- ☐ Admit patient into monitoring program
- ☐ Provide phone notification to patient to introduce daily home monitoring
- ☐ Explain benefits of home monitoring, discuss location of monitor, and identify scheduled daily monitoring time(s)
- ☐ Evaluate appropriateness of home monitor based on diagnosis/secondary diagnoses, family dynamics, and home situation
- ☐ Customize monitor with programmed subjective questions and/or peripheral medical devices for individual patient need(s)
- ☐ Install and instruct patient on use of HomeMed monitor and transmit baseline vital signs
- ☐ Provide written monitor instructions
- ☐ Verify vital sign transmission, set patient-specific vital sign parameters (alert limits), and activiate "CHF alert" within central station

Patient/Caregiver/Family Education

- ☐ Provide basic disease process educational information: *What is Congestive Heart Failure?*
- ☐ Give diet, sodium, and fluid recommendations based on patient condition
- ☐ Provide medication education: Indications, dosage, timing, route, adverse effects
- ☐ Stress importance of maintaining MD appointments
- ☐ Educate patient about basic vital sign awareness, appropriate ranges, and when follow-up occurs based on vital sign values
- ☐ Teach patient recognition of common signs and symptoms
- ☐ Explain when, how, and whom to notify when symptoms occur
- ☐ Explain goals and benefits of daily home monitoring
- ☐ Instruct patient on answering disease-specific questions and the purpose of subjective questions

CARE MANAGEMENT OVERVIEW: DAILY MONITORING

Daily Review and Response of Clinical Data

- ☐ Patient objective and subjective data monitored daily by a skilled clinician
- ☐ Review of color-coded, triaged (stratified), and trended clinical data to determine follow-up
- ☐ Contact patient for further assessment if vital signs dictate
- ☐ Provide education, positive reinforcement, and follow-up to patient during phone contact to enhance behavior modification
- ☐ Facilitate visit to clinic, home, hospital, or other based on data gathered from home monitor

Ongoing Review and Response of Clinical Data

- ☐ Evaluate patient status and identify subtle changes in condition via weekly trend review
- ☐ Reinforce patient teaching, medication compliance, etc.
- ☐ Provide early detection and intervention as needed
- ☐ Work collaboratively with healthcare personnel to maximize efficiency
- ☐ Review vital sign parameters (alert limits) based upon patient condition
- ☐ Evaluate clinical progress and response to teaching via periodic documentation review

nursing agencies may use this sample as a template for better managing these chronic disease patients and use it as a template to design other in-house protocols for telemanaging patients living with other chronic diseases. These protocols will provide a focused start for nurses to learn and use home telehealth correctly and consistently.

Clearly, by using the protocol for patients who regularly use telehealth equipment for tracking their status, nurses will receive a good deal more targeted information than is possible by scheduled, in-person visits. And as a result, the use of telehealth tools, together with clinical oversight/practice, allows for more efficient and effective clinical management by allowing the patients' needs to drive the care. As home telehealth protocols are utilized more extensively, the improved clinical and operational efficiencies may ultimately impact the home care agencies' bottom lines.

Let's understand this clinically driven, as-needed approach to care services more fully so that it is not misunderstood as providing less care. In the following case study, a proactive, patient-centered approach enabled a home healthcare agency to identify early exacerbations in a patient's condition and take appropriate action.

Case Study: Home Telemonitoring of Multiple Chronic Illnesses

The focus patient is a 71-year-old male patient who suffers with stage 4 cardiomyopathy/pulmonary hypertension, atrial fibrillation, COPD, and type 2 diabetes mellitus. This patient has been an active patient with a home healthcare agency in Michigan since November 28, 2000, with an admitting diagnosis of CHF.

Initially, the patient was seen three times a week by an RN for CHF assessment and management. The patient's history included frequent hospitalizations for exacerbation of CHF and uncontrolled atrial fibrillation. He encountered a total of four hospitalizations in the year prior to placing a telemonitoring system in his home, after about 6 months of receiving conventional home care.

Ever since he was placed on a telemonitoring system for daily tracking more than 8 months ago, he has not been rehospitalized. The telemonitoring interactions with his nurse have made him very conscientious of the role that his medications, diet, and fluid restrictions play in his overall health status.

In addition, the telemonitor has proven its benefits to local physicians. The patient's family physician, cardiologist, and pulmonologist all were able to better care for their patient with the tabular and graphical trends that were elicited from the daily vital signs monitor. This information aided in the titration and addition of the various medications needed to control the patient's CHF/atrial fibrillation. The physicians were able to ascertain the response to the medication adjustments as well as other treatment modalities such as O_2 titration. At the start of care, the patient's weight was 196 pounds and is now at a stable 187 pounds, with the symptoms more controlled than they have ever been.

The patient's nurses, meanwhile, have peace of mind knowing they can keep an eye on their patient daily while making additional visits as needed, with the documentation to justify the additional nursing visit. This tool can also be incorporated into the nurses' care plan, enabling a higher standard of care to the patient.

At present, the patient is being case managed by nursing staff visits of once per month. He now enjoys a newfound peace of mind and security as well as an improved state of health—something this patient has not experienced in over a year.

LEGAL, ETHICAL, AND REGULATORY ISSUES

Telehealth is affected by certain legal, ethical, and regulatory issues of which nurses should be aware. In the United States, interstate practice of telenursing, for example, requires attending nurses to be licensed to practice in all of the states in which they provide telehealth services. Legal issues such as accountability for practice and the potential for and definition of malpractice are still largely unresolved concerns that are difficult to address, according to attorney and medical doctor Barry Cepelewicz (2003). Nurses must be vigilant about keeping extensive documentation of their visits on-site and off. Charges of negligence, for instance, can be countered by nurses' providing documented evidence of visits and interventions made to their patients, particularly when the nurses were located off site.

In addition, there are many considerations related to patient confidentiality and safety of clinical data. Precautions that simply must be taken include ensuring that patients sign informed consent releases to receive telehealth services. When the patient is presented with the informed consent form, the nurse must assure the patient that physiological data such as blood pressure readings that will be transmitted over telephone lines or other public communication means will be kept confidential and protected. In addition, for safety considerations, pointed efforts must be continually undertaken by the nurses' agencies to upgrade information systems to ensure that a high level of data security is provided at all times.

A DAY IN THE LIFE OF A HOME TELENURSE

Within the range of available telehealth tools, telenurses must choose tools that are appropriate to the patients' needs and capabilities. A very important consideration is whether the patient can perform what is expected. Take, for instance, an automated weight scale to be used daily to track an elderly CHF patient's weight status. Simple procedures for patients using these devices are typically unplugging the telephone from the household telephone jack, plugging in the scale to the phone jack, stepping on the scale, pushing a send button, and replugging the telephone. Weight readings received at a central nursing station are accurate and timed on the patient's stored record.

Certainly the procedure is automated and low touch. However, there is also ample room for patient/nurse contact, most particularly if a weight gain is noted by the patient's nurse. The following is an example of usual telephone contact procedures made by one telenurse, Mary Bondmass, who responds to her CHF patients' 2-pound weight gain in the past 24 hours with what she calls "teaching opportunities" (quoted in Kinsella, 1998).

> Typically, Bondmass reports, she asks patients who showed a weight increase: "What did you have for dinner last night?" Then, "Tell me what you've been eating this week." Hmm, Chinese take-out again.
>
> She might then say, "Sounds like a lot of salt," which would then lead into the "teaching opportunity" about salt intake and fluid retention that the patient should have heard at least once before. Mary, the nurse, might say: "Look at your ankles," which may be swollen with retained fluids; or, if she noted a shortness of breath, indicating fluid in the lungs, she would point that out. Patients would then get an immediate, practical lesson in cause, effect, and correctable actions for managing and preventing fluid retention. (p. 47)

This case well illustrates one nurse's contention (Bernier, 2001) about the value of home telehealth: she notes that with home telehealth, nurses are working "at a distance but not in the dark" (p. 640). Nurses can see how patients are managing from the data sent and identify the interventions that might be needed to correct problems.

Many telenurses have their patients' weight information and alerts of gains automatically transferred to their pagers and use the telephone to call the patient and reinforce details for, say, CHF patients' newly learned dietary routines. At that time, the nurses may also request an order from a physician for a diuretic for the patient, doing so in a more timely manner than would likely be the case with less frequent patient–nurse in-person contact. In fact, with relatively long periods (days) between in-person visits, many patients seek help at emergency rooms for troubled breathing and pain—symptoms that might well be identified and corrected more speedily through telehealth interventions.

THE PATIENT'S ROLE IN TELEHEALTH

The range and sophistication of home telehealth tools is expanding regularly, and a concern by nurses when choosing appropriate tools for their patients is to ask, will my patient use this device? Elderly patients may find the monitoring technology that may speak to them in their homes and videocameras to assist in wound care tracking a daunting introduction to home health care. To assuage the possible discomfort, these and other such tools have undergone much iteration so that they are easier to use and the capability to be turned on and off assured. When patients are scheduled for a televisit, these devices can be turned on and used. This use by patients is key, of course, so that the information we need about them will be gathered and transmitted so that needs can be acted upon by telenurses.

The importance of ensuring patient satisfaction with home health service delivery was predicted to be a megatrend in 2007 (Remington, 2007). Data gathered from the Hospital Consumer Assessment of Health Providers and System (H-CAHPS) survey tool will measure consumer satisfaction, which, in turn, will enable patient satisfaction to become a performance measurement for every provider across the healthcare delivery system. For this reason, nurses must pay attention to the many examples of studies in home telehealth indicating a great deal of patient satisfaction with telehealth, particularly those that note a preference for telehealth—not conventional care. One example reports on patients' indicating that the telehealth monitor helped them change the way they performed self-care (Chetney, 2006). Other studies also note that patients seen with telehealth have a better understanding of their own disease process and note the ease with which patients are able to manage self-care and so enjoy an improved quality of life (Sanderson, 2007). By patients' achieving a good understanding of and performing self-care by the end of their home health admission periods, an important goal of home telehealth has been attained.

However, when we move beyond issues of technical ease of use and look more closely at patients' preferences for privacy or at their desires to use the telehealth devices according to their own schedules, we are moving head-on toward the growing trend of consumer-directed health care. This is the new reality in health care. In part, the baby boom generation, many of whom are educated and comfortable with technology, are driving this trend toward as-needed, when-wanted care. Challenges of scheduling and possibly even reengineering telehealthcare services may be a concern (or an opportunity!) for tomorrow's home telehealthcare nurses. That is because we are only now beginning to learn how to care differently for this new generation of patients—with telehealth care on their own terms.

THE FOUNDATION OF KNOWLEDGE MODEL AND HOME TELEHEALTH

We have much to learn about usual home telehealthcare service delivery, particularly to the elderly and chronically ill, and for this important purpose, using the Foundation of Knowledge model is key to learning how to use telehealthcare tools with our typical patients (elderly, needing pointed care) and operate effectively as telenurses.

To understand the mechanics and effectiveness of home telehealth delivery within the Foundation of Knowledge model, we must begin with a typical home telehealth case from which we can learn the telenurse's role in this model.

Case Study: The Role of a Home Telehealth Nurse

Mrs. A is an 84-year-old woman recently discharged from the hospital with a diagnosis that includes an exacerbation of CHF. She also has diabetes and hypertension. Mrs. A was discharged from the hospital on multiple medications and lives alone.

Home care services were initiated with skilled nursing care visits, some home health aide support, and orders to include daily telemonitoring of her vital signs. The telehealth device will remotely monitor her BP, heart rate, O_2 saturation, and weight. In addition, the patient will answer customized questions about her disease on a daily basis. This information will then be transmitted daily to the home care agency where the telehealth nurse/clinician can determine appropriate clinical actions based on the data trends and preset baseline alerts that indicate when set parameters have been exceeded.

Knowledge Acquisition

In the previous case study, knowledge acquisition involves the nurse's receiving the information from the telehealth devices via a variety of communication modes. For example, the nurse receives the patient's vital signs taken in the home and the patient's responses to customized questions. All of this information is transmitted to a remote server or site (a central station or Web site) that is easily accessible to the nurse.

Knowledge Processing

As a result of the nurse's knowledge acquisition, the next step to be followed is knowledge processing (i.e., understanding a set of information and ways it can be useful to a specific task). In the case study, the nurse assesses the patient's vital signs along with subjective data received from the patient as a result of customized questions that she is asked. For example, she might be asked if she feels more short of breath today compared to a normal day. The nurse then combines this information with the overall patient history and diagnosis to get an up-to-date view of the patient's status and asks where this information fits into the clinical picture being presented for this patient.

As an example, the nurse notes:

> Postacute heart failure patient shows trended data with weight gain of 5 pounds over 2 days. Elevated BP, decreased O_2 sats, and answers yes to questions about increased shortness of breath and increased fatigue.

After processing all of the current information, the nurse is able to target the appropriate next steps involving knowledge generation and knowledge dissemination.

Knowledge Generation

By using her own nursing skills and clinical knowledge of the disease process, the nurse considers all of the data as it applies to Mrs. A and decides which is the best course of action to take and acts on the data. The nurse may, in addition, ask a variety of questions to insure that a complete and accurate decision about next steps for the patient is made. These questions may include:

- Do I need to gather additional data?
- Do I need to call the patient?
- Do I need to call the physician and inquire about a change in care plan?

Knowledge Dissemination

Finally, the nurse determines how the knowledge will be used and disseminated. Various questions that were posed in the knowledge generation stage are acted upon, including:

- Calling the doctor
- Obtaining a change in medication order
- Calling the patient and instructing her in medication change
- Reviewing activities that could have led to the changes (e.g., eating salty foods)
- Educating the patient on disease process, symptom management, and self-management techniques
- Continuing to monitor the patient on an ongoing basis

SUMMARY

Telehealth is a rapidly developing mode of health service delivery in which nurses can expect to play a key role. The most promising area of concentration for nurses is in home telehealth care, an area which is expected to provide extensive care to the burgeoning numbers of American elderly persons living with challenging chronic diseases and conditions. Many telecommunications-ready tools to assist nurses in delivering this care are available, and their effectiveness in maintaining or improving patients' health outcomes is well documented. Today's nurses can play a very significant role in providing telehealth services to typical home care patients (elderly, needing regular and targeted care) and operate effectively as telenurses. The practice of telehealth will provide opportunities for telenurses to play a key role in care management across the healthcare continuum.

Parting Thoughts for the Future and a View Toward What the Future Holds

Consumers will drive the way health care is delivered in the future. Consider that tomorrow's healthcare facility might have no walls. The evolving role of the Internet, personal health records and telehealth all will support a more integrated healthcare model. This convergence of trends and solutions will continue to expand with new business practice models such as retail clinics and concierge care.

The care continuum will need to be supported by a clinical and caregiver structure that will use data collected to make better and more informed healthcare decisions. Health parameter data could be used by the end user for personal direct care decision making, or it may be used by a member of the healthcare community to determine appropriate healthcare interventions.

Technology of today will be different from technology of tomorrow as access to broadband communications systems, acceptance of technology, and mobility and data transfer evolve. As a result of emerging needs, many companies will enter the market and offer a wide range of information technology tools from embedded and worn sensors to remote monitoring devices. We will continue to see different user interfaces to receive customized health services, such as the TV, cell phones, and perhaps someday the iPod.

Clearly, by making key information readily accessible, there will be solutions across all areas—home health, hospitals, and a range of other settings—that facilitate collaboration in care delivery and health information.

Products that integrate into consumers'/patients' everyday lives to improve the quality of life will continue to emerge. As we move forward, you will surely see the important role that telehealth and telenursing will play in improving quality of life and care for the patients we serve.

Foremost, we must be open to change and be willing to embrace ever-evolving practice models. We should always use tools to improve our care delivery models to make more targeted contact with and about our patients.

THOUGHT-PROVOKING Questions

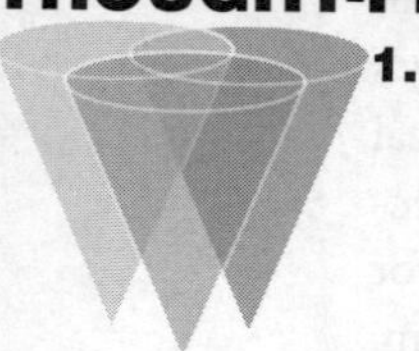

1. Will the increased use of these telehealth technology tools be viewed as dehumanizing patient care, or will they be viewed as a means to promote more contact with healthcare providers and new ways for people to stay connected (as in online disease support groups), thereby creating better long-term disease management and patient satisfaction?

2. As telehealth technology advances towards seamless data access regardless of distance or health system, how can we protect patient privacy rights and the confidentiality of personal medical data?

References

Allan, R. (2006, June 29). A brief history of telemedicine. *Electronic Design.* Retrieved September 7, 2007, from http://www.elecdesign.com/Articles/Index.cfm?AD=1&ArticleID=12859

American Association for Retired Persons (AARP). (1996). *Understanding senior housing into the next century: Survey of consumer preferences, concerns, and needs.* Washington, DC: AARP.

American Heart Association. (2007). *Statistics you need to know: Statistics on medication.* Retrieved September 7, 2007, from http://www.americanheart.org/presenter.jhtml?identifier=107

American Nurses Association (ANA). (2001). *Developing telehealth protocols: A blueprint for success.* Washington, DC: ANA.

American Telemedicine Association (ATA). (2002). *Home telehealth clinical guidelines.* Retrieved September 7, 2007, from http://www.americantelemed.org/icot/hometelehealthguidelines.htm

American Telemedicine Association (ATA). (2007). *Defining telemedicine.* Retrieved April 28, 2008, from http://www.atmeda.org/news/definition.html

Bernier, L. (2001). Assessing respiratory status from a distance. *Home Health Care Nurse, 19,* 632–640.

Centers for Disease Control and Prevention. (2005). *Chronic disease overview.* Retrieved September 7, 2007, from http://www.cdc.gov/nccdphp/overview

Cepelewicz, B. (2003). Legal issues in telemedicine. In A. Kinsella (Ed.), *Home healthcare: Wired and ready for telemedicine, the nurses' and nursing students' edition* (pp. AI–IX). Kensington, MD: Information for Tomorrow.

Chetney, R. (2006, July/August). What do patients really think about telehealth? In-depth interviews with patients and their caregivers. *The Remington Report, 26,* 28–29.

Hoffman, C., Rice, D., & Sung, H-Y. (1996). Persons with chronic conditions: Their prevalence and costs. *JAMA, 276,* 1473–1479.

Institute of Aging, University of California at San Francisco. (1996). *Chronic care in America: A 21st century challenge.* Princeton, NJ: Robert Wood Johnson Foundation.

Kinsella, A. (1998). *Home healthcare: Wired and ready for telemedicine, the second generation.* Sunriver, OR: Information for Tomorrow.

Kinsella, A. (2002a). Predicting home healthcare needs: A next step in patient monitoring. *Home Health Care Nurse, 20,* 725–729.

Kinsella, A. (2002b). Wound care and telehealth. *Telehealth Practice Report 3,* 9.

Kinsella, A. (2004). "*Obesity and new applications for home telehealth care.*" Home Health Care Technology Report 1 (3): 36;45.

National Pharmaceutical Council. (2003). *Infos and facts about [medication] non-compliance.* Retrieved September 7, 2007, from http://www.m-pill.com/index.php?browse=compliance

Pennsylvania Homecare Association and Pennsylvania State University. (2004). *2003–2004 telehealth project evaluation year two: The impact of telehealth on nursing workload and retention.* Unpublished report.

Quality Insights of Pennsylvania. (2005). *Home telehealth reference 2005.* Unpublished report.

Remington, L. (2007, January/February). Healthcare MegaTRENDS, predictions and forecasts. *The Remington Report 15,* 5–10.

Sanderson, S. (2007, July/August). Cardiopulmonary disease management: A patient-focused approach to home health care. *The Remington Report, 15,* 46–47.

Skiba, D. J. (1998). Health-oriented telecommunications in nursing informatics. In M. J. Ball et al. (Eds.), *Where caring and technology meet* (pp. 40–53). New York: Springer.

Stern, D. J. (2007, January/February). Intuitive system monitors resident behavior patterns. *Assisted Living Consult,* 21–25.

U.S. Dept. of Commerce, Bureau of the Census. (1993). *Sixty-five plus in America.* Washington, DC: GPO.

U.S. Department of Health and Human Services. Health Resources Services Administration [HRSA]. Bureau of Health Professions. (2002). *Projected supply, demand, and shortages of registered nurses: 2000–2020.* Retrieved September 7, 2007, from http://www.ahca.org/research/rnsupply_demand.pdf

U.S. Department of Health and Human Services. Health Resources Services Administration [HRSA]. Bureau of Health Professions. (2004). *The registered nurse population: Findings from the 2004 National Sample Survey of RNs.* Retrieved September 7, 2007, from http://www.bhpr.hrsa.gov/healthworkforce/rnsurvey04

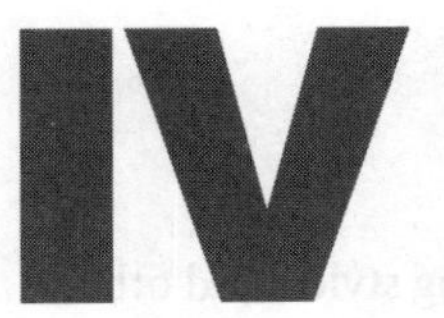

section

Nursing Informatics Applications: Nursing Research and Nursing Education

Nursing informatics (NI) provides us with more tools and capabilities than we can imagine at times. Just as NI has changed the way we administer and practice nursing, it has also dramatically impacted our research and educational practices.

Nursing research has evolved with the technologies. In the era of evidence-based practice, we must continue to critically think about our actions. What is the science behind our interventions? We must no longer do things one way just because they have always been done that way. Research the problem. Utilize your evidence-based resources. Critically select your electronic and nonelectronic references. Consolidate the research findings and combine and compare the conclusions. Present your findings and propose your solution. You may be the first to ask why, and thus become a key player in making change happen. Nursing informatics enhances and facilitates collaboration; improves access to online libraries; provides research tool transparency for collection, analysis, and dissemination of research knowledge; and facilitates the development of a common data language. NI provides organizational and informational support to advance translational research, helping to fill the gap between research findings and practice implementation. Repeat studies are needed to provide meaningful meta-analyses and systematic reviews of evidence to advance practice. Technology advancement in the area of incorporating evidence into clinical tools must continue. Removing the barriers to knowledge-seeking behavior and providing access to evidential resources will promote knowledge use and, in the end, improve patient outcomes.

Nursing education is evolving with the integration of nursing informatics tools to promote learning. The tools that are available must be used prudently by reflecting on and applying knowledge on teaching styles, learning styles, and other pedogogical concerns. As informatics capabilities continue to expand, a phenomenal amount of potential for virtual reality-embedded education looms on the horizon. Once the purview of gamers and geeks, virtual reality has exploded onto the academic scene. The use of virtual reality has the potential for cross-pollination between fields of inquiry across the curriculum, the university, and even learning systems. Many university departments will experiment with virtual reality in the hopes of staying current and appealing to their young and demanding "generation next" constituency. However, we must realize that much of society loves the feel of books too much to dismiss them as archaic. We believe that there is room for both books and technology in education. In other words, let's not throw the baby out with the bathwater! Students, educators, and administrators will ultimately return to a modified form of face-to-face classroom teaching, even with the availability of newer and more adventuresome teaching technologies. Further, once the fast, high-burn technologies stop flooding the marketplace, and big business provides opportunities for proprietary online universities, modified traditions will take their place, creating new spaces for nontraditional students, as well as members of the 'net generation, both anxious for technology use in the classroom for very different reasons.

As you are aware, the material in this book is placed within the context of the Foundation of Knowledge model (Figure IV-1) to meet healthcare delivery systems', organizations', patients', and nurses' needs. Nursing research is conducted to generate knowledge. In relation to the model, the nurse researcher is involved with every aspect from acquiring (collecting) and processing (analyzing) data and information, generating knowledge, and disseminating the results or findings (knowledge). Through this work, the researcher generates knowledge for the nursing profession. Knowledge generation is extremely important in the advancement of nursing science. Nursing education promotes scholarship and evidence-based teaching and learning. Through the sound integration of information management and technology tools, teaching and learning strategies promote the social and intellectual growth of the learner. As teachers and learners quest for knowledge, the pursuit of lifelong learning is instilled. Teachers and learners involved in the process of education are also involved with all of the levels of the model. Typically they acquire and process data and information and generate and disseminate knowledge within the frame of reference of their educational institution. Their knowledge generation is on a limited, individual/course/school basis unless they become involved with developing publications and educational research that will inform others in the nursing profession.

FIGURE IV-1
Foundation of Knowledge model. (Designed by Alicia Mastrian.)

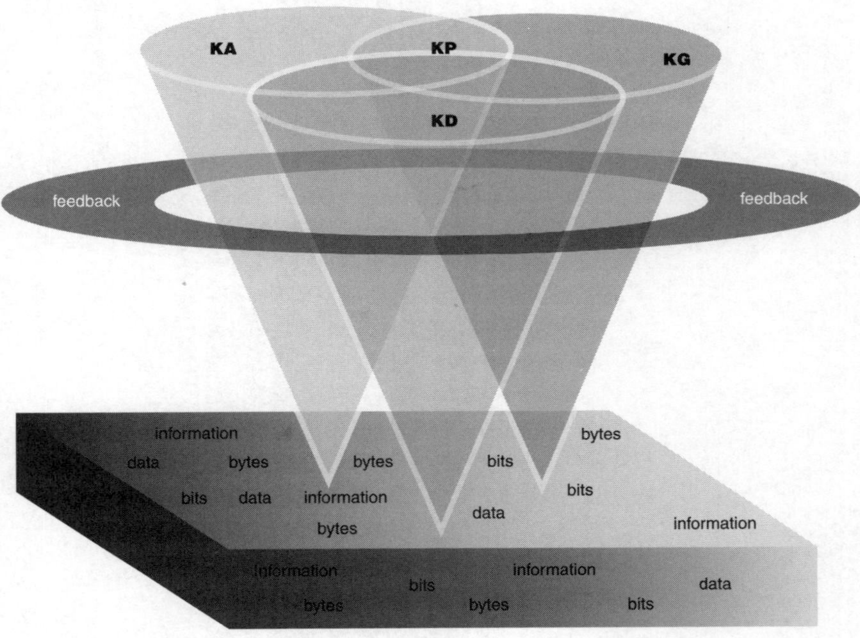

KA- Knowledge Acquisition
KD- Knowledge Dissemination
KG- Knowledge Generation
KP- Knowledge Processing

As you read through this section, we challenge you to ask yourself the following questions:

- How can I apply the knowledge I gain from my practice setting to benefit my patients and enhance my practice?
- How can I help my colleagues and patients understand and use the current technology that is available?
- How can I use my wisdom to help create the theories, tools, and knowledge of the future?

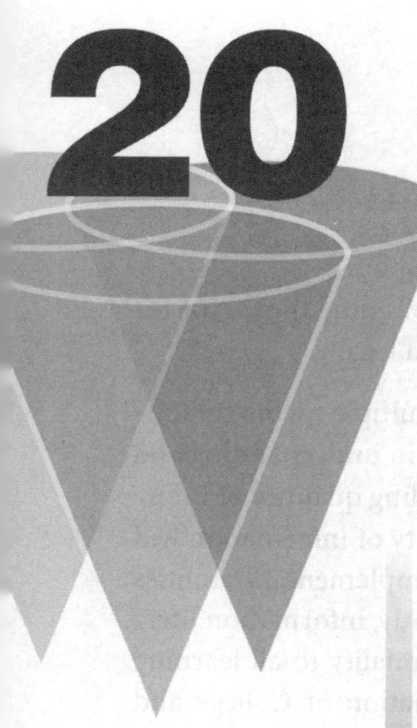

Nursing Research: Data Collection, Processing, and Analysis

Sylvia M. DeSantis

Objectives

1. Describe nursing research in relation to the Foundation of Knowledge model.
2. Explore the acquisition of previous knowledge through Internet and library holdings.
3. Assess informatics tools for collecting data and storage of information.
4. Compare tools for processing and analyzing quantitative and qualitative data.

Key Terms

American Library Association (ALA)
Cumulative Index to Nursing and Allied Health Literature (CINAHL)
Educational Resources Information Center (ERIC)
Foundation of Knowledge model
Information literacy
MEDLINE
Personal digital assistant (PDA)
PsycInfo

INTRODUCTION: NURSING RESEARCH AND THE FOUNDATION OF KNOWLEDGE MODEL

The **Foundation of Knowledge model** suggests that the most important aspect in information discovery, retrieval, and delivery is the ability to acquire, process, generate, and disseminate knowledge in ways that help those managing the knowledge reevaluate and rethink the way they are understanding and utilizing what they know and have learned. These goals closely reflect the Information Literacy Competency Standards for Higher Education, presented by the **American Library Association (ALA)** in 2003 in response to changing perceptions of how information is created, evaluated, and used.

According to the ALA (2000), an information literate individual is able to:

- Determine the extent of information needed
- Access the needed information effectively and efficiently

- Evaluate information and its sources critically
- Incorporate selected information into one's knowledge base
- Use information effectively to accomplish a specific purpose
- Understand the economic, legal, and social issues surrounding the use of information and access and use information ethically and legally

In addition, because information is available through multiple media (graphical, aural, and textual), new challenges arise for individuals in understanding and evaluating it. This uncertain quality, coupled with an expanding quantity of information, has created unforeseen challenges. The sheer quantity of information will not by itself create a more informed citizenry without complementary abilities necessary to use this information effectively. Most significantly, information literacy forms the basis for lifelong learning, forming a commonality to all learning environments, disciplines, and levels of education (Association of College and Research Libraries, 2000).

KNOWLEDGE GENERATION THROUGH NURSING RESEARCH

Information literacy is an intellectual framework for finding, understanding, evaluating, and using information—activities that may be accomplished in part through fluency with information technology and sound investigative methods, but most importantly, through critical reasoning and discernment. The Association of College and Research Libraries (2000) has suggested that "information literacy initiates, sustains, and extends lifelong learning through abilities which may use technologies but are ultimately independent of them" (p. 5)

Because nursing informatics combines all aspects of clinical practice, research, administration, and education (Ball, Hannah, & Douglas, 2000), the ability to recognize the need for a specific kind of information and locate, evaluate, and effectively use it (ALA, 1989) within the nursing informatics paradigm will catapult nurses ahead of other healthcare professionals in applying and engaging various facets of technology. However, because so few nurses have formal training in technology but still represent a disproportionate number of users, the ways in which nursing research integrates technology and health care within nursing informatics creates a heretofore unseen challenge (McHaney, 2007). This potentially enormous impact on the future of health care and technology will inform the success of information-literate nurses, those who will have learned how to learn and who will understand the intricacies of how knowledge is organized, retrieved, and used in such a way that others can learn from them (ALA, 1989). Whether a nurse fills the role of administrator, manager, educator, or staff, integrating technology has become a necessity for every nurse in today's technological marketplace (McHaney, 2007).

ACQUIRING PREVIOUS KNOWLEDGE THROUGH INTERNET/LIBRARY HOLDINGS

In an environment of rapid technological change coupled with an overwhelming proliferation of information sources, nurses face an enormous number of options when choosing how and from where to acquire information for their academic studies, clinical situations, and research. Because information is available through so many venues—libraries, special interest organizations, media, community resources, and the Internet—in increasingly unfiltered formats, healthcare practitioners must inevitably question information authenticity, validity, and reliability (Association of College and Research Libraries, 2000). Often, the retrieval of reliable research and information may appear to be a daunting task in light of the seemingly ubiquitous amount of information on the Web. Focusing on specific information venues will not only aid this search but will also assist in negotiating the endless maze of resources, thus allowing a nursing practitioner to find the best and most accurate information efficiently.

Professional Online Databases

Professional databases contribute to the invisible Web—a source of online information generally invisible to all Internet users except those with professional or academic affiliations, such as faculty, staff, and students. Databases range from specific to general and act as collection points by aggregating information like abstracts and articles from many different journals; two such databases include the **Cumulative Index to Nursing and Allied Health Literature** (**CINAHL**) and **MEDLINE.** CINAHL, for example, specifically includes information from all aspects of allied health, nursing, alternative medicine, and community medicine, while the MEDLINE database contains more than 10 million records, maintained and produced by the National Library of Medicine. Other databases such as **PsycInfo**, from the American Psychological Association, and the **Educational Resources Information Center** (**ERIC**) database may also benefit nursing needs. Many databases also offer full-text capabilities, which means that entire articles are available online. The articles and abstracts contained within these databases have already passed the rigors of publication in professional journals and are thus considered viable and authentic peer-reviewed sources.

Libraries with subscriptions to databases often employ library professionals able to help patrons through the vast amounts of available electronic information; utilizing the expert research capabilities of a health science librarian at one's local university is the best way to learn how to conduct database searches that will yield the most efficient and useful results. Also useful are Web sites that provide tutorials on best searching practices specifically for medically oriented databases, such as the Nursing Informatics Competency Project (http://library.med.nyu.edu/library/instruction/tutorials/nursing/index.html), which assists nursing students and professionals in using CINAHL's search engine efficiently.

Search Engines

Search engines allow users to surf the Web and find information on nearly anything, although many researchers steer clear of search engines because of the vast amounts of unsubstantiated information. Since no legitimacy needs to be provided for any information that appears on the Web, an author can make claims, substantiated or not, and still use the Web as a publishing venue. Despite the pitfalls associated with search engines in general, they may still yield a bounty of useful information when used with discretion, such as the following:

- Different search engines will produce different results for the same research. For example, one popular search engine ranks its results by number of hits a page or site has received. Consider that while the uppermost research results will be relevant, the order in which results appear does not indicate quality or viability of the source.
- Different Web address (domain) suffixes—.com, .edu, .org, .gov, etc.—can indicate who is responsible for creating the Web site. While an .edu site is hosted by an educational institution and for that reason may seem legitimate, consider that it could belong to a student stating personal opinion, gossip, or guesswork. In contrast, .gov sites are maintained by the government and will nearly always have professional contact information. Web hosts develop new domain suffixes constantly, so while looking at the suffix could be useful, it cannot be the only deciding factor when choosing to trust information.
- When possible, check the last updated dates (how old is the page?), contact information (is there an available bibliography or sources?), links to external sources (do they seem relevant?), and previous attained knowledge from other reputable sources (is the information too unbelievable?) before trusting information found on a Web page.
- Fees and information retrieval charges should be approached with skepticism. Private companies do offer information aggregate services for a fee. In these cases, users pay a flat monthly fee for access to collections of articles in a particular field. What users—especially those affiliated with an academic institution—may not realize is that they likely have access to the same—if not more complete—information through their institution's library system for free.
- Some legitimate databases and traditional newspapers who maintain a Web presence do provide access for a small fee, but just as many others simply ask

users to register in order to see articles for free. Many nursing students and professionals affiliated with a university may find that their university library has already purchased access for the student body.

Electronic Library Catalogs

Nearly all higher education institutions have their library catalogs online. While this is an obvious convenience for many students, some nursing professionals unused to working completely online may be intimidated by an e-catalog. Both the tiniest university and the busiest community college have library professionals able to demonstrate how to navigate a basic search of its catalog. Asking for assistance in learning how to access the vast assortment of journals, books, databases, and other resources available at one's college library is an excellent idea. Those in nursing programs at larger universities will likely find free classes that specifically teach users how to navigate and use the online catalog. If smaller colleges and universities do not offer these services, one should take advantage of the library's online tutorials, help pages, frequently asked questions (FAQ) pages, and online reference service (if available). Many times, local public libraries will have subscriptions to popular databases as well and will offer free classes to patrons on searching techniques, providing another free access point to the best information for one's research needs. Making full use of available library resources serves to strengthen information literacy skills, thus enabling learners to master content and extend their investigations, become more self-directed, and assume greater control over their own learning (Association of College and Research Libraries, 2000).

INFORMATICS TOOLS FOR COLLECTING DATA AND STORAGE OF INFORMATION

Nurses are already intimately familiar with data collection as daily agents of patient care documentation, patient monitoring, and interview data (Chang, 2001). In this way, formal nursing data sets are actually made up of gathered information such as healthcare definitions, classification, and nursing information. Before data can be analyzed or critically reviewed to determine outcomes or assessment, it must be collected and aggregated.

Nurses may generate and record data from their own observations or with the assistance of various devices. In this way free text—informational data such as drug dosages administered, resources used, problems diagnosed, etc.—is recorded manually. Free text is then interpreted and organized by some standardizing principle, either manually or by computer. In this way, data (often qualitative data that cannot be traditionally measured) can be organized and processed. Data actually becomes information when these separate components are interpreted, organized, combined, and structured within a specific context to convey particular meanings (Hovenga & Sermeus, 2002).

Software designed to collect, sort, organize, store, retrieve, select, and aggregate data are database management systems (DBMSs), and nursing and health data may be separated into four basic types: resource data (e.g., financial information); patient/client demographics; activity data (clinical data); and health service provider data. These primary data are recorded manually or collected electronically, with manual collection providing a greater opportunity for error. Data that has been electronically recorded follows a programmed set of instructions built into the software, thus cutting down substantially on collection error. Of paramount importance in the collection process are the data collection form and computer interface used for inputting the data; these will affect completeness, consistency, and accuracy (Hovenga & Sermeus, 2002).

Quantitative data collection tools or instruments include questionnaires, interviews, surveys, quizzes, assessments, e-mail interviews, and Web-based surveys. Questionnaires, one of the most popular forms of data collection, can be administered in hard copy, on paper, or programmed into a Web site where individuals may answer the questions electronically (Chang, 2001). Other electronic data collection tools include **personal digital assistants (PDAs)** and on-site laptops. A benefit of using electronic data collection is the ability to transmit data to another computer directly for compilation and analysis, thereby cutting down on error (Hebda, Czar, & Mascara, 2005).

An excellent example of innovative electronic data collection is the system used by the participants in the Nightingale Tracker System pilot study, in which nursing students traveling to rural clinical sites submitted information into handheld devices while miles away from their preceptor-supervisors. Results suggest that, despite some technical challenges associated with the hardware, using the handheld technology enhanced students' learning (especially in the area of physical assessment), increased their confidence in practicing in community-based settings, and provided efficient data input capabilities (Ndiwane, 2005).

Harder to measure, nonnumerical qualitative data can be collected electronically, as well, in the form of a narrative or diary-like entry. Much in the way free text is analyzed and sorted; this narrative dialogue is assessed and then sorted according to the data collection's organizing principle (Chang, 2001).

TOOLS FOR PROCESSING DATA AND DATA ANALYSIS

Data analysis is the process by which data collected during the course of a study is processed to identify trends and patterns of relationships. Descriptive statistics allows the researcher to organize information meaningfully, thus facilitating insight by describing what the data show (Hebda et al., 2005). There exist a range of tools to facilitate analysis including specialized databases, word processing/spreadsheet/database applications, as well as statistical packages (Hovenga & Sermeus, 2002).

Quantitative Data Analysis

Quantitative data focuses on numbers and frequencies rather than experience and meaning. While the kind of data generated by quantitative collection is fairly straightforward and easy to analyze—responses to questionnaires, experiments, and psychometric tests—quantitative data analysis has come under criticism. Psychologists prefer to use a combination of quantitative and qualitative data, backing up research participants' explanations with statistically reliable information obtained by numerical measurement (*Quantitative and Qualitative Data,* n.d.).

In quantitative studies, variables represented by data are collected in numerical form. These values are then entered into specific fields that have predetermined meanings or are coded. Various quantitative data analyses can be applied to nursing research, such as intervention research, quality improvement studies, and outcomes research. One of the most common statistical packages on the market available for this kind of analysis is the Statistical Package for Social Sciences. Depending on the research goal, the researcher may use different types of analysis. Different statistical goals may require hypothesis testing, model building, descriptive/exploratory analyses, and others. For example, hypothesis testing is based on assumptions regarding the relative truth of the hypothesis, so a data analysis would compare actual outcomes with purported hypotheses (Chang, 2001).

Qualitative Data Analysis

Extremely varied in nature, qualitative data can include nearly any information that can be captured and is not numerical (Trochim, 2006a). Qualitative data is more concerned with describing meaning than in drawing statistical inferences; what is lost in reliability (faulty transcription, forgotten details, etc.) is gained in validity (*Quantitative and Qualitative Data,* n.d.). Although qualitative data relies upon judgments, it can still be manipulated numerically, much in the same way quantitative data can be open to judgment (Trochim, 2006b).

Some major types of quantitative data include in-depth interviews, direct observation, and written documents. Interviews include individual and focus group interviews and may be recorded in some way. Interviews differ from direct observation in their interactive nature. Direct observation differs from case to case and often means the researcher does not make contact with the respondent. Written documents might include a variety of written materials including memos, newspaper clippings, conversation transcripts, books, etc. (Trochim, 2006a).

Computers can aid greatly in the storage, tabulation, and retrieval of qualitative data by acting as the equivalent of an electronic filing cabinet (Hebda et al., 2005). Data analysis can also be aided by simple data management programs, such as Excel, in which a user can categorize data and link categories with key words (Chang, 2001). Data can be converted into information and knowledge by either inductive or deductive reasoning. Most qualitative methods utilize an inductive approach in which one generates hypotheses (versus a deductive approach in which hypotheses are tested). Data analysis includes statistical analysis in which samples and populations are compared, in order to discern whether the sample is biased or reflective of a true situation. Another aspect of analysis includes seeking relationships between a variable and events (Hovenga & Sermeus, 2002).

SUMMARY

In this chapter, you learned the value of information literacy and its relationship to knowledge and lifelong learning. You were acquainted with informatics tools useful to acquiring and assessing previous knowledge, as well as tools useful for collecting and storing and analyzing information. **One thought I'd like to leave you with is that** information literacy and informatics tools used to find and process information into usable knowledge is a critical skill set for living in the 21st century.

THOUGHT-PROVOKING Question

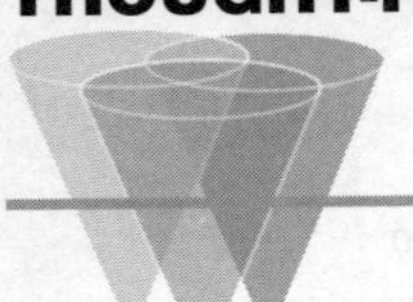

How will the advent of information literacy affect nursing informatics in the 21st century?

References

American Library Association (ALA). (1989). *Presidential committee on information literacy: Final report.* Retrieved on June 22, 2008 from http://www.ala.org/ala/acrl/acrlpubs/whitepapers/presidential.cfm

American Library Association (ALA). (2000). *Information literacy competency standards for higher education.* Chicago, IL: Author.

Association of College and Research Libraries. (2000). *Information literacy competency standards for higher education.* Retrieved on June 22, 2008, from http://www.ala.org/ala/acrl/acrlstandards/standards.pdf

Ball, M. J., Hannah, K. J., & Douglas, J. V. (2000). Nursing and informatics. In M. J. Ball, K. J. Hannah, S. K. Newbold, & J. V. Douglas (Eds.), *Nursing informatics: Where caring and technology meet* (pp. 6–14). New York: Springer.

Chang, B. L. (2001). Computer use in nursing education. In V. Saba & K. McCormick (Eds.), *Essentials of computers for nurses: Informatics for the new millennium* (3rd ed., pp. 445–456). New York: McGraw-Hill.

Hebda, T., Czar, P., & Mascara, C. (2005). *Handbook of informatics for nurses & health care professionals* (3rd ed.). Upper Saddle River, NJ: Prentice Hall.

Hovenga, E. J. S., & Sermeus, W. (2002). Data analysis methods. In J. Mantas & A. Hasman (Eds.), *Textbook in health informatics: A nursing perspective* (pp. 113–125). Amsterdam: IOS Press.

McHaney, D. F. (2007, June–August). Embracing the integration of technology and care. *The Alabama Nurse, 34*(2), 1.

Ndiwane, A. (2005). Teaching with the Nightingale Tracker technology in community-based nursing education: A pilot study. *Journal of Nursing Education, 44*(1), 40–42.

Quantitative and qualitative data. (n.d.). Retrieved November 18, 2007, from http://www.holah.karoo.net/quantitativequalitative.htm

Trochim, W. M. K. (2006a). *Qualitative data.* Retrieved November 17, 2007, from www.socialresearchmethods.net/kb/qualdata.php

Trochim, W. M. K. (2006b). *Types of data.* Retrieved November 17, 2007, from www.socialresearchmethods.net/kb/datatype.php

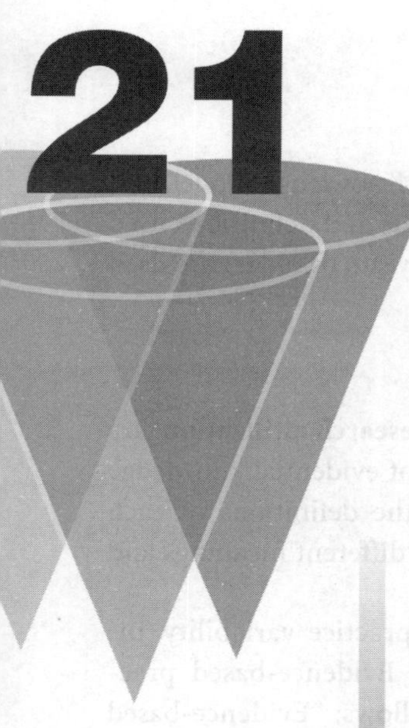

21 Translational Research: Generating Evidence for Practice

Jennifer Bredemeyer and Ida Androwich

Objectives

1. Clarify the differences between evidence-based practice and translational research.
2. Describe models for introducing research findings into practice.
3. Identify barriers to research utilization in practice.

Key Terms

Agency for Healthcare Research and Quality (AHRQ)
Context of care
Evidence
Evidence-based practice (EBP)
Iowa model
Meta-analysis
National Guideline Clearinghouse (NGC)
Open Access Initiative
Qualitative study
Quantitative study
Research utilization
Research validity
Translational research

INTRODUCTION

Mr. James is an 87-year-old gentleman with osteoarthritis in his knees. He is frail, very thin, and requires assistance getting out of bed. Mary, RN, is a brand-new nurse and is making her rounds with her team members and nurse's aide, Mark. Realizing Mr. James is at risk for skin breakdown and falls, she reviews the agency policy manual regarding pressure ulcer prevention and fall prevention. What other resources could Mary consult if she wanted more information on preventing these issues? If Mary wanted to know what current research suggests about preventing each of these conditions, how would she obtain this information?

The objective of this section is to introduce the reader to the concept of translational research and its role in **evidence-based practice (EBP)** with specific emphasis on nursing informatics. Prior to pursuing the content in this section, the reader should already have an understanding of nursing research, the Foundation of Knowledge model, and knowledge generation through nursing research. Key words and definitions used in this text are described briefly below. Classic sources (5 years or older) are used to enhance the reference base.

CLARIFICATION OF TERMS

Evidence-based practice, **translational research**, and **research utilization** are all terms that have been used to describe the application of evidential knowledge to clinical practice. The following paragraphs explore the definitions of each topic, which, although the terms are related, have slightly different meanings and applications.

In evidence-based practice, the goal is to decrease practice variability, increase patient safety, and eliminate unnecessary cost. Evidence-based practice as defined by Goode and Piedalue (1999) is as follows: "Evidence-based clinical practice involves the synthesis of knowledge from research, retrospective or concurrent chart review, quality improvement and risk data, international, national, and local standards, infection control data, pathophysiology, cost effectiveness analysis, benchmarking data, patient preferences, and clinical expertise" (p. 15).

Research utilization is a subset of evidence-based practice. Research utilization is often mistakenly interchanged with the term *evidence-based practice.* It is the utilization of original findings from a disciplined study in a practical application unrelated to the original research study (Polit & Beck, 2004, p. 673), and it is a subset of evidence-based practice.

Translational research is used to describe the translation of medical, biomedical, informatics, and nursing research into bedside clinical interventions. The goal in translational research is focused on the generation of more research. It is easy to see where the confusion lies in the terminology, since, although the goals remain the same, there are slight nuances to each definition. Problems with translational research exist when the scientific aspects of the bedside application are poorly understood by the clinician and the human subject concerns are poorly understood by the scientist. Difficulties in translating research exist when research applications do not fit well with the clinical context or practical considerations constrain the application. Since negative results are not popular for scientific publication, studies that reveal negative results may be avoided (Manrincola, 2003). Translational research is complicated by the follow-up analysis, practice, and policy changes that occur when adopting the research into practice (Titler, 2004). An organizational culture positively or negatively affects changes to a clinical application and establishes the groundwork as well as the support for change-making activities.

History of EBP

Research results are crucial to furthering evidence-based practice. The concept of using randomized control trials and systematic reviews as the gold standard against which one should evaluate the validity and effectiveness of a clinical intervention was introduced by Archie Cochrane, a scientist and a physician, in 1972. Cochrane was a prisoner of war in World War II and was given the position of medical officer at the time of his internment. His experiences led to his belief that not all medical interventions have been needed or that some have caused more harm than good. Cochrane viewed the randomized clinical trial as means of validating and determining reliability of clinical interventions. He saw the need to limit interventions to those that were scientifically based and effective, and that they were not just based on hunches.

Cochrane's colleague, Iain Chalmers, was heavily influenced by Cochrane's ideas and developed a comprehensive clinical trials registry of 3,500 clinical trial results in the field of perinatal medicine. In 1988, the registry became available electronically. Eventually, the National Health Service in England, recognizing the value of and need for this work, developed the Cochrane Center, so named in honor of Archie Cochrane. Under the direction of Iain Chalmers, the Cochrane Center expanded to encompass a more global vision. The Cochrane Collaboration was initiated in 1993 and expanded internationally to maintain systematic reviews in all areas of health care (Dickersin & Manheimer, 1998).

Evidence

Discussion abounds in the area of what constitutes **evidence**. The randomized control trial (RCT) is considered the most reliable type of trial. The updated Stetler model of research utilization (Stetler, 2001) identifies internal and external forms of evidence. External evidence originates from research and national experts and internal forms of evidence originate from nontraditional sources such as clinical experience and quality improvement data.

Evidence includes standards of practice, codes of ethics, philosophies of nursing, autobiographical stories, esthetic criticism, works of art, **qualitative studies**, and the patient and clinical knowledge (Melnyk, Fineout-Overholt, Stone, & Ackerman, 2000). French (2002) summarizes evidence as "truth, knowledge (including tacit, expert opinion and experiential), primary research findings, **meta-analyses** [boldface added] and systematic reviews" (p. 254). Nurses may additionally draw upon evidence from the **context of care** such as audit and performance data, the culture of the organization, social and professional networks, discussion with stakeholders, and local or national policy (Rycroft-Malone et al., 2004, p. 86).

There has been concern from nurse theorists that nurses are being influenced too much by the medical model in accepting the randomized control trial as the only true source of evidence, thereby "reverting to the medical perspective" rather than incorporating "theory-guided evidence and diverse ways of knowing" (Fawcett, Watson, Walker, & Fitzpatrick, 2001, p. 115). The context change from medicine to nursing requires nurses to apply other knowledge as well as nursing theory. Utilizing research results alone as a basis for clinical decision making ignores other types of evidence inherent in nursing practice (Scott-Findlay & Pollock, 2004).

In order to use evidence in practice, the weight of the research, also called **research validity**, must be determined. Evidence hierarchies have been defined to grade and assign value to the information source. An example of an evidential hierarchy by Stetler, Brunell et al. (1998) prioritizes evidence into six categories:

1. Meta-analysis
2. Individual experimental studies
3. Quasiexperimental studies
4. Nonexperimental studies
5. Program evaluations such as quality improvement projects
6. Opinions of experts

The hierarchy identifies meta-analysis as the best quality evidence since it utilizes multiple individual research studies to come to consensus. It is interesting to note that opinions of experts are the least significant and yet nurses most often seek the opinion of a more experienced colleague or peer when seeking information regarding patient care (Pravikoff, Tanner, & Pierce, 2005).

Qualitative research allows us to understand the way in which the intervention is experienced to the researcher and to the participant as well as the value of the interventions to both parties (O'Neill, Jinks, & Ong, 2007). Qualitative research is not always considered in evidence-based practice, primarily due to the fact that methods for synthesizing the evidence do not currently exist. A method for synthesizing qualitative research is still being defined. The Cochrane Qualitative Research Methods Group (CQRMG) is attempting to develop search, appraisal, and synthesis methodologies for qualitative research (Joanna Briggs Institute, n.d.).

BRIDGING THE GAP BETWEEN RESEARCH AND PRACTICE

The time between research dissemination and utilization may be significant, and as Cochrane realized, the delay in utilization may adversely affect patient outcomes. Bridging the gap between research and practice requires an understanding of the key concepts and barriers, accessibility to research findings, access to clinical mentors for research understanding, a reinforcing culture, and a desire on the part of the clinician to implement best practices (Melnyk, 2005; Melnyk, Fineout-Overholt, Stetler, & Allen, 2005). In the **Iowa model** of evidence-based practice, research and other critically reviewed evidential sources are adopted, with the support and involvement of system resources directly in the practice setting with the potential goal of developing a standard of care (Titler, 2007). Stetler indicates that the groundwork required to create a conceptual framework supportive of an evidence-based practice includes workplace culture change and support of the change through leadership (Stetler, Brunell et al., 1998). Beliefs and attitudes, involvement in research activities, information seeking, professional characteristics, education, and other socioeconomic factors were identified by Estabrooks, Floyd, Scott-Findlay, O'Leary, and Gushta (2003) as potential determinants of research utilization; however the meta-analysis pointed out that there was too much original research and not enough repetition of previous studies to advance the knowledge base regarding research utilization. Developing countries are constrained economically from accessing research sources. Organizations such as the Cochrane Collaboration provide free reviews in order to fill this void. Still, knowledge dissemination strategies and education are required (The Cochrane Collaboration, 2004).

Barriers

Barriers to the application of evidence-based practice are lack of time, lack of access to libraries within a facility, lack of technology confidence, lack of knowledge on how to search for information, and lack of value assigned to using research in practice (Pravikoff, Tanner, & Pierce, 2005). Additionally, in an observational study of the information-seeking behaviors of on-duty nurses, McKnight (2006) noted that nurses did not feel ethically comfortable with taking time from patient care to read publications, nor was much time available. Nurses may see the job of interpreting research as too complex or may see the organizational culture as a barrier to implementation (McCaughan, Thompson, Cullum, Sheldon, & Thompson, 2001).

THE ROLE OF INFORMATICS

Computers are used in all areas of research such as (1) literature search databases, like CINAHL; (2) online literature reference lists such as RefWorks; (3) data coding; (4) data analysis; (5) model building; (6) meta-analysis; (7) qualitative analysis; and (8) dissemination of results (e.g., via e-mail or Internet Web site) (Saba & McCormick, 2001). The collaborative component of research is supportive of informatics science. Technology has become so important to research that the National Institutes of Health has invested in reengineering of the clinical research enterprise as part of its road map initiative for medical research (National Institutes of Health, 2007).

The time-critical nature of patient care interventions and lack of time to investigate research questions is a problem ripe for an informatics solution. An informatics infrastructure is critical to supporting a clinician's access to information in a clinical setting. Research in the area of advancing access to evidence using technology is ongoing. Giuse et al. (2005) describe the evolving role of the clinical informationist as a partner on the healthcare team for the purpose of providing timely clinical evidence into the clinical workflow. Though not specific to nursing informatics, the National Institutes of Health provides awards under its Clinical and Translational Science Award (CTSA) program to accelerate the transfer of research to the clinical setting.

As an example of the integration of informatics and the medical record, Matter (2006) describes the positive effects of a successful integration of referential links with EBP clinical content in the clinical pathway on patient outcomes. The pilot started in 2005 at Pinnacle Health in Pennsylvania, involved two vendors, and combined the power of the electronic medical record with evidence-based electronic reference links to create a point of care tool that allowed clinicians to combine nursing care plans supported by the corresponding evidential link. Gains in the development of institutional guidelines, clinical collaboration, and 76% compliance with pain assessment 2 hours after administration were realized.

The Cochrane Collaboration showed an increasing need to improve on the speed of knowledge acquisition and access to evidence. With the goal of promoting the use of research findings and tool use based on these findings, the **Agency for Healthcare Research and Quality (AHRQ)** became an active participant in pushing evidence forward into practice. The AHRQ is a government-sponsored organization with the mission of reducing patient risk from harm, decreasing healthcare cost, and improving patient outcomes through the promotion of research and technology applications focused on evidence-based practice. In 1999, AHRQ implemented its Translating Research into Practice Initiative (TRIP) in order to generate knowledge about evidence-based care (Agency for Healthcare Research and Quality, 2001). In the second TRIP initiative (TRIP-II), focus was on collaboration and bringing research to practice with focus on the underserved. As part of an AHRQ initiative, the **National Guideline Clearinghouse (NGC)** was developed. NGC is a comprehensive database of evidentially based clinical practice guidelines and related documents that are regularly published through the NGC electronic mailing list and are available on the NGC Web site (National

Guideline Clearinghouse, 2007). The NGC Web site allows users to browse the Web site for the clinical guidelines, view abstracts and full-text links, download full-text clinical guidelines to personal digital assistive (PDA) devices, obtain technical reports, and compare guidelines.

In addition, there are a growing number of printed and electronic resources available to assist in creating guidelines and offering information about evidence-based practice. A sampling of existing Web sites is shown in Table 21-1.

TABLE 21-1
Online Evidence-Based Resources

Web Site	Description
The Agency for Healthcare Research and Quality www.ahrq.gov	The agency for Healthcare Research and Quality contains a wealth of information regarding healthcare quality. There is no charge for access to the site or its resources.
Cinahl http://cinahl.com	Cinahl information systems offers a multitude of online services, which include Web site link sources, Cinahl's online nursing and allied health database, document delivery, and search services.
BMJ Publishing http://www.bmjpg.com	The BMJ publishing group provides clinical databases by prescription. The BMJ Clinical Evidence site allows the download of some clinical papers and some interesting risk tools without charge.
The Cochrane Collaboration http://www.cochrane.org	The Cochrane Collaboration provides reviews for free, but full-text articles are by subscription.
World Views on Evidence-Based Nursing http://blackwellpublishing.com/wvn	Through Blackwell Publishing, this magazine, sponsored by Sigma Theta Tau, is dedicated exclusively to evidence-based nursing articles. The magazine is also offered online by subscription.
Entrez PubMed http://www.ncbi.nim.nih.gov/sites/entrez	Entrez PubMed is a service provided by The National Library of Medicine (NLM). The NLM was developed by the National Center for Biotechnology Information (NCBI), which provides access to life science journals and MEDLINE citations. Some of the journal links are free and some require a subscription.
PubMed Central http://www.pubmedcentral.nih.gov	PubMed Central (PMC) is a free digital archive of science-related articles managed by the NCBI. BioMed Central (an open-source online archive) may be accessed here.
The Joanna Briggs Institute http://www.joannabriggs.edu.au/about/home.php	The Joanna Briggs Institute was established in 1996 as a resource for best care practices. Joanna Briggs was first matron of the Adelaide Hospital in Australia and is recognized for her financial and organizational support. The Joanna Briggs Institute is a leader in developing evidence-based practices.

DEVELOPING EVIDENCE-BASED PRACTICE GUIDELINES

There have been several models developed to guide organizations into translating research into practice. Brief descriptions of the several models are listed in Table 21-2. As an example, Titler (2007) identifies the steps in the Iowa model for translating research into practice as (1) identifying the problem, issue or topic in nursing practice; (2) research and critique of related evidence; (3) adaptation of the evidence to practice; (4) implementation of the evidence-based practice; and (5) evaluation of patient outcomes and care practices. Careful analysis and discussion of the research and/or other forms of evidence in this scenario may reveal that given the context, implementation may not be practical. Following implementation, results must be monitored to determine if the application works for the context. Thoughtful discussion of the findings will help the clinical team determine if further research is warranted or if further change is needed.

Information technology is important in synthesizing the research regardless of the model. Bakken (2001) recommends "1) standardized nomenclature required for the electronic health record (standardized terminologies and structures), 2) digital sources of evidence, 3) standards that facilitate health care data exchange

TABLE 21-2
Comparison of Model Approaches to Evidence-Based Practice

Stetler model (Stetler, Bunell et al. 1998)	ACE Star model (Stevens, 2004)	The Iowa model of evidence-based practice to promote quality care (Titler et al., 2001)
1. Preparation 2. Validation 3. Cooperative evaluation 4. Decision making 5. Translational application 6. Evaluation	1. Discovery 2. Evidence summary 3. Translation 4. Integration 5. Evaluation	1. Select the trigger as impetus for practice (knowledge focused or practice focused) change. 2. Determine if the topic is worth pursuing for the organization and if not, pursue new trigger. 3. Determine if there is significant research base. If so, change, otherwise conduct research, or seek more research. 4. If change is appropriate for practice, implement change. 5. Monitor results. 6. Disseminate results.

among heterogeneous systems, 4) informatics processes that support the acquisition and application of evidence to a specific clinical situation, and 5) informatics competencies" (p. 1999). Bakken's recommendations encourage an infrastructure that creates a database of experiential clinical evidence.

META-ANALYSIS AND GENERATION OF KNOWLEDGE

Systematic reviews combine results from multiple primary investigations in order to obtain consensus on a specific area of research. Studies are discarded from the review if they are not considered sound, thereby creating a reliable end result. The strength of the systematic review is its ability to corroborate findings and reach consensus. Systematic reviews show the need for more research by revealing the areas where quantitative results may be lacking or minimal. Bias may occur if selected studies are inadequate, if all sources of evidence are not investigated, or publications selected are not adequately diverse (Lipp, 2005).

Meta-analysis, a form of systematic review, uses statistical methods to combine the results of several studies (Cook, Mulrow, & Haynes, 1997). **Quantitative studies** are typically used. According to Glass (1976), meta-analysis is "the statistical analysis of a large collection of analysis results from individual studies for the purpose of integrating the findings" (p. 3).

Kraft (2006) describes the documentation search strategy for meta-analysis as beginning with the identification of the studies through a search of bibliographic databases, identification of meta-analysis articles that match search criteria, elimination of articles that do not match search criteria, review of the reference lists in the meta-analysis for other articles that may relate to the topic, and review of each article for the quality and content. Additional sources should include unpublished works such as conferences and dissertation abstracts with the goal of obtaining as many relevant articles as possible. Gregson, Meal, and Avis (2002) identify the steps of a meta-analysis as (1) defining the problem followed by protocol generation, (2) establishing study eligibility criteria followed by literature search, (3) identifying the heterogeneity of results of studies, (4) standardizing the data and statistically combining the results, and (5) conducting sensitivity testing to determine if the combined results are the same. The often cited criticism of meta-analysis is that emphasis is on quantitative studies, not qualitative. Additionally, the analysis is only as good as the studies used in the analysis (Gregson, Meal, & Avis, 2002). Collection and dissemination of these meta-analysis and systematic reviews are available in paper and on the Internet, although many such databases require a subscription.

The term *open access* refers to a worldwide movement to make a library of knowledge available to anyone with Internet access. The **Open Access Initiative** came about in response to the tremendous cost of research library access. Libraries pay large fees for journal subscriptions and the richness of library references are limited to what the budget allows. The cost of keeping current with research has caused library subscriptions to decline (Yoitis, 2005). Open access adds to the controversy with some journals charging authors for publications, which in itself may provide a financial barrier to publication of this form.

According to Suber (2004), open access refers to digital literature that is available to anyone with Internet access free of charge. There are two vehicles for open access: (1) archives and (2) journals. Open access journals are generally peer reviewed and freely available. The publishers of open access journals do not charge the reader but obtain funds for publishing elsewhere. Open access journals may charge the author for publishing. The Public Library of Science at http://www.plos.org/ charges $2,750 to publish but waives the fee if the author claims financial hardship. Other sources of funding may include donations, grants, advertising, and other private funding sources.

SUMMARY

We live in amazing times. Technology has taken us faster and further than we ever thought we could go. Our jobs have become more technical and more complicated. In some ways technology has increased our margin for error. Some of us will continue to rely on our little scraps of paper and our systematic methods to keep us and our patients safe. Sometimes we become so tied to these things we close our minds to new innovations. The evolving quality culture and patient safety are dragging us forward. For the benefit of our patients, we must move forward.

Collaboration, improved access to online libraries, research tool transparency, a common data language, organizational and informational support, and continued research are a short list of needed items to advance translational research. Repeat studies are needed to provide meaningful meta-analysis and systematic reviews. Technology advancement in the area of incorporating evidence into clinical tools must continue. Removing the barriers to knowledge-seeking behavior and providing access to evidential resources will promote knowledge and in the end improve patient outcomes.

In the era of evidence-based practice, we must continue to critically think about our actions. What is the science behind our interventions? We must no longer do things one way just because they have always been done that way. Research the problem. Utilize your evidence-based resources. Critically select your electronic and nonelectronic references. Consolidate the research findings and combine and compare the conclusions. Present your findings and propose your solution. You may be the first to ask why, and you may be a key player in making change happen.

The Future

Titler (2007) indicates that future priorities should include development of theoretical formulations to guide research and systematic reviews so that they may be grouped by organizational context (such as primary care, outpatient, etc.). Focus on other forms of research such as qualitative research should also be incorporated into systematic reviews. **The most important thought we'd like to leave you with is that** the technology is available now to incorporate evidence into reference links in clinical care plans. Incorporation of personalized clinical desktops to allow each clinician to have appropriate references (similar to Internet adbot technology) provided to them may be possible. Time, research, and technology will tell.

THOUGHT-PROVOKING Questions

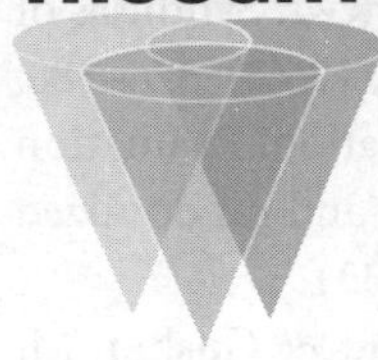

1. Twelve-hour shifts are problematic for patient and nurse safety, and yet hospitals continue to keep the 12-hour shift schedule. In 2004, the Institute of Medicine (Board on Health Care Services & Institute of Medicine, 2004) published a report that referred to studies as early as 1988 that discussed the negative effects of rotating shifts on intervention accuracy. Workers with 12-hour shifts realized more fatigue than workers on 8-hour shifts. In another study done in Turkey by Ilhan, Durukan, Aras, Turkcuoglu, and Aygun (2006), factors relating to increased risk for injury were: age of 24 or less, less than 4 years of nursing experience, working in the surgical intensive care units and working for more than 8 hours. As a clinician reading these studies, what would your next step be?
2. The use of heparin versus saline to maintain the patency of peripheral intravenous catheters has been addressed in research for many years. The American Society of Health System Pharmacists (ASHSP) published a position paper in January 2006 (American Society of Health System Pharmacists, 2006) advocating its support of the use of 0.9% saline in the maintenance of peripheral catheters in nonpregnant adults. It seems surprising that their position paper references articles that advocate the use of saline over heparin dating from 1991. What do you feel are some of the barriers that would have caused this delay in implementation?

References

Agency for Healthcare Research and Quality. (2001, March). *AHRQ profile: Quality research for quality healthcare.* Retrieved July 29, 2007, from Agency for Healthcare Research and Quality Web site, http://www.ahrq.gov/about/profile.htm

American Society of Health System Pharmacists. (2006). ASHSP therapeutic position statement on the institutional use of 0.9% sodium chloride injection to maintain patency of peripheral indwelling intermittent infusion devices. *American Journal of Health System Pharmacy, 63,* 1273–1275.

Bakken, S. (2001). An informatics infrastructure is essential for evidence-based practice. *Journal of American Medical Informatics Association, 8,* 199–201.

Board on Health Care Services & Institute of Medicine. (2004). *Keeping patients safe.* Washington, DC: The National Academies Press.

The Cochrane Collaboration. (2004). Bridging the gaps across the income divide: A review of the Collaboration's efforts to date and recommendations for the future. Retrieved September 14, 2007, from http://www.cochrane.org/colloquia/abstracts/ottawa/O-006.htm

Cook, D. J., Mulrow, C. D., & Haynes, R. B. (1997). Systematic reviews: Synthesis of best evidence for clinical decisions. *Annals of Internal Medicine, 126*(5), 376–380.

Dickersin, K., & Manheimer, E. (1998). The Cochrane Collaboration: Evaluation of health care services using systematic reviews of the results and randomized control trials. *Clinical Obstetrics and Gynecology, 41*(2), 315–331.

Estabrooks, C. A., Floyd, J. A., Scott-Findlay, S., O'Leary, K. A., & Gushta, M. (2003). Individual determinants of research utilization: A systematic review. *Journal of Advanced Nursing, 42,* 73–81.

Fawcett, J., Watson, J., Walker, P. H., & Fitzpatrick, J. J. (2001). On nursing theories and evidence. *Journal of Nursing Scholarship, 33*(2), 115–119.

French, P. (2002). What is the evidence on evidence-based nursing? An epistemological concern. *Journal of Advanced Nursing, 37*(3), 250–257.

Giuse, N. B., Koonce, T. Y., Jeronme, R. N., Gahall, M., Sathe, N. A., & Williams, A. (2005). Evolution of a mature clinical informationist model. *Journal of the American Medical Informatics Association, 12*(3), 249–255.

Glass, G. V. (1976). Primary, secondary and meta-analysis of research. *Educational Research, 5*(10), 3–8.

Goode, C. J., & Piedalue, F. (1999). Evidence-based clinical practice. *Journal of Nursing Administration, 29*(6), 15–21.

Gregson, P. R., Meal, A. G., & Avis, M. (2002). Meta-analysis: The glass eye of evidence-based practice? *Nursing Inquiry, 9*(1), 24–30.

Ilhan, M. N., Durukan, E., Aras, E., Turkcuoglu, S., & Aygun, R. (2006). Long working hours increase the risk of sharp and needlestick injury in nurses: A need for new policy implication. *Journal of Advanced Nursing, 56*(5), 563–568.

Joanna Briggs Institute. (n.d.). *Joanna Briggs Institute.* Retrieved September 3, 2007, from the University of Adelaide and the Joanna Briggs Institute Web site, http://www.joannabriggs.edu.au/cqrmg/about.html

Kraft, M. R. (2006). Meta-analysis: A research tool. *SCI Nursing Journal, 23*(2). Retrieved September 25, 2007, from United Spinal Association Web site, http://www.unitedspinal.org/publications/nursing/2006/08/27/research-corner/

Lipp, A. (2005). The systematic review as an evidence-based tool for the operating room. *Associate of Operating Room Nurses Journal, 81*(6), 1279–1287.

Manrincola, F. M. (2003). Translational medicine: A two-way road. *Journal of Translational Medicine, 1,* 1–2. Retrieved August 18, 2007, from BioMed Central Ltd. Web site, http://www.translational-medicine.com/content/1/1/1

Matter, S. (2006). Empower nurses with evidence-based knowledge. *Nurse Management, 37*(12), 34–37.

McCaughan, D., Thompson, C., Culllum, N., Sheldon, T. A., & Thompson, D. R. (2001). Acute care nurses' perceptions of barriers to using research information in clinical decision-making. *Journal of Advanced Nursing, 39*(1), 46–60.

McKnight, M. (2006). The information seeking of on-duty critical care nurses: Evidence from participant observation and in-context interviews. *Journal of the Medical Library Association, 94*(2), 145–151.

Melnyk, B. M. (2005). Advancing evidence-based practice in clinical and academic settings. *Worldviews on Evidence-Based Nursing, 3,* 161–165.

Melnyk, B. M., Fineout-Overholt, E., Stetler, C., & Allen, J. (2005). Outcomes and implementation strategies from the first U.S. evidence-based practice leadership summit. *Worldviews on Evidence-Based Nursing, 2*(3), 113–121.

Melnyk, B. M., Fineout-Overholt, E., Stone, P., & Ackerman, M. (2000). Evidence-based practice: The past, the present, and recommendations for the millennium. *Pediatric Nursing, 26*(1), 77–80.

National Guideline Clearinghouse. (2007). *National guideline clearinghouse.* Retrieved July 29, 2007, from National Guideline Clearinghouse Web site, http://www.guideline.gov/

National Institutes of Health. (2007). *NIH roadmap for medical research.* Retrieved August 8, 2007, from Office of Portfolio Analysis and Strategic Initiatives at the National Institutes of Health Web site, http://nihroadmap.nih.gov/

O'Neill, T., Jinks, C., & Ong, B. N. (2007). Decision-making regarding total knee replacement surgery: A qualitative meta-synthesis. *BMC Health Services Research, 7*(52). Retrieved September 3, 2007, from PubMedCentral Web site, http://www.pubmedcentral.nih.gov/articlerender.fcgi?artid=1854891

Polit, D. F., & Beck, T. C. (2004). *Nursing research: Principles and methods* (7th ed.). Philadelphia: Lippincott Williams & Wilkins.

Pravikoff, D. S., Tanner, A. B., & Pierce, S. T. (2005). Readiness of U.S. nurses for evidence-based practice. *American Journal of Nursing, 105*(9), 40–51.

Rycroft-Malone, J., Seers, K., Titchen, A., Harvey, G., Kitson, A., & McCormack, B. (2004). What counts as evidence in evidence-based practice? *Journal of Advanced Nursing, 47*(1), 81–90.

Saba, V. K., & McCormick, K. A. (2001). *Essentials of computers for nurses: Informatics for the new millennium* (3rd ed.). New York: McGraw-Hill.

Scott-Findlay, S., & Pollock, C. (2004). Evidence, research, knowledge: A call for conceptual clarity. *Worldwideviews on Evidence-Based Nursing, 1*(2), 92–97.

Stetler, C. B. (2001). Updating the Stetler model of research utilization to facilitate evidence-based practice. *Nursing Outlook, 49*(6), 272–279.

Stetler, C. B., Brunell, M., Giuliano, K. K., Morse, D., Prince, L., & Newell-Stokes, V. (1998). Evidence-based practice and the role of nursing leadership. *Journal of Nursing Administration, 28*(7/8), 45–53.

Stetler, C. B., Morsi, D., Rucki, S., Broughton, S., Corrigan, B., Fitzgerald, J., et al. (1998). Utilization-focused integrative reviews of nursing service. *Applied Nursing Research, 11*(4), 195–206.

Stevens, K. R. (2004). *ACE star model of EBP: Knowledge transformation.* Retrieved July 10, 2007, from the University of Texas Health Science Center at San Antonio Web site, http://www.acestar.uthscsa.edu/Learn_model.htm

Suber, P. (2004). *A very brief introduction to open access.* Retrieved September 14, 2007, from Earlham College Web site, http://www.earlham.edu/~peters/fos/brief.htm

Titler, M. (2007). Translating research into practice: Models for changing clinician behavior. *American Journal of Nursing, 107*(6), 26–33.

Titler, M. G. (2004). Methods in translation science. *Worldviews on evidence-based nursing, 1,* 38–48.

Titler, M. G., Kleiber, C., Steelman, V., Rakel, B., Budreu, G., Everett, L., et al. (2001). The Iowa model of evidence-based practice to promote quality care. *Critical Care Nursing Clinics of North America, 13*(4), 497–509.

Yoitis, K. (2005). The Open Access Initiative: A new paradigm for scholarly communications. *Information Technology & Libraries, 24*(4), 157–162.

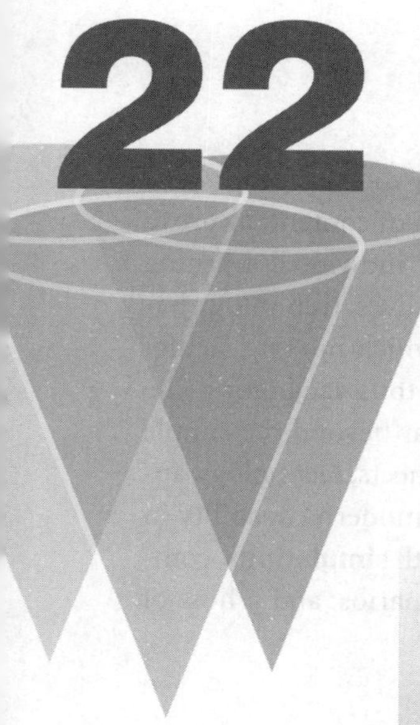

Nursing Informatics and Nursing Education

Sylvia M. DeSantis

Objectives

1. Describe nursing education in relation to the Foundation of Knowledge model.
2. Explore knowledge acquisition and sharing.
3. Assess technology tools and delivery modalities used in nursing education.
4. Compare and contrast knowledge assessment methods.

Key Terms

Advocate
Asynchronous
Audiopods
Avatars
Blended
Blogs
Case study
Chats
Collaboration
Compact disc read-only memory (CD-ROM)
Computer-assisted instruction (CAI)
Computer-based
Continuing education
Digital versatile disc or digital video disc (DVD)
Digital pen
Distance education
E-learning
E-mail
Electronic mailing list
Face to face
Foundation of Knowledge model

INTRODUCTION: NURSING EDUCATION AND THE FOUNDATION OF KNOWLEDGE MODEL

Nursing informatics facilitates the integration of information, data, and knowledge to support nurses, patients, and other providers in their various settings and decision-making roles (Carty & Ong, 2006). The **Foundation of Knowledge model** specifically prompts nurses to extend theoretical and metaphorical knowledge into practical, holistic determinations based on a variety of factors and contexts. Because competencies in informatics include but are not limited to **information literacy**, computer literacy, and the ability to use strategies and system applications to manage data, knowledge, and information (as cited in ANA, 2000), the ability of nursing students to use computer-mediated communication skills is essential to success in the nursing field.

The rise of telecommunications, computer-mediated communications, and virtual technologies has opened up opportunities for improving communication and extending care within the healthcare industry (Barnes & Rudge, 2005). Proponents of instructional

Key Terms *Continued*
High fidelity
Hybrid
Hypertext
Information literacy
Instant message (IM)
iPod
MP3 aggregator
Multimedia
'Net generation
Online
Personal digital assistant (PDA)
Podcast
Portal
Portfolio
Problem based
Really simple syndication (RSS)
Resource description framework (RDF)
Real time
Role playing
Scenario
Second Life
Simulation
Smartphone
Tutorial
Videopods
Virtual reality (VR)
Web-based
Web-enhanced
Webcasts
Wi-Fi
Wiki

applications of computer technology view it as a way to erase geographical boundaries for students, enhance the presentation of content, improve learning outcomes, and even tailor instruction to individual learning needs. When carefully matched with curricular objectives, technology becomes an efficient and affordable avenue through which nursing faculty may provide useful knowledge to their students, thus facilitating the learning process (Hebda, Czar, & Mascara, 2005). Far beyond the simple applications of word processing software or spreadsheets, technology applications have evolved greatly, taking advantage of modern capability in providing nursing and related healthcare students with **simulations**, complex **multimedia**, virtual reality-assisted clinical scenarios, and a host of information and literature-gathering Internet tools.

Knowledge Acquisition and Sharing

The shift from computer literacy to information literacy and management has drawn attention to interactivity and design as the most important components of interactive Web-enhanced/Web-based courses in providing effective learning environments. Thurmond (as cited in Carty & Ong, 2006, p. 523) discusses the four types of interactions related to Web-enhanced courses; these include learner–learner, learner–content, learner–instructor, and learner–interface interactions. In traditional learner–learner exchanges, students interact with one another to troubleshoot, work out challenges, and exchange solutions generated from different perspectives. Traditional and familiar, both learner–content and learner–instructor interactions expect students to work directly with course content and/or the faculty member and then participate in relevant course activities, such as tests and reviews. Learner–interface interaction includes the ways students access their coursework and their ultimate success or failure in finding, retrieving, and utilizing what they need (Carty & Ong, 2006). When **Web enhanced**, these interactions include **online** chats, forum discussions, participation in electronic mailing list groups, instant messaging, blogging, and using **e-mail**, all of which ask the student to engage, digest, utilize, and disseminate information in new ways.

Hardware and Software Considerations

In the 21st century, nursing informatics has begun to rely especially heavily on technology usability, functionality, and accessibility. **Computer-assisted instruction (CAI)** has had an enormous impact on nursing informatics, with many CAI programs offering individualized instruction in the form of customizable scenarios, frameworks, and programs for study. Additionally, CAI contributes to better understanding of material by supporting all learning styles, types, and paces. Consequently, nursing skills have presented endless development potential for software development, making the effective use of software and hardware by educators and students a prime necessity (Riley, 1996).

Software is used to describe the instructions that direct a computer's hardware to work, while hardware describes physical computer components, like a mouse, keyboard, and monitor. Software essentially translates commands into computer language, allowing the hardware to perform its functions. Without hardware and software, computer technologies would be moot, and without software, hardware does not function (McHugh, 2006). Applications software refers to the various programs individuals use to communicate with others, do work, play games, or watch multimedia on a computer. The most common software package sold with computers is an office package that generally includes a word processing program, spreadsheet capability, a presentation graphics program (like PowerPoint), and some kind of database management system. Software packages are available on **compact disc read-only memory (CD-ROM)**, **digital versatile disc** or **digital video disc (DVD)** or through the Internet, allowing the user to download the software directly from a vendor's Web site (McHugh, 2006).

When evaluating software or hardware for purchase, careful assessment of the products and services will help an educator, administrator, or student to make the best choices. Most important when evaluating software is understanding how congruently the software's functionality compares to learning goals and objectives. While many programs are available for assisting a nurse practitioner who is evaluating software for particular learning purposes, the main criteria concern *content* (Is the information accurate? Is it relevant?), *format* (How is information visually presented? Is it in frames? Does it come with graphics?), *documentation style* (What's the tone? Is it scholarly and applicable?), and *strategies* (Is the software useful for all students, including remedial students and accelerated students?) (Edwards & Drury, 2000).

Hardware decisions will depend upon the way a computer system will be used, in addition to cost, ease of use, and durability (Clochesy, 2004). Systems purchased for personal use may differ dramatically from those purchased for online learning labs or smart classrooms. Because the technology inherent to workstations, servers, and computers in general tends to change so rapidly, discussing large system decisions with an information technology expert will yield a better informed decision. Some factors to consider include where the system will be stationed (at home for personal use or in a learning lab for use by many students), how many desktops there will be (one or a few dozen), if it will be networked to a school's internal system, if printing will be available, and the level of security needed (Hebda et al., 2005).

Delivery Modalities

Nursing educators are discovering that current students are not responding in the same ways the educators did during their own tenure as students. Technology-laden students from the millennial age demand instant information delivered in an entertaining fashion, an expectation built upon extensive exposure to e-mail, text messaging, online chatting, and the Internet (Ridley, 2007). Additionally, many nursing departments are facing an increase in student enrollment as well as a corresponding growth in faculty. While new nursing faculty bring significant clinical experience to their academic positions, also apparent for some is an underlying tension and unfamiliarity with technological advances, outcomes-based accreditation initiates, and teaching itself. Schools of nursing are scrambling to provide professional development for busy nursing faculty and introducing them to best practices in teaching (Shaffer, Lackey, & Bolling, 2006).

Learning is a multispatial function, and in the age of technology innovation, instructional delivery can inhabit many forms in both physical and virtual spaces. Spaces in academia are no longer defined by a class or its content, but instead by the learning the class is trying to promote. To this end, learning spaces should support multiple modes of learning and delivery, including reflection, discussion, and experience, as well as facilitate **face-to-face** and online interaction within and beyond classrooms. Truly innovative delivery—whether face-to-face classroom interaction, online engagement, or a blended hybrid of technology and traditional classroom teaching—supports learning activities, rather than standing independently of them (Oblinger, 2005).

Face-to-Face Delivery

Ridley (2007) suggests that although it is the most widely used teaching method among nurse educators, traditional face-to-face lecture yields only a 5% information retention rate over a 24-hour period, compared with demonstration (30%), discussion groups (50%), practice activities (75%), and peer teaching (90%) (as cited in Sousa, 1995).

Additionally, the inability of physical space to keep pace with learning models also inhibits the benefits gained from face-to-face interaction between teacher and student. For example, collaborative learning grinds to halt when class is held in a room with chairs bolted to the floor, facing a lectern (Oblinger, 2005); this kind of spatial arrangement prohibits a sense of classroom community by inhibiting easy peer interaction, reducing students' ability to see each other, and concentrating all attention on the professor.

Conversely, in a collaborative learning environment, the professor guides conversation and sets up discussion, acting less as classroom authority and more as facilitator, helping students maintain focus, gently guiding discussion, and ultimately empowering students to push knowledge boundaries in a safe and secure atmosphere of peer support. This inductive, epistemological approach promotes active, critical thinking skills and assists students in learning not just facts, but *how to learn*. As future healthcare professionals determined to rely upon quantification and rationale, nursing students would benefit from face-to-face classroom interaction that hones student ability to manufacture new personal truths through interaction with people and ideas in ways that cannot always be measured and counted.

Ridley (2007) suggests that such interactive, cooperative learning strategies might include gaming, **role playing,** and **problem-based** learning. Because games are nonthreatening and fun, they promote critical thinking and teamwork by pushing students to work together in groups to find answers and achieve success. Role playing is similar in that it allows students to try on real-life **scenarios** by filling either prescripted or ad-libbed roles (doctor, nurse, patient, clinician, etc.) without the fear or pressure of putting another's life at risk while trying to determine the best course of action or find a solution to a fictitious patient's health issue.

Problem-based learning, a well accepted form of interactive learning, takes assignments out of a contextual vacuum and applies real-life scenarios to problems or challenges. Students work in groups to solve the dilemma presented by real patient cases and build on prior knowledge, using higher level thinking skills and progressive inquiry to resolve the problem (Ridley, 2007).

Online Delivery

E-learning, online learning, and **Web-based** education have caused a significant shift in student–teacher relationships in nursing education, and, according to Phillips (1999), "the Internet will offer a chance to make real profits from education, while offering students a choice about who will educate them and at what price" (¶ 14). According to Oblinger (2005), not only are learning spaces no longer physical or formal, especially on campuses with wireless capabilities but nursing students are also expecting to make use of wide ranges of cutting-edge technology during their academic tenure, exchanging the traditional sage on the stage for a technologically-savvy guide on the side (as cited in Leasure, Davis, & Thievon, 2000) who gives up the role of gatekeeper and instead promotes and facilitates dialogue as central to teaching–learning (Aquino-Russell, Maillard Strüby, & Reviczky, 2007).

Student-centered and no longer limited to the domain of the classroom, lab, or even a patient's bedside, online learning allows educators to translate theory into practice, creating a virtual classroom space that promotes **collaboration**, engagement, discussion, and analysis.

Detractors of online learning initiatives suggest, however, that sharing an online space undermines the student–teacher relationship, makes building peer relationships difficult, and generally disrupts the normal classroom dynamic, thus creating an unfamiliar, uncomfortable atmosphere. Despite these concerns, studies show that not only do Web-based courses continue to gain in popularity, but they also enhance learning in ways that encourage students to share personal experiences and support. Researchers cite many factors that make online learning laudable, with accessibility and convenience two of the most frequently cited issues (Aquino-Russell et al., 2007).

The **asynchronous** and time-independent elements of Web-based courses answer a huge need for flexible class times by today's growing population of nontraditional learners. Additionally, Web-based and place-independent learning allows participation by anyone, anywhere in the world, with access. Related to this issue is the democratizing effect of online learning, such that all students have the same opportunity to participate without judgment. And, finally, Web-based classes provide an easily accessible permanent record, a convenience for both teachers and learners (Aquino-Russell et al., 2007).

Online learning has the capability to reenvision classroom interaction, and depending on the specific delivery mode, can even change basic pedagogical concepts. The best online delivery—whether through a **chat**, **blog**, or class—will, just like traditional classes in a physical space, adhere to solid teaching parameters that assure student investment and success. These include providing students a clear set of learning activities and expected outcomes, relating content to real situations using **case studies** and simulation (problem-based learning), building in collaborative activities, such as team projects, building in an instructor's personality and presence, and setting up technology such that users build their confidence rather than experience failure and frustration (Winfield, Mealy, & Scheibel, 1998). Refer to Box 22-1.

Hybrid or Blended Delivery

Traditional courses are more frequently being offered as online, virtual classes, i.e., **distance education**—learning that occurs elsewhere than in the traditional classroom and consequently, requires special course, design, planning, techniques, and communication. A hybrid of this delivery mode includes learning in which tradi-

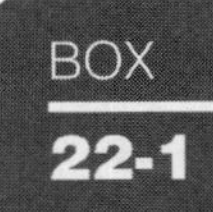

A Day in the Life

Eric Doerfler

Sometimes these days, I feel like I can't get away from technology. I teach three classes that I keep tabs on through our course management system. It's a great system, but when the network is down, it's hard to get anything done. I am a teaching assistant in another university, and that program is all online, too. Every work day, I'm spending time in this electronic world of my students. Of my own courses I can say this: at least every 2 weeks I see their nonvirtual faces. I have a handheld computer for my schedule and my address book. I use software for my finances, and that synchronizes to the handheld computer. I type my patient notes into a word processor. When someone calls with a problem, I can boot up my laptop and get a reminder of what I did and why.

That's the upside. Although I sometimes feel too dependent on complex machines for what was once simpler, the access I have and the options I am offered have changed my daily life. Online discussion boards offer reticent students a less threatening environment in which to participate, so I see more class participation. Posting articles online reduces my department's copying costs—and logistical aggravation. If I see a good article, I don't need to print it, send it down to the copy center, and wait. My calendars are backed up—if one computer doesn't work, another one does, and in fact there's no way for me to ever lose my address book, check register, or other key documents!

It's more expensive to live this way, though. Computers, peripherals, and ink cartridges all cost money. Life was cheaper when I bought a day planner each December and retired the last. Electronic health records almost drove my practice budget into deficit until I went back to typing them into the laptop and saving/printing them. As I make my way through each day, I do sometimes find myself wondering how and when this can all become less bothersome, disjointed, and complex, and more simple, interconnected, private, and reliable—without driving me and all of us into the poorhouse! And although I teach informatics, as I go along I find that less technology is more, and I have started to walk by all the latest gadgets, waiting for the inevitable evolution that will marry me to my machines without spoiling my humanity or my peace of mind.

tional classroom time is enhanced or broken up with online components, thereby creating a class in which **blended** learning occurs. Some forms of **hybrid** learning include Web-enhanced learning and learning that takes place in and makes use of smart classrooms, for example, teaching in a wired room equipped with classroom learning technologies such as the Blackboard Learning System.

Web-enhanced instruction—such as asking students to blog responses to a reading or class discussion—allows technically ambivalent institutions to participate in the technology revolution without huge budgetary expenditure and also addresses a preference by some faculty for a way to include innovation and technology in classes without giving up traditional classroom engagement. *Syllabus* magazine has reported that most distance learning courses used up to five media to reach students, including chats, telephone calls, forums, student Web pages, and group pages, in addition to print materials from lab manual study guides and textbooks, and samples of student work, quizzes, and tests (Hibbison, 2001). Faculty are reaching for multiple media and hybrid approaches to encourage student-centered learning, maximize teaching effectiveness, and take advantage of the best on-campus and online teaching and learning (Black & Watties-Daniels, 2006). See Box 22-2.

BOX 22-2

Open Source and Moodle, a Course Management System

Dee McGonigle and Kathleen Mastrian

Open source is being used in business and health care. Open source refers to standards and guidelines for writing software open source code. The power comes in the fact that it is often free to use and "Open source is a development method for software that harnesses the power of distributed peer review and transparency of process. The promise of open source is better quality, higher reliability, more flexibility, lower cost, and an end to predatory vendor lock-in" (Open Source Initiative, 2007, ¶ 1). Graham (2005) adds that "Ten years ago there seemed a real danger Microsoft would extend its monopoly to servers. It seems safe to say now that open source has prevented that. A recent survey found 52% of companies are replacing Windows servers with Linux servers" (¶ 1). Open source is changing the way health care and education are conducting their business. Educators are looking to open source software to help manage their online courses since they can have flexibility, reliability, and lower costs.

Moodle, Modular Object-Oriented Dynamic Learning Environment, is an open source course management system (CMS) or learning management system (LMS). *About Moodle* (2008) describes Moodle as open source software for "producing Internet-based courses and web sites" (¶ 1). *What is Moodle?* (n.d.) describes Moodle as a "learning management system that lets you provide documents, graded assignments, quizzes, discussion forums, etc. to your students with an easy to learn and use interface. Moodle is developed by a worldwide effort of over 75,000 students,

BOX Continued
22-2

faculty, and staff at over 6500 institutions around the world" (¶ 1). Munoz and Van Duzer (2005) compared Blackboard and Moodle. They describe Moodle as "Open source (free!). Customizable by programming staff. Flexible for the instructor and developer. Supported by programmers world-wide" (¶ 2).

Open source code and the promise of free and/or low-cost globally supported software continues to gain appeal. As more and more people turn to open source, the more robust it will become, since it is a community effort between users and programmers.

References

About Moodle. (2008). Retrieved January 31, 2008, from http://docs.moodle.org/en/About_Moodle

Graham, P. (2005). *What business can learn from open source.* Retrieved January 31, 2008, from http://www.paulgraham.com/opensource.html

Munoz, K., & Van Duzer, J. (2005). *Blackboard vs. Moodle: A comparison of satisfaction with online teaching and learning tools.* Retrieved January 31, 2008, from http://www.humboldt.edu/~jdv1/moodle/all.htm

Open Source Initiative. (2007). *Home.* Retrieved January 31, 2008, from http://www.opensource.org/

What is Moodle? (n.d.). Retrieved January 31, 2008, from http://www.humboldt.edu/~moodle/whatis.html

Smart classrooms, also known as digital and multimedia classrooms, integrate computer and audiovisual technologies by providing a ceiling-mounted projector with an access point at the front of the room, an instructor podium/workstation, sound, and network access. An enhanced smart classroom would also provide networked student workstations instead of traditional desks, allowing students to follow along online and perform network or Web searches, chat, blog, or myriad other activities as dictated by the professor. For example, at the CSU School of Nursing, users access announcements, course materials, faculty information, Web sites, and other tools through Blackboard, enabling the nursing faculty to extend learning beyond the physical classroom walls.

Surveys by WebCT, an online virtual learning environment system created in 1995 and now slowly being phased out in favor of other systems, confirm the growing realization among faculty that traditional campus courses can benefit from the interactive components of a Web site, forums, and chat, etc., and that online courses also benefit from face-to-face contact. In another survey, faculty showed strong preference for Web-enhanced classroom instruction over either traditional classroom-only instruction or online-only distance education, observing that student achievement is maximized in courses that combine online and classroom elements (Hibbison, 2001).

Technology Tools

The **'net generation** or millennial generation—students who have grown up inside a wired world of instant access and online everything—are connected, digital, experiential, and social. Working in teams comes naturally to this peer group, and interacting in peer-to-peer situations is a familiar and common learning mode. These students desire information immediately, are skilled multitaskers, and are, according to Oblinger in a 2005 Educause learning initiative, "no longer the people our educational system was designed to teach" (as cited in Prensky, 2001). Certain social trends emerging from the morass of both traditional and innovative technology tools include the use of technologies attempting to meet the needs of these new learners; through the utilization of software, hardware, drivers, dedicated servers, plug-ins, and an Internet connection, students can chat, collaborate, play a game, or interact electronically with a peer in some way, all with little to no learning curve or effort. Because visual media is now the vernacular of a highly digital culture, students and faculty are also embracing technology tools that allow for the creation and interpretation of visual images (Oblinger, 2005). These tools might take the shape of interactive tutorials, a created city within a virtual reality landscape, or even a multimedia action maze that prompts users to choose different outcomes within a scenario. Regardless of the particular tool, technology can only perform as well as the pedagogy that drives it, thus creating a need for integration, support, and sustainability within nursing education programs willing to implement new instructional and assessment strategies (Bassendowski, 2005). Refer to Box 22-3.

BOX 22-3

Digital Pen Technology Tool

Dee McGonigle, Kathleen Mastrian, and Nedra Farcus

Digital pens are actual writing implements that can also digitally capture handwriting or drawings. They are battery operated and generally come with a universal serial bus (USB) cradle that permits uploading captured materials to the desktop, laptop, or palmtop computer. Scribes can use them as a ballpoint pen and write on regular paper just as they would with a normal pen. If one would like to capture what he is writing or drawing digitally, he needs to purchase digital paper to write on. This paper

BOX Continued
22-3

is different from regular paper in the fact that there are small dots that permit the digital pen to see what one is writing or drawing so it can be captured digitally. Some manufacturers are trying to create digital pens that use regular paper. If one decides that she wants to capture what she is working on, she needs to instruct the pen to save her work. There are memory limitations; the memory will generally hold around 40 pages of captured digital paper.

Digital pens have been around for a while, and some of the former models are probably still collecting dust in someone's office. This new resurgence in the digital pen, however, is reflective of the advances in technology. Fried (2008) states that,

> One thing all the new products have going for them is that they come at a time where Windows' support for digital ink has never been better. With Windows XP, only the stylus-based Tablet PC edition really supported pen input. With Windows Vista, though, the operating system supports more kinds of ink, including that from tablets like those from Wacom, as well as things like Iogear's Digital Scribe (¶ 22).

Some of these new marvels are using Bluetooth wireless technology that can send captures directly to a computer. The file formats vary by manufacturer but are typically GIF or JPEG, making them easily shared and supported.

Think of the educational applications for being able to capture 40 pages of material and upload it to a computer, share it, and exchange it. What about the impact on patient care? The city of Stockholm is slated to use digital pens in its healthcare delivery system. According to *City of Stockholm to Use Anoto's Digital Pen to Improve Elderly Care Services* (2007),

> The Anoto digital pens will primarily be used to facilitate documentation and information transfer, in order to improve the quality of elderly homecare in the city (¶ 4).
>
> The technology has already been deployed successfully in Solna and Sundbyberg, two towns north of Stockholm, where homecare nurses use the digital pen to register their arrival and departure times on each visit and tick off the services delivered to each patient, on a digital form (¶ 5).

The Logitech io digital pen system can be used to document assessments. A digital camera in the pen captures a watermark pattern when the user writes on interactive paper. The pen is then set in a USB cradle, and the data is uploaded into the computer where it is converted to text. The use of a digital pen system enables students to complete an assessment in the home with pen and paper and share the information with their professor and/or a research team for analysis within a short period of time.

The digital pen is being used for many applications in education and healthcare. Would this be something you would use?

continues

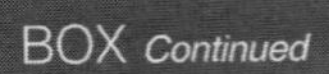

BOX 22-3 *Continued*

References

City of Stockholm to use Anoto's digital pen to improve elderly care services. (2007, September). *Wireless News, 1.* Retrieved January 25, 2008, from ABI/INFORM Trade & Industry database (Document ID: 1343068491).

Fried, I. (2008). *Is the digital pen mightier?* Retrieved on January 25, 2008, from http://www.usatoday.com/tech/products/cnet/2007-08-24-digital-pen_N.htm

Tutorials

Academic institutions face a multitude of challenges in trying to satisfy the information needs of users who are inundated daily by tons of information as part of their regular Web use. In addition to facing a technological revolution, it appears that academia is facing a pedagogical one as well, trying to meet their students' needs in innovative and engaging ways. One solution to providing students not only information, but the skills to find, evaluate, understand, and apply this information comes in the form of online **tutorials** (Bracke & Dickstein, 2002).

Modern tutorials attempt, to some extent, to mimic lectures by guiding users through a series of objectives or tasks, usually allowing the user to do the work at his or her own pace (Edwards & Drury, 2000). Tutorials generally stand alone as autonomous multimedia that may use animation, text, graphics, sound, questions, and different kinds of interactivity to engage and intrigue the user. They tend to promote active learning by prompting the user to answer sets of questions, follow clickable **hypertext**, or complete quizzes. For example, users might be asked to fill in worksheets after reviewing anatomy concepts, take a quiz, post an answer to a question, or even click through a scenario by choosing the best course of action in a mock clinical situation.

Some tutorials, such as those employed by the medical students at the Morgan Stanley Children's Hospital of New York, are designed to be brief (10 minutes), interactive, very focused, and immediately relevant. In this case, medical students bustling through a busy clinical rotation who accessed the tutorials actually raised examination grades (Pusic, Pachev, & MacDonald, 2007).

Because most students benefit from being able to contextualize a lesson's framework and purpose, the most effective tutorials provide users with understandable navigation, like a table of contents at its beginning, or additional navigational aids, such as icons, buttons, or text that indicate where and how they need to progress (Dewald, 1999). For example, Penn State University Libraries offers a nursing tutorial specifically designed to teach the tenets of evidence-based practice (http://www.libraries.psu.edu/instruction/ebpt-07/index.htm). While any piece of the tutorial may be accessed at any time, it prompts the user to follow a linear path in applying the four basic steps of evidence-based practice in order to make the process easier and more understandable.

Effective tutorials surpass the simple presentation of information in a Web-based format; they instead address certain pedagogical and student-centered needs by identifying and taking into consideration specific factors such as instructional content, the educator's purpose and teaching goal, the initiative's overall purpose, the potential need for special conceptual input, the learners' ultimate objectives in completing the tutorial, and the standards that determine what qualifies as successful completion of the tutorial (DeSantis, 2002).

And while most tutorials are created to stand alone, some may also benefit and supplement face-to-face instruction, such as the interactive information skills tutorial developed at the Institute for Health and Social Care Research in Salford, United Kingdom. This tutorial divides a traditional lecture series into chunks, incorporating questions that would normally arise during the session into the text, and providing hyperlinks as well. This allows users to browse to different parts of the tutorial, open a database in a new window in order to perform a practice search, and access other features (Grant & Brettle, 2006). Tutorials, in all their iterations, urge students to hone and develop effective critical thinking skills.

Simulations

Used within healthcare circles for more than 15 years, the use of simulations in nursing training has experienced a recent upsurge in popularity due, in part, to the new availability of high-quality simulation equipment and a reduction in price for this technology. Ranked by fidelity, or the level of realism the equipment resembles, simulation may take various forms, from **computer-based** simulation, in which software is used to simulate a subject or situation (for example, an interactive tutorial featuring a nurse–patient situation), to full-scale simulation, in which all the elements of a healthcare situation are recreated using real physiology, people, and interaction in an attempt to resemble an environment as closely as possible in order to immerse students in the experience (Seropian, Brown, Gavilanes, & Driggers, 2004).

Task and skill training ranks as the most popular form of simulation, during which students hone repetitive skills through interaction with a wide range of equipment, including products such as low-fidelity plastic IV arms to **high-fidelity** virtual reality trainers. The expectation is that students will learn to respond to a situation through a repeated practice-and-learn model of knowledge acquisition; however, because even basic nursing skills, like administering an injection, require both technical skill *and* interpersonal skill, task and skill training enjoys only limited usefulness within the Foundation of Knowledge model without additional clinical exposure or high-fidelity simulation. Even reasonable anatomical fidelity cannot simulate accurately the intensity and vagaries inherent in clinical situations, thus making it difficult for the student to accurately assess and integrate one's clinical judgment, knowledge, and acquisition of skills (Seropian et al., 2004).

The most useful teaching simulations combine high-fidelity equipment with **real-time** demonstrations of simulated medical emergencies, such as those enacted by the patient simulator lab at the Patient Safety Institute, a training subcenter of the North Shore-Long Island Jewish Health System (NS-LIJHS). Home to programmable human simulator mannequins (including an infant) that can exhibit a variety of symptoms resembling various patient scenarios, the patient simulator lab tests and trains nurses and staff responding to simulated medical emergencies using real-time demonstrations and gives immediate feedback on their video-recorded activities. Intended to help improve both clinical and decision-making skills, the mannequins mimic human responses such as breathing, coughing, and speaking, and are anatomically accessible in their ability to be intubated, catherized, and auscultated (Spillane, 2006). The richest and most educationally useful simulation training for students will result as a combination of best practices, current pedagogy, appropriate choice of simulation, clinical experience, and theory (refer to Box 22-4).

BOX 22-4

Simulations in Education

Dee McGonigle and Kathleen Mastrian

There are human simulators for every patient that we care for ranging from the neonate, to pediatrics, to adults, and even simulators for birthing. The realism comes from the lifelike actions and reactions that the mannequins exhibit. Through the programming in the software, these simulated patients can speak to us, have reactive pupils, palpable pulses, heart and breath sounds, react to drugs we administer, enter into arrhythmias, and even have a cardiac arrest.

When we engage in simulations, it helps us to hone our skills for application in our real clinical situations. As we review our performance in the simulation, the software programming provides a debriefing. This reflection allows us to spend time critically thinking about our clinical decision making as well as how we interact with our patients. Simulations provide a means to enhance our clinical skills in a safe environment.

Virtual Reality

In traditional **virtual reality (VR),** the user receives multiple sensory inputs, either mediated or generated by a computer, through visual stimulation (glasses, goggles, screens), audio input (earphones, microphones, synthesizers), and touch (smells, gloves, bodysuits). A form of simulation training and once considered a science fiction technology of the future, virtual reality healthcare training has been widely used by medical students and surgeons in training, allowing individuals to practice an operation before working on the patient (Turley, 2000). The most current spotlight in virtual reality systems focuses on **Second Life,** an online virtual world created by San Francisco-based Linden Lab in 2003 with multiple teaching applications.

Virtual worlds are online environments in which the residents are **avatars** who, in turn, represent individuals participating online. Virtual world participants have an opportunity to design nearly every aspect of their environment, from their avatars' clothing, gender, and appearance (EDUCAUSE, 2006), to more complex elements that openly lend themselves to teaching approaches supported by the Foundation of Knowledge model, such as how the avatars communicate, move, interact, and create. Because virtual worlds are so versatile in their setup, and preselected environments are highly customizable, healthcare instructors have the opportunity to create learner-led scenarios, rather than outcome-based models of knowledge development (EDUCAUSE, 2006), thus creating opportunities for "mediated immersion" (Dede, 2005), a "neomillennial learning style" (Skiba, 2007b, p. 156) that encourages the ability to negotiate multiple media and simulation-based virtual settings and communal learning, providing an important and valuable balance among experiential learning and guided mentoring (Dede, 2005).

No longer limited to the purview of computer geeks, virtual worlds like Second Life have not only gained the attention of large organizations like The American Cancer Society and the Centers for Disease Control and Prevention (CDC), but also educational institutions such as Penn State University, Dartmouth College, and Harvard University, among others (Skiba, 2007b). Because virtual worlds foster unintentional learning through gamer-like technology in which students discover and create knowledge in order *to accomplish something,* rather than experiencing traditional outcome-based learning, their experiences result in greater comprehension and deeper knowledge. In a virtual clinical scenario, for example, a simulated, immersive environment presents invaluable learning opportunities for the student assuming the role of healthcare provider. Faculty can monitor the interaction and interrupt as necessary to provide advice or suggestions, while the students negotiate the real and virtual world components of the scenario and their avatar patients, thus becoming aware of how, why, and when to apply specific skills within a clinical setting (EDUCAUSE, 2006).

Because so much of the data nurses rely upon is complex, and so many patient cues lack concrete language or responses, virtual worlds' animated, immersive, 3D environment allows students to practice skills, try new ideas, and learn from their mistakes while receiving feedback from educators within a globally networked classroom environment. While some students may struggle to participate in virtual communities for various reasons, increasing comfort with multidisciplinary learning among students and educators will encourage the refinement of best practices for effective integration of these tools into mainstream education (EDUCAUSE, 2006).

Internet Tools: Webcasts, Searching, Instant Messaging, Chats/Online Discussions, Electronic Mailing Lists, and Portals

The general consensus in nursing education suggests that any technology that allows users to interact and engage both materials and each other is useful. More specifically, the Foundation of Knowledge model would qualify this observation with the caveat that technology must display user-friendly capabilities to provide benefits to its users, thus allowing students to not just find information and each other online, but also engage, challenge, and institute their discoveries. Providing nursing students easy, free Internet tools for reaching the first step of this equation—gaining access to materials and peers—has been addressed by a proliferation of communication technologies available to any user with an Internet connection. Beyond the gadgetry, with the development of new strategies, practices, applications, and resources in technology comes the need for instructional strategies that not only appeal to this newer generation of students but also enhance learning. These strategies, coupled with easily accessible and functional tools, encourage nursing students to see beyond the right answer, and instead seek out information that will encourage them in developing approaches to issues and resolutions for problems (Bassendowski, 2005).

Webcasts » Webcasts, typically live presentations delivered via the Web, offer great potential for students and faculty to engage both information and each other globally, tapping students' multiple intelligences in order for them to access what they need. Because of the growing ease in producing streaming video and subsequently delivering it via larger bandwidth, Webcasts have grown in popularity and are especially favored by programs that feature distance education components. While some institutions are creating their own Webcast delivery system, most users rely on a few standard providers who, in turn, present the Webcast online. Although often delivered live, allowing audience members to participate, many instructors use Webcasts as an access point for prerecorded archives of lectures and presentations by experts their students would not otherwise have the opportunity to see or hear. Studies show that students enthusiastically embrace Webcast technology, accessing archived presentations more repeatedly than traditionally filmed sessions of guest lecturers; this dynamic level of engagement aids students in better grasping the subject manner. Like much dynamic technology, Webcasts provide an innovative component that keeps students engaged but tend to work best when learners are provided with learning outcomes before viewing (Bell, 2003).

Searching » One of the most common and proliferate search tools in technology today is the **wiki**. Wikis are Web sites or hypertext document collections that allow users to edit and add content in an open-ended forum. The appeal of (and objection to) wikis lies in their ability to let anyone with an interest and an Internet connection participate in a once-exclusive community of knowledge creators and seekers. As an environment that encourages practice and learning, wikis support learning communities where students collaborate online (Skiba, 2007a). Higher education has evolved from a place of straightforward knowledge transmission to a place where one strives to become a member of an expert community, and wikis promise to create opportunity for individuals to participate in this community in heretofore untapped ways. Most objectionable about wikis is their lack of organizing principle (many are organized alphabetically) and the ability for anyone to edit entries, the latter of which creates new intellectual property right challenges. Wikipedia, for example, the best known wiki project on the Web, is an online encyclopedia of sorts whose open access policy regarding its content keeps educators and professionals wary of inaccurate information (Skiba, 2007a). For additional search information, see "Search Engines" in Chapter 20.

Instant Messaging » Instant messaging, one of many collaborative Web chat tools available to any user with a computer and Internet access, continues to establish itself as a working, useful tool for informatics learning, providing instant access to and communication between people, information, and technology. While some **instant message (IM)** services even provide voice and video, all IM clients (of which the three leading are Yahoo! Messenger [Y!M], AOL Instant Messenger [AIM], and MSN Messenger) provide real-time text, allowing users to interact in the form of an on-screen conversation through a technology that is free, already quite popular with users, Web based, doesn't require additional hardware or software, and has a very low learning curve for those few who are unfamiliar with it. Beyond having a real-time conversation, IMing an individual also allows the user to share links, pictures, and files. This kind of easy accessibility allows students, when logged on, to collaborate, seek real-time help from professors or librarians, and engage others working on questions, studying for clinical exams, or reviewing information or notes (Chase, 2007).

Chats/Online Discussions (Blogs) » Real-time chats occur all over the Internet, at each hour of every day. The best-known chat tools are instant messenger clients, but *chatting* also refers to real-time discussion venues in which users meet in virtual chat rooms to engage in conversations by posting messages; this provides a comfortable, recognizable way of communicating for 'net generation students used to surfing the Web and interacting online. In a chat, students can meet, discuss, and engage each other over any given topic. Chats take various forms, the most complex of which involve highly evolved virtual communities in which users step into various rooms where they interact with any other individuals in the room at the same time. Initially the exclusive purview of gamers and/or hardcore programmers creating private online communities, chat rooms now exist for a wide variety of topics and interests.

Web logs, also known as blogs, have emerged as low-investment and easy-to-use writing tools that, through their very setup and appearance, enhance health professionals' communication, writing, reading, information-gathering, and collaboration skills (Maag, 2005). Blogs are a kind of online journal, created by individuals who then invite comments from visitors to that Web space. Compared to technically complex online projects, like tutorials and various multimedia, blogs are immediate, free to set up and access with an Internet connection, and even easily negotiable by the technically ambivalent. Since, by nature, blogs present a built-in discussion area to the user, they are especially useful for study groups interested in reflecting on material and evaluating ideas in a collective, collaborative way (Shaffer et al., 2006).

Electronic Mailing Lists » One low-investment information-gathering tool for use by nursing professionals includes membership in an **electronic mailing list**. These electronic discussion groups that use e-mail to communicate promote communication and collaboration with others interested in a particular field of study (Hebda et al., 2005). Electronic mailing lists require very little to participate, usually just a free subscription and e-mail capability. Electronic mailing lists are available on any subject but most share common features such as the need to subscribe and then log in to participate. The moderators of an electronic mailing list will have specific instructions on how to post messages and how to set subscription controls. Posting information means that when one replies to a topic thread, one generally has sent information to every member of the list. Like other technologies, the capabilities of electronic mailing lists will continue to change and expand, providing ongoing viability for use in nursing education.

Portals » Similar to electronic mailing lists in the way they deliver specific information to one's e-mail, a **portal** allows the personalization of a specific Web site. Portals organize information from Web pages into simple menus so that the user may choose what they want to view and how they want to view it (Hebda et al., 2005). For example, WebMD is one of the most popular and best-known portals, allowing users to create accounts, bookmark their favorite information, sign up for e-mail notifications, and more. Portals, like most Web technologies, require an Internet connection and a free subscription that will allow one to log in.

Podcasts: Audiopods and Videopods

Podcasts are audio recordings linked to the Web that are then downloaded to an MP3 player (Gordon, 2007) or computer where the listener accesses the recording or video. An outgrowth of the Apple **iPod** market frenzy, podcasts are developed and delivered by way of the Internet and require minimal investment, which includes a microphone, an Internet connection, and (often free) editing software. Although most listeners use an MP3 player (of which iPod is but one brand name) to access podcasts, a desktop computer will work just as well (Oblinger, 2005).

Beyond possibilities for global accessibility to whatever information one may record, podcasts also allow for automatic updates in the form of a **really simple syndication (RSS)** (also known as **resource description framework (RDF)** site summary) feed that lets subscribers receive automatic notification whenever a podcast is updated (Gordon, 2007). Refer to Box 22-5.

Podcasts

Jackie Ritzko

A basic Web search using the search term *nursing podcast* produced 1,220 hits on one search engine. But what does this mean in the context of nursing informatics? The implication is that there are many resources on the Internet that somehow involve podcasts with a nursing focus. How these sites might be of use to a professional in the nursing field is the focus of this box. But before any discussion of the educational uses

continues

BOX Continued
22-5

of a technology tool can take place, there needs to be an understanding of the hardware, software, training, and support that is required in order to use the tool.

Podcast is a term coined from the words *iPod* and *broadcast.* The word *iPod* is the name given to a family of portable MP3 players from Apple Computer. MP3 is a common file format for electronic audio files. Audio files, or in particular, MP3 files, can contain verbal speech, music, or a combination of both. MP3 files can be played or listened to using an MP3 player. MP3 players can be portable devices such as the iPod, or an MP3 player can simply be software that is installed and used on a computer. We can now see that a podcast is simply an MP3 file that can be played on an MP3 player. Broadcast, in its simplest usage, refers to the ability to send out. In terms of podcast, broadcasting is the ability to share MP3 files in such a way that the files are delivered to the user whenever new versions are available through a subscription. This ability to share resources and access the most up-to-date resources is a great advantage especially for the educational community.

We will now discuss podcasts in terms of function ranging from the more basic to the more advanced—finding podcasts, listening to podcasts, creating podcasts, and sharing podcasts. Finding podcasts at a minimal level requires only an Internet connection and a Web browser. As indicated at the beginning of this box, a basic Web search for the term *nursing podcast* found many sites. Performing a basic Web search, however, may provide a user with only limited search capabilities. An **MP3 aggregator** is a program that can facilitate the process of finding, subscribing to, and downloading podcasts. A commonly known aggregator is Apple Computer's iTunes, which is a free program available as a download from apple.com. While iTunes is common, keep in mind that it is not the only program of this type. Using a program such as iTunes gives one the ability to search for podcasts based on many criteria including category, author, or title. The iTunes program provides access to audio downloads that may be either songs or podcasts. In both cases, users will find downloads that are free as well as those that require payment.

Since podcasts are MP3 audio files, an MP3 player is needed in order to listen to a podcast. As noted, this can be done on a computer with an MP3 player or on a portable MP3. There are two ways in which podcasts can be downloaded. They can be manually downloaded, or a user can subscribe to a podcast. In the case of a subscription, once a new track is added to the podcast, iTunes will automatically deliver it to a computer. Continuing to use iTunes as an example, once a podcast is found, it can be downloaded from iTunes to a computer. Once on the computer, it can be listened to or transferred to a portable device.

One may also choose to produce or record podcasts. As with most technology solutions, there are typically hardware and software requirements. The hardware for recording a podcast can vary. In a stationary setup, a microphone can be connected to a desktop or laptop computer. Standalone audio recorders can also record podcasts, and some MP3 players have built-in recorders. Free recording software is available for most computer platforms.

BOX *Continued*
22-5

There may be times when a podcast is created for the sole use of the creator. But more often, a podcast is created with the intention of being shared and listened to by others. Podcasts can be stored on Web servers for distribution and can also be shared via tools such as iTunes. A common area within iTunes where educational institutions are able to host podcasts is iTunesU.

Podcasts have many uses in education in general and more specifically in nursing education. As mentioned at the beginning of this box, simple searches on the Web produce many hits for nursing podcasts. Informal learning can take place when a nursing student listens to podcasts. Listening to or creating podcasts may be a formal class assignment, providing new ways to interact with course material.

Short discussions of what is new in the field may appear as podcasts on the Internet, in particular in news and research sites. Learners may rely on the portability of MP3 players to take learning on the road. Commuters as well as walkers and joggers are often seen listening to MP3 players. Since creating podcasts is relatively easy and inexpensive, they can be produced by students as review files for common terms or they can be used for students to self-assess their ability to discuss topics. The uses of podcasts from an educational perspective are limitless.

We need to bring the discussion of podcasts back to the Foundation of Knowledge model. For each task or process in the model, we can see how podcasts can fit. Podcasts can be used to acquire new knowledge from sources on the Web. Listening to podcasts provides learners with another tool for learning in addition to readings and lectures, thus reaching a wider audience with varying learning styles. Since podcast creation is simple and inexpensive, podcasts are an ideal way to generate and disseminate knowledge.

Audiopods » **Audiopod** is a term used to describe a traditional or audio-based podcast. Participating in podcasting can exercise not just basic technology skills, but also writing, editing, and speaking skills as well. Writing scripts for a podcast can be an excellent exercise in critical thinking and information delivery, while the technology itself allows global access to information by faculty, teachers, and students anywhere, at any time (Gordon, 2007). Both faculty and students can create audiopods with little difficulty, and most often use podcasts to share additional class materials, updates, and even entire lectures (Oblinger, 2005).

Videopods » Similar to audiopods in set-up and accessibility, a **videopod** is a podcast that provides video in addition to audio functionability. Faculty might use videopodcasts to demonstrate concepts, interview experts in the field, and even assess student progress (Gordon, 2007). Libraries and other institutions have even begun using the videopod as a learning alternative to the ubiquitous and often mocked information video, finding that highly mobile students are more readily embracing this technology (Oblinger, 2005).

Multimedia

As technologically savvy students continue to demand accessible, interactive learning tools to keep them engaged, an increasing number of instructors are experimenting with and incorporating multimedia into their courses. Generally, multimedia refers to a computer-based technology that incorporates traditional forms of communication to create a seamless and interactive learning environment, such as interactive tutorials, streaming video, and problem-solving programs. Nursing education has long relied on traditional multimedia such as slide presentations, overheads, and training videos for **continuing education** of staff, classroom learning, and patient education (Edwards & Drury, 2000), but new advances in multimedia now allow faculty to add innovations such as simulations and virtual reality to their healthcare training, providing a way for students to learn procedural skills such as insertion of needles and physical assessment without any risks to an actual patient.

Research suggests that the seeing, hearing, doing, and interacting afforded by multimedia facilitates learning retention, with multimedia at least as effective as traditional instruction, but with the benefit of greater learner satisfaction. Authoring software—programs that allow users of varied technical skill to design and create Web pages and movies—has greatly facilitated the use of multimedia by faculty (Hebda et al., 2005), although the most effective multimedia relies on the careful and pedagogically appropriate combination of textual material, graphics, video, animation, and sound (Edwards & Drury, 2000), a distinctly separate skill set from teaching and instructing.

Beyond providing a flexible method of delivery for instructional information, multimedia promises to motivate students by requiring them to analyze evidence in ways that require higher-order thinking and problem-solving skills. Similarly, faculty can begin to think about their classes in new ways and accommodate different student learning styles (Oblinger, 2005). Refer to Box 22-6.

Promoting Active and Collaborative Learning

Because of the shift within the teaching/learning context from the individual seeking answers to the group trying to construct new knowledge from available information, the most effective learning solutions will require new digital communication skills, new pedagogies, and new practices (Costa, 2007). A collaborative, student-centered approach utilizes the best tenets of inductive teaching by imposing more responsibility on students for their own learning than the tradi-

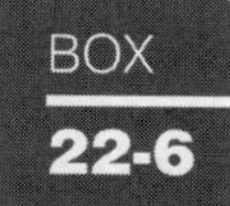

Personal Digital Assistant

Dee McGonigle and Kathleen Mastrian

INTRODUCTION

The personal digital assistant (PDA) is a handheld or palmtop computer. PDAs have gained appeal due to their small size; they are usually designed to fit in a pocket, making them easily portable with impressive performance capabilities that allow one to store, access, and organize information such as calendar entries, documents, spreadsheets, databases, notes, and to-do lists. The capabilities and access are limited by the processing speed and memory, and of course, the faster and more robust the memory capabilities are, the more the unit costs. As one considers purchasing a PDA, it is important that the prospective buyer reflects on his or her current and future needs. One would want to be able to expand capabilities as needed without having to replace the PDA. Therefore, it is important to review all of the PDAs currently available prior to selecting one. Interactive comparisons of various PDA's are available at (CNET, 2008a) and reviews of various models are available at (CNET, 2008b). Softpedia (2007a) provides the latest news on handhelds and is typically updated daily and an opportunity to download a user's manual and view PDA reviews (Softpedia 2007c).

Most of today's PDAs' operating systems are either Linux, PocketPC (Windows), or PalmOS (Palm). Since they can be used in networked environments including wireless configurations, they can theoretically keep the clinician in constant access to patient information, colleagues, and other necessary resources.

The applications available provide a wide range of functionality from simple to highly complex software tools. Nurses can use dosage calculators, drug and specialty databases, educational applications, or clinical forecasting tools; take dictation; or practice telenursing all from a PDA. Since the PDA is compact and one uses a stylus or scroll bars to manage information from inputting, accessing, and output, there are many add-ons available to enhance functionality as well as ease of use.

HOW TO USE A PDA

The PDA could have the following equipment: a display/touch screen, infrared (IR) port, USB connector, secure digital (SD) memory slot, clock icon, menu icon, sync icon, find icon, Web browser button, navigator button or pad, calendar icon, home icon, contacts icon, scroll button/bar, headphone jack, internal Bluetooth, internal **Wi-Fi**, speaker, multiconnector, reset button, stylus, microphone, and/or cell phone capabilities. The configuration of the PDA will affect its performance and one's ability to use it. The navigation buttons and scroll functions allow the user to see, access, and open applications, files, and documents. Depending on the PDA selected, how one inputs data and commands will vary. There are handwriting and voice recognition

continues

BOX Continued
22-6

capabilities available but generally users employ a mixture of a plastic stylus, touch screen, and handwriting recognition software. The handwriting software that recognizes the characters one writes and transfers them to letters and numbers is Graffiti on Palms and Block Recognizer for Pocket PCs. The Transcriber software used on the Pocket PC will recognize legible normal handwriting, printing, or a combination of writing and printing. Thus, users do not have to remember the character codes for the letters and numbers. Users can also type input using the soft keyboard, a small keyboard on the screen, or add-ons such as a small or full-size peripheral keyboard using a Bluetooth or USB connection.

Almost all of the current PDAs come with an expansion slot enabling the owner to increase storage space or memory. Secure digital (SD) is a common type of card that provides additional memory relatively inexpensively. For those thinking about purchasing a PDA, an expansion slot is a must-have item in today's environment.

Most PDAs come with office applications, sync software, Bluetooth, cables, and an IR port. The office applications could include word processing, spreadsheets, database, and/or presentation software. The sync software is short for synchronize and functions to sync or match and update information on both a computer and PDA. Bluetooth is a form of wireless connectivity that is commonly used in cell phones, although it usually does not provide Internet access, it does facilitate file transfer between a PDA and a computer. One can purchase an adaptor if one has a PDA without Bluetooth. Cables are an inexpensive way to connect to a computer, essentially plugging the PDA into a computer. The downside of using cables is that the user must be near the computer in order to connect. The IR beams of light are used as a unidirectional means to wirelessly transfer select data or entire programs to other PDAs. The data and information are not exchanged or traded but rather transferred in only one direction. If someone had something that was needed in hard copy, she could also beam a document to an IR-enabled printer. Most commonly, people beam their business cards. For example, if one attended a career fair or conference and visited exhibitor booths, he could beam his business card into a vendor's PDA. In order to beam across platforms, additional software would be required.

As PDAs continue to evolve, so do their capabilities and connectivity. The Internet connectivity (Web browser and e-mail) provides the clinician with communication capabilities and constant access to real-time online data and information. Since the PDA is portable, connectivity must be ready whenever and wherever it is needed. One way to establish connectivity is through the use of Wi-Fi. The Wi-Fi compatibility provides for use at hot spots throughout the country such as cafes, coffee shops, hotels, restaurants, and universities. It can also use the existing wireless network in an agency or office. This feature can be added to a PDA by purchasing a Wi-Fi adaptor.

Some cell phones, called **smartphones**, have limited PDA capabilities, while some PDAs are phone enabled. Smartphones have limited PC functionality; they have an op-

BOX *Continued*
22-6

erating system and facilitate the use of e-mail and other applications. Based on one's practice setting, the addition of the phone features could be an important consideration.

APPLICATIONS

As nurses, there are tremendous advantages to using a PDA in our practice. They can be used to track patients, as point-of-care (POC) devices, or calculators. The PDA could take dictation at the bedside or on the go as the user travels between patients or appointments. As reference tools, they can provide ready access to clinical and/or drug databases, electronic textbooks and reference materials, online journals in real time such as *MEDLINE,* the *Online Journal of Nursing Informatics (OJNI),* and educational tools such as study guides and care planning documents such as those found in Dykes Library (2008) and PDA Cortex (n.d.). Users can transfer information within a network even when they are in the field. Using the network, they could send a note to a case manager, update a physician on the status of patients they visited in their homes, or even send prescriptions to the pharmacy. The PDA allows users to maintain their schedules or calendars and receive reminder alarms. One can even use a PDA for professional development such as continuing education offerings or furthering academic education online. Whether one is an avid PDA user, is beginning to use a PDA, or is just contemplating purchasing one, it is best to get involved and participate in the list that discusses PDA use in nursing at http://www.rnpalm.com/nursing_pdas_listserv.htm.

The PDA can enhance the health care for our patients as well. We can monitor our patients and send surveys and questionnaires; they can submit their responses to us as their healthcare provider or to the healthcare institution. The PDA can enhance their access to their clinicians, especially for patients who are mobile; the PDA can go where they go and they can keep in touch via e-mail/phone/fax/instant messaging, or text messaging. They can maintain their appointment and medication schedule as well as receive patient education materials and access clinician recommended Web sites/electronic mailing lists.

The educational arena has embraced this technology. Nursing instructors are communicating and sharing information with their learners and clinical settings using PDA technologies. Using wireless connectivity in class, instructors can receive instant feedback as to the understanding of their learners. PDAs can even assist with discussions and provide study aids, interactive exercises, and quizzes. For a nursing student, the reference materials and podcasts available for coursework could be stored on a PDA for easy access. Students could upload and download clinical documents and information with an instructor and clinical setting staff. In the clinical setting, the easy access to robust reference tools and materials such as dosage calculators helps to reduce errors. The educational applications will continue to expand as more software and capabilities become available.

This is certainly not an exhaustive list of PDA applications or equipment, and the truth of this information era is that the current will be the past by the time this is in

BOX *Continued*
22-6

print. PDAs continue to evolve and become smaller and more robust (About.com, n.d.; Seko, 2005; Softpedia, 2007a; Softpedia, 2007c). As this future continues to unfold, so will our applications of PDAs in nursing.

References

About.com (n.d.). *Palmtops/PDAs: Fossil wrist PDA FX2008 with Palm OS review.* Retrieved on January 12, 2008 from http://palmtops.about.com/od/palmhardware/fr/FossilWristPDA.htm

CNET. (2008a). *PDA—CNET reviews.* PDAs matching "PDA" Retrieved January 12, 2008, from http://reviews.cnet.com/4244-5_7-0.html?query=PDA&tag=srch&target

CNET. (2008b). *CNET Reviews: What to look for in handhelds.* Retrieved January 12, 2008, from http://reviews.cnet.com/4520-3127_7-5021319-1.html?tag=wtlf%5C%22%3Ehttp://computers.cnet.com/hardware/0-1087-8-20549052-1.html?tag=wtlf

Dykes Library. (2008). *Popular freeware for PDAs.* Retrieved January 12, 2008, from http://library.kumc.edu/resources/PDAFreebies.htm

PDA Cortex. (n.d.). *The Journal of Mobile Informatics and PDA resources for health-care professionals.* Retrieved January 12, 2008, from http://www.rnpalm.com/

Seko, S. (2005). *IR watch Ver 0.3: The version only for WristPDA.* Retrieved January 12, 2008, from http://www.pamupamu.com/soft/irmoniw/irw.htm

Softpedia. (2007a). *Handhelds area and latest handheld devices (RSS).* Retrieved January 12, 2008, from http://handheld.softpedia.com/#devices

Softpedia. (2007b). *Headline news: Handhelds news and latest handhelds news.* Retrieved on January 12, 2008, from http://news.softpedia.com/cat/Telecoms/Handhelds/

Softpedia. (2007c). *Handhelds area and PDA manual 1.0 download (for the PocketPC).* Retrieved January 13, 2008, from http://handheld.softpedia.com/get/Documents-E-Books/Pda-Manual-36435.shtml

tional lecture-based deductive approach. These constructivist methods are built on the widely accepted principle that students are constantly constructing their own realities rather than simply absorbing versions presented by their teachers. Collaborative methods will often involve students' discussion of questions and in-class problem solving, with much of the work (in and out of class) done by students in groups rather than individually (Felder & Prince, 2007).

Johnson and Johnson (1990) have identified five significant elements for successful collaborative learning. These include:

1. Face-to-face interaction between students, thus allowing them to build on each other's strengths
2. Mutual learning goals that, in turn, prompt students to exhibit positive interdependence rather than individualized competition
3. Equal participation in the work process as well as personal accountability for the work one contributes
4. Regular debriefing sessions as a group after meetings or presentations during which time feedback is shared and observations analyzed
5. Use of cooperative group process skills learned in the classroom

And while collaborative learning relies heavily on student investment and participation, institutions must ultimately create the best settings—both physical and electronic—where collaboration is encouraged. This can be achieved with a sound educational and technological infrastructure, reliability on proven working models, adaptable physical spaces, and even pedagogical support in the form of preceptors or mentors.

Especially useful for nursing students is the collaborative fieldwork model in which two or more students share a clinical setting and the same fieldwork educator. In this model, learning happens in a reciprocal fashion, with students constructing knowledge from watching each other and exchanging ideas. The most effective fieldwork experiences will be highly structured with clear outlines of responsibilities, duties, and expectations, insuring that the experience matches learner expectations. All activities performed by students, such as performing evaluations, are done jointly, so that peers might provide each other objective feedback, leading to eventual increased self-confidence (Costa, 2007). In this way, suggests Costa (2007), individuals with different viewpoints and experiences create a space where new knowledge emerges and existing knowledge can be restructured (as cited in Cockrell, Caplow, & Donaldson, 2000).

Libraries have also begun to recognize their role in students' success with and predisposition to collaborative learning with redesigned spaces that reflect students' need to huddle in small groups, sit closely together without barriers, chat about their work, and view digital information without physical hindrances like carrels or work stalls. A leader in this movement has been Indiana State University, whose new information commons features completely overhauled furniture, software, monitors, processing power, and wireless access to the university's network. Students can now collect as a group at kidney-shaped tables, better see the information loaded on the flat-screen monitors, make use of brainstorming, design, and planning software, and discuss their work in a chat-friendly zone. Some faculty have even scheduled classes at the learning stations, and students, including those in nursing, have responded enthusiastically to the evolved space (Gabbard, Kaiser, & Kaunelis, 2007).

In addition to adaptable physical spaces that encourage discussion and group work, students also require a supportive infrastructure that provides essential elements necessary to successful research and scholarship. These include professional development support in the form of workshops that help students acquire or refresh skill sets, presentation opportunities, and hardware, software, and resource support. One such example includes participation by nursing students at the University of Texas medical branch school of nursing in the scholarly talk about research series (STARS) in which students and faculty give presentations of their work before presenting at professional conferences (Froman et al., 2003), thus eliciting collegial feedback, collaborative troubleshooting, and shared research ideas.

Consider that simply adopting a collaborative, inductive method of learning will not necessarily lead to better learning and more satisfied students. As with any form of instruction, collaborative teaching methods need skilled and careful implementation. Because students are often resistant to instruction that makes them more responsible for their own learning, those who attempt an inductive learning method should adhere to best practices, such as providing adequate scaffolding-extensive support and guidance when students are first introduced to the method and gradual withdrawal of support as students gain more experience and confidence in its use (Felder & Prince, 2007).

Nursing preceptors and mentors, for example, can provide this kind of scaffolded support, filling roles as clinically active role models (Armitage & Burnard, 1991) and problem-solving **advocates** and collaborators (Gagen & Bowie, 2005). Primarily concerned with the teaching and learning aspects of the relationship, preceptors help students learn by acting as clinical practitioner role models from whom the students can copy appropriate skills and behaviors. Kramer (1974) introduced the concept of nurse preceptor to address the disparity of the theory–practice gap—the difference between what is taught in class and what actually happens in nursing practice. Preceptors enhance clinical competence through direct role modeling, especially valuable in a field where competence and clinical ability are paramount (Armitage & Burnard, 1991). Mentors, similar to preceptors, provide equally valuable assistance to nursing students in the form of a facilitator. Mentors are most often employed in nursing and education to support new professionals trying to fulfill the rigors of a new position while negotiating the stress inherent to a new environment (Gagen & Bowie, 2005). Mentors tend to address student needs through open conversation, student advocacy, feedback on student progress, facilitation, teaching, and general support (Neary, 2000).

Generally, these and other forms of institutional support promote students' adoption of a meaning-oriented approach to learning, as opposed to a surface or memorization-intensive approach. Collaborative, inductive learning promotes intellectual development that challenges the dualistic thinking that characterizes many entering college students, which holds that "all knowledge is certain, professors have it and the task of students is to absorb and repeat it" (Felder & Prince, 2007, p. 55). Further, this kind of learning helps students acquire the self-directed learning and critical thinking skills that characterize the best scientists and engineers (Felder & Prince, 2007). The active, engaging elements of collaborative learning increase self-confidence, promote autonomy in students, and foster a commitment to lifelong learning (Costa, 2007), all necessities for the success of a new millennial information-literate student.

KNOWLEDGE ASSESSMENT METHODS

An integral and critical component of educational programming is the evaluation of different learning methods. An evaluation process relies upon actions taken to measure outcomes, such as the attainment of learning. Process or formative evaluation takes place over the lifespan of a program and is ongoing, while summative evaluation is enacted at the end of a program or learning activity.

Both administrators and nursing educators across various programs are responsible for evaluating their programs; beyond gathering feedback from participants and learners—an important but ultimately one-dimensional evaluative tool—effective program evaluation should be considered in relation to successes, failures, and how program revision might reinstate a program's effectiveness (Menix, 2007). Dickerson (2005) suggests that evaluation constitutes a substantial part of the work of the nurse educator as defined in the *Scope and Standards of Practice for Nursing Professional Development* (Dickerson, as cited in American Nurses Association, 2000).

Papers/Projects

When one is looking for feedback and assessment of a particular learning activity, data are best collected during and at the completion of the activity. During the activity, different factors assist in determining how well a teaching strategy is working; these factors might include participant engagement (Are students listening? Is there notetaking? Does anyone have questions or comments?), ease of use of equipment and resources, and time required to complete an activity. Much in the way nursing practitioners modify care plans in the midst of an unsuccessful treatment, so should educators change course when it appears the learning experience is not progressing as planned (Dickerson, 2005).

Evaluation by participants at the end of a project is also valuable since learners can provide information related to the attainment of objectives and the teaching effectiveness of both the faculty and the learning materials while the experience is still fresh and memorable. Learner input, though sometimes considered biased and unreliable (such as student evaluations refuted by many faculty as useless), actually represent useful feedback to the success of a project or assignment (Dickerson, 2005). Faculty at the University of Colorado at Boulder address this issue by choosing samples of student work for evaluation by faculty or external reviewers to see how well students are meeting program skills and goals. Because these papers and projects are graded by an instructor as part of the course, this form of embedded assignment ensures that the students are still expending effort without having to do extra assessment-specific assignments (University of Colorado at Boulder, Office of Planning, Budget and Analysis, 2001).

When a paper assignment or project does fail, the outcome provides a valuable learning opportunity for all educators to look closely at the pedagogy, structure, goals, outcomes, and expectations of success of the proposed activity and determine what needs revising or reevaluating in order for what the educator would term "successful" completion. While many educators and researchers evaluate programs for effectiveness and to maintain certain standards (Dickerson, 2005), most innovative is the educator who evaluates and observes superficial failures as learning opportunities to improve pedagogy and delivery.

Discussions

While traditional in-class discussion seems almost outdated in light of the stunning advances in technology that allow learners to participate in every kind of activity from computer-guided online quizzes to interactive simulations, the educator as facilitator still holds value and importance in a traditional or even blended classroom. In one study, students exposed to competency-based, written self-learning modules and students exposed to competency-based, didactic lecture modules performed equally. A sample was selected from a group of registered nurses who attended a mandatory yearly review of standards from the Occupational Safety and Health Administration (OSHA) and the Joint Commission on Accreditation of Healthcare Organizations (JCAHO). The 67 subjects were given pretests, were exposed to the same content material through two different kinds of presentations, and were then posttested. Results indicated no significant differences among scores of either group. This suggests that advantages of one teaching method versus another lie, ultimately, in the educator (Schlomer, Anderson, & Shaw, 1997). Self-direction, independence, and a willingness to collaborate all mark the millennial learner, but without guidance, pedagogical grounding, and even a basic contextualized introduction to concepts and materials, even self-motivated, highly information-literate learners will flounder without assistance. Refer to Box 22-7.

A Typical Week

Patricia Sweeney

My responsibilities as a nursing faculty member and my use of technology in support of education vary in a typical week. I am usually in the classroom 1 day a week, on clinical rotation with students 2 days a week, and at meetings 1 day a week; and I spend the remainder of the time preparing for class and reviewing my clinical or classroom skills.

Class, clinical, and office days involve a variety of activities. Class days begin after I check my e-mail, usually from my home in the morning. I then review my lecture notes, handouts, and any planned classroom activities. I typically teach for 2–4 hours, taking two 10-minute breaks. I use the technology available in the nursing classroom, which includes a computer station with Internet access, a document camera for showing paper overheads or textbook documents, PowerPoint presentations displayed using the projector, and Blackboard display software. I usually use the computer to display PowerPoint presentations and try to incorporate at least one other dynamic activity to enhance the students' understanding of the day's content. When class is finished, I spend a few more hours in my office meeting with students, updating lectures, writing exam questions, reviewing student assignments, preparing for meetings, and answering phone or electronic messages. At the end of my day, I take my university laptop home so that I can continue working from home. I can access my e-mail, our course management system, and the Internet from home. I can grade assignments, view who has taken required online exams, or communicate with students.

My clinical day is what most people would anticipate. I meet with students at 7 a.m. Preconference time is spent reviewing the care of assigned patients. I always want to be sure that students are prepared and understand priorities of care, potential problems, treatments, and medications. I spend the next 6 to 7 hours monitoring students and patients, collaborating with staff nurses, assisting with documentation, and demonstrating or helping with any treatments or skills. Postconference time is used to clarify information from the day and discuss interesting findings or problems. I often give students information that relates to course content as it applies to patients that we've taken care of during clinical experiences. I use the Internet to identify the most recent evidence-based reports for the topics and use that information to discuss advances in patient technology and patient care. I end my day by going to my office after the clinical rotation to check my regular mail and phone messages or to attend

continues

BOX *Continued*

22-7

any scheduled meetings. I also keep track of students' clinical progress and learning needs and types of patients and procedures each student has experienced on an electronic template. I can then show students their progress and use the form for the students' final clinical evaluations.

One day a week is devoted to meetings. The school of nursing has all of its major committee work scheduled on the same day each week, while campus committee meetings are usually scheduled during the noon hour. I have two school of nursing meetings a month and four campus meetings. Each meeting lasts between 1 and 2 hours. I'm able to prepare and review for these in the morning prior to the scheduled meeting time. Current agendas, previous minutes, and any individual committee assignments are posted in the course management system for the school of nursing committee work. I link to these meetings using video or phone conferencing. Local campus meeting information is sent via e-mail and I attend those meetings in person.

I have 1 office day a week. Students have access to my office hours information and availability in our course management system. Students are encouraged to meet with me during these times to chat about their progress or so I can answer questions about an upcoming exam. I also see about 20 of my advisees at midsemester when it is time to register for the next semester. I use the online course registration supports such as the electronic audit of student progress and electronic schedules. I spend a part of every semester using campus and university resources to keep updated on technology. I've attended many programs on how to use the course management system, develop tests for the Web, and perform more effective computer library searches. Most of these programs are offered by our campus IT department or the tech support specialist. Faculty is often asked to test new technology in the classroom. Currently, a student response system is being evaluated. This is a system similar to what is used to poll the audience on the *Who Wants to Be a Millionaire* game show. I know I'll use this system in the future to identify student understanding of class content. I could display sample test questions and ask students to respond. This system will benefit students in several ways. First, students can participate and remain anonymous. Students would not feel embarrassed by showing they don't know something. I could use it to ask questions during lecture by surveying the class. I could identify what percent of the class selects the most appropriate answer and grasps key information in each lecture.

I hope that you can see how diverse and challenging life is for a nursing educator. I don't really know how I would manage all of the necessary activities without technology. As a teacher for more than 20 years and an RN for more than 25 years, I did not grow up during the computer age. I was forced into it. I often learned about technology along the way. I was quite hesitant initially about the power of computers and then the Internet. As a novice faculty member at the university in 1992, I was asked to be one of the first persons from our campus to participate in a new program involving 1 week of intense daylong courses on the use of technology for teaching. I implemented new ideas slowly, but now a day doesn't go by that I don't use technology for some aspect of

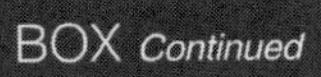

BOX 22-7 Continued

my career. I feel lost when the IT staff takes my laptop for a day of servicing. I now take advantage of every learning opportunity related to technology and teaching.

LESSONS LEARNED

If I had to offer some guidelines for the use of technology in nursing education based on my own experience, I would provide the following:

1. Know your school's resources. Identify the key people who can help you access those resources.
2. Use what works for your courses. There are so many different ways that technology can be used. Select the tools that help to meet your students' needs.
3. Try something new each semester. It's important to learn how to incorporate new ideas for classroom and clinical instruction into a course.
4. Evaluate your instructional methods. Use what works and change what does not work.
5. Make technology work for you. Select the technologies that help you to be organized and track information or student progress.

FUTURE TRENDS IN EDUCATION

I can only imagine how technology will change teaching, advising, service, and research. I anticipate that almost every type of undergraduate class may move to an online format. This is already occurring for certain majors, but is more difficult for nursing as an applied science. Nursing classes can be conducted online, with an instructor available as needed at a local campus. Technology already allows faculty to place most materials on the Internet, including word-processed documents, instructor PowerPoint presentations, video and other digital data, and links to library resources. As more students attend classes online, the faculty workload may change. Planning and implementing online classes is more time consuming than resident instruction since all materials must be developed for the Internet. Presentation of the information must also be detailed and organized. Internet connectivity may improve to the point that students can sit at their computer at a designated time and be in a live class with other students and the faculty member.

Nursing students will always need clinical experience, with a major portion of clinical practice devoted to caring for real patients. It seems that clinical faculty will always be needed, though the role may change. In the future, students may be assisted by staff and monitored by clinical faculty through some remote access. Clinical practice will also involve the use of more simulations. Clinical sites for certain specialties, such as pediatrics and obstetrics, are already becoming scarce. There are national seminars and entire companies devoted to the use of mannequin simulations and other technology for nursing students. Instructors can use simulations to demonstrate high-tech clinical environments or emergency situations. Companies are already developing case studies to correspond with equipment that they sell. Students can practice with these "patients" in a more controlled environment—a virtual hospital.

continues

BOX Continued
22-7

I also foresee that the technological advances in advising systems will minimize the need for academic advisors. All advising materials are already available online. Students are becoming more comfortable looking for information, scheduling classes, and reviewing graduation requirements. The students who will continue to seek out faculty advisors will be those who are uncertain of their major or looking for career advice.

Research and service to a university will also change. Faculty already has access to some full-text journals and books online. The number of these available will continue to increase, and eventually almost any material will be available in full text and online. This will make it easier to access materials, though it may be more time consuming to perform a library search. Faculty service roles will probably not change much, though they may take a different form. Faculty will be asked to serve on new committees devoted to online learning and technology. Faculty will spend more time learning to use technology as it continues to develop and change.

I often comment that as a nursing instructor my role is as an assistant to the student. Teaching nursing in the future will probably evolve more into a coaching role. Teachers will help students identify information and resources and utilize those resources in an appropriate manner. I hope that I will always learn to use new technology to make learning easier for students and to help me accomplish my own personal and professional goals.

Testing

With legal and financial implications of employee and student performance a major concern for all providers and healthcare organizations, multiple requirements for competence in nursing practices within the healthcare system have been established by national agencies and associations, like those suggested by the American Nurses Association. Of specific concern to educators and administrators is the gap exhibited by test takers who, while scoring exceptionally well on exams, are, conversely, unable to perform a clinical procedure or recognize a warning sign in a patient experiencing difficulty. Use of traditional testing as an evaluative tool has been in existence for decades, though research shows that criterion-based performance better measures skill levels while also identifying deficiencies (Redman, Lenburg, & Walker, 1999).

As a result, some schools, such as the University of Colorado's school of nursing, have redesigned their curricula as well as the competency-based curricular outcomes for their educational programs. These substantial programmatic changes have resulted in a unique approach to nursing at both the undergraduate and graduate levels, with a new focus on such competency-based outcomes as "competent effective reflective practice" (Redman et al., 1999, p. 3) and "generation of nursing knowledge and leadership and social change for improved health of individuals, communities, populations, and global environments" (Redman et al., 1999, p. 3).

Additionally, faculty at the University of Colorado at Boulder use embedded testing to assess outcomes, with goals built into exams or other assignments. Student performance regarding these items is part of an outcomes assessment, and it is graded accordingly by an instructor as part of the course (University of Colorado at Boulder, Office of Planning, Budget and Analysis, 2001). Such changes promise to deliver substantial changes in the way nursing is taught, perceived, and executed.

Case Scenarios

Professional organizations are increasingly recommending performance-based assessments of students in professional degree programs, and enacting case scenarios provides an opportunity for students to practice procedural responses. Case scenarios, a form of problem-based learning, are now even available through simulation software or virtual reality programming. This kind of testing, in which students must respond within context to a perceived situation rather than a theoretical or fact-based question, allows educators to gauge procedural knowledge—in other words, it allows them to gauge *how* a student executes a skill or applies concepts and principles to specific situations (Garavalia, 2002). For example, in a clinical context, a student could explain how to change a dressing, insert an IV, or intubate an individual, but the knowledge would be declarative rather than procedural and, thus, for some evaluators, not as valuable. Conditional knowledge is often reflected in procedural knowledge as well, demonstrating a student's ability to know when and why action is or is not taken, and how.

The best assessment strategies are identified through consideration of the cognitive level of the objective, the nature of the task, and the best context for the assessment. Performance assessments can be used throughout a curriculum, not just as a final component of a practical or clinical experience. Most important is insuring that the assessment tool and task matches the instruction and the stated learning objective (Garavalia, 2002).

Other: Portfolios

Viewed in the 1980s as realistic evaluative tools of student accomplishment and learning, **portfolios** in nursing education are rising in popularity as useful tools for documenting students' exposure to educational experiences. A nursing portfolio allows a student to document a variety of sometimes unquantifiable skills, such as creativity, communication, and critical thinking. Further, portfolios can reflect achievement of goals, self-evaluation, and professional development, also providing a way for returning students to log and document past work or life experiences in a creative but structured way without taking a standardized test. The usefulness of a portfolio for an undergraduate in a nursing program depends upon a structured system of organization: an identification page with resume, a table of contents, separate and clearly marked sections, etc. In this way portfolios can monitor program outcomes, positively influence employment and graduate school admission, and provide a clear snapshot of a student's strengths and abilities (Alexander, Baldwin, & McDaniel, 2002).

KNOWLEDGE DISSEMINATION AND SHARING

Sharing stories and experience from a clinical point of view accomplishes much more than simply promoting camaraderie or empathy (although this kind of engagement is infinitely valuable in its own way); sharing experiences of clinical learning can help convey lifesaving information to other clinicians in a way that is more memorable and palatable and less imposing than warnings delivered outside a social context. Clinical and caring knowledge, often rooted in everyday exchanges, become socially embedded such that those with experience in particular clinical settings share common knowledge and understanding. The social embeddedness of caring and clinical knowledge is a result of shared and shaped collective understanding of practice and sometimes provides an alternative view.

The power of pooled knowledge in combination with knowledge produced in dialogue with others helps to limit tunnel vision and is a powerful strategy for maximizing the clinical knowledge of a group. Whether the nurse is networking, presenting, or seeking continuing education or recertification, an understanding of socially embedded knowledge coupled with the multiple perspectives of skilled practitioners allows for a rich and vibrant opportunity to apply nursing skill effectively (Benner, Tanner, & Chelsa, 1997).

Networking

Considered crucial to career development because of opportunities for collaboration and information exchange, networking encourages professional support by making successful professionals accessible to their colleagues. Further, developing interactive professional networks between academic and clinical nurses can benefit practice in diabetes, stroke, and mental health care, as well as in community nursing wherein practitioners are encouraged to collaborate (Gillibrand, Burton, & Watkins, 2002).

The value of networking to members of male-dominated professionals such as law, business, and medicine resides in opportunities to make contact with fellow professionals, and in turn, further careers. This observation is especially poignant for nursing—a predominantly female profession—which, until recently, has rarely reaped the benefits of formal networking (Nicholl & Tracey, 2007).

Because nurses tend to gather their information from personal networks such as colleagues or professional meetings, the increased availability of technology to assist in networking has greatly facilitated information exchange. Blogs, e-mail, Web sites, electronic mailing lists, and other communicative technologies have made collaboration and networking possibilities endless, allowing nurses to access and learn from colleagues' experiences. Using the Internet allows for the discovery of information heretofore unavailable through traditional information sources (Pravikoff & Levy, 2006), helping nursing professionals decide if, for example, pursuing research opportunities or collaboration on specific professional projects seems viable.

Formal networks, such as the International Nurse Practitioner/Advanced Practice Nursing Network (INP/APNN), unveiled in 2000, promote the exchange of knowledge, resources, and expertise in order to enhance the presence of nursing in primary health care. Created in response to the globalization of nurse practitioner and APNN roles, the network enables the enhancement and advancement of practice both for countries just beginning to initiate APN roles and for those with experienced practitioners (Affara, Cross, & Schober, 2001).

Membership and participation in professional associations also provide ways to network and advance one's profession. Professional associations provide venues through which members may set standards for professional practice, establish codes of ethics, become involved in advocacy, engage in continuing education opportunities, access job banks, subscribe to professional journals, and act as a common voice for the profession. For example, the American Nursing Association of Occupational Health Nurses is instrumental in maintaining healthcare issues on the political agenda. Research shows that nurses hesitate to join professional organizations due to barriers associated with cost, distance to meetings, lack of activities in one's geographic area, and inability to attend meetings. Because networking creates fertile areas for the development of new ideas, partnership, jobs, and strategies, both national and state associations would benefit from creating greater opportunities for healthcare practitioners to earn continuing education credit and network with others in their field (Thackeray, Neiger, & Roe, 2005).

Presenting and Publishing

Much in the way the American Association of Colleges of Nursing (AACN) maintains standards for nursing education, professional journals also hold their contributors to similarly rigorous standards and provide a valuable venue in which nursing professionals might share ideology and innovations in the field. With the proliferation of online journals and nursing information available in multiple medias, publishing remains an excellent way to participate in the dissemination of professional information. Both nursing magazines and journals reach considerable audiences; journals' distinctions lie in their authorship and audience. While journal articles are written by and for scholars, with refereed or peer-reviewed journals requiring a blind review by a group of reviewers in order to eliminate bias, magazine articles may be written by a professional in the field, an editor, freelancer, or other author. Publishing provides excellent opportunities to extend knowledge and share research.

Similar to publishing, making presentations at contemporary professional conferences allows nursing educators and students to gain experience and share scholarship with colleagues. Presentations must meet certain standards for an audience to find them credible and effective. Since an audience will retain 50% of what they see and hear in a presentation versus 20% if they only hear it, experts suggest the use of audiovisual aids in making professional presentations most effective (Bergren, 2000). A noteworthy presentation could involve multiple levels of complexity, from a simple PowerPoint to an animated tutorial. Because technology and well-designed visuals will not make up for lack of preparedness or research, presenters should be aware of their target audience and details of the research being presented. Regardless of media or presentation style, audiovisual presentations should be designed consistently and simply, using easy-to-read and understand colors and fonts and audience-appropriate language.

Conferences often host poster presentations to share research findings, innovations and exemplar programs in a low-investment but visually captivating way. Because posters are primarily visual, with little or no verbal supplementation, most important for consideration are room elements such as size, space limitations, and lighting. The best nursing practitioner posters will feature consistent visual components, like appropriately sized, readable font and simple colors, and will be based on a research concept or clinical objective (Berg, 2005). A high-tech alternative to a paper poster is an electronic poster—a continuously running PowerPoint presentation either projected for larger audiences or left to run from a laptop or desktop for smaller audiences (Bergren, 2000). Both publishing and presenting provide opportunities for the nursing practitioner to disseminate new knowledge and stay abreast of information in her field.

Continuing Education/Recertification

Nationally, nursing employers and institutions have, due to budgetary constraints, begun to eliminate continuing education (CE) programs traditionally reliant on classes, conferences, and workshops; consequently, reliance upon outside agencies and technology have increased to meet this need. The traditional approach to obtaining CE credits has included home study offered by professional journals and organizations in which the client reads articles, answers related questions, and sends in the test form and fee. While fairly straightforward, this technique provides little in the way of peer interaction (Hebda et al., 2005).

With the ubiquitous technology influx and the accessibility it affords, obtaining CE credits through e-learning is considered a beneficial delivery method for mandatory educational programs as well as other programs that provide employees with opportunities to maintain and/or improve skills. Benefits of e-learning for CE training include the ability to access information at any time (thus creating a flexible schedule) and experience instant feedback and individualized instruction by seeking out specific, additional information as needed.

E-learning can also benefit administrative support of CE credits by providing instantly accessible computerized records and other tracking features such as records of success and completion, associated costs of program development, and staff productivity. Allowing nursing professionals to complete mandatory training on demand represents a huge benefit of e-learning, with the best programs allowing for customization to accommodate program revisions and regulation changes (Hebda et al., 2005).

In some cases, acquiring CE credits may help one achieve recertification as well. Available through myriad professional organizations, recertification ensures that nurses are staying current in their fields and some specialties; for example, the field of pediatric nursing requires annual recertification in order to maintain professional status. During recertification, the Pediatric Nursing and Certification Board offers each certified pediatric nurse (CPN) options for ensuring she or he is maintaining national standards within the specialty of pediatric nursing (Pediatric Nursing Certification Board, 2007).

As an added benefit, some hospitals provide extra allowances to nurses who maintain certification, with recent studies showing those who are certified having a salary of $8,000–$10,000 more than uncertified colleagues. Additionally, 90% of nurse managers indicate they would hire a certified nurse over a noncertified nurse. Research shows that the trend in magnet hospitals to encourage, reward, and promote certified nurses is spreading to other facilities and healthcare settings, with retirement centers and home health agencies now beginning to seek certified nurses for perceived extra benefit to their customers and a marketing advantage in hiring nurses with guaranteed levels of competence (Peterson, 2007).

One such program that facilitates educational programs for medical professionals around the nation and helps nurses reach recertification goals is the innovative Wake Area Health Education Center (AHEC) registered nurse (RN) refresher program designed to return registered nurses to practice. Nurses participate in a series of medical/surgical didactic models, participate in clinical practicums, and work one-on-one with an RN preceptor who provides instruction and evaluation of skills over the course of 160 hours. Most notable about this program is the initiation of handheld devices for use by the refresher students who, as a result, more actively used the medical library and experienced great self-confidence with both knowing how to use technology and in their return to nursing practice. As of 2006, more than 50 healthcare organizations were partnering with Wake AHEC in providing the clinical practicum portion of the RN refresher program, and more than 1,100 RNs had enrolled since its inception in 1990 (Colevins, Bond, & Clark, 2006). For information on continuing education, visit the American Nurses Association continuing education page at http://nursingworld.org/ce/cehome.cfm.

SUMMARY

The future holds a phenomenal amount of potential for virtual reality-embedded education. Once the purview of gamers and geeks, virtual reality has exploded onto the academic scene with potential for cross-pollination between fields of inquiry across the curriculum, university, and even learning systems. All kinds of university departments will experiment with virtual reality in the hopes of staying current and pleasing to their young and demanding constituency; however, much in the way society loves the feel of a book too much to make it archaic, so too will students, educators, and administrators ultimately return to a compromised form of face-to-face classroom teaching, even in the face of newer and more adventuresome teaching technologies. Further, once fast, high-burn technologies stop flooding the marketplace and making education an even bigger business for proprietary online universities, modified traditions will take their place, creating new spaces for nontraditional students as well as the 'net generation, both anxious for technology use in the classroom for very different reasons.

The most important thought I would like to leave you with is the following suggestion: much in the same way you would hesitate to leave a project, syllabus, or concept unexplained, work against the assumption that technology runs itself. Consider that flash is not substance, and drama is not depth; technology only performs as well as the pedagogy that undergirds and sustains it. Plan for and use technology with care so that its best features consequently enrich yours as an educator or learner.

THOUGHT-PROVOKING Questions

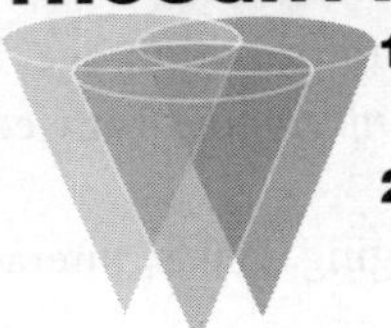

1. What are some of the forces behind the push toward a more wired learning experience in nursing education?
2. What technology do you find most beneficial to use in your practice or education setting? Why do you find this tool useful? From your perspective, how could this tool be enhanced?

References

Affara, F., Cross, S., & Schober, M. (2001). Discovering resources—Making global connections, international networking. *Journal of the American Academy of Nurse Practitioners, 13*(10), 445–448.

Alexander, J. G., Baldwin, M. S., & McDaniel, G. S. (2002). The nursing portfolio: A reflection of a professional. *The Journal of Continuing Education in Nursing, 33*(2), 55–59.

American Nurses Association. (2000). *Scope and standards of practice for nursing professional development.* Washington, DC: Author.

Aquino-Russell, C., Maillard Strüby, F. V., & Reviczky, K. (2007). Living attentive presence and changing perspectives with a Web-based nursing theory course. *Nursing Science Quarterly, 20*(2), 128–134.

Armitage, P., & Burnard, P. (1991). Mentors or preceptors? Narrowing the theory-practice gap. *Nurse Education Today, 11*, 225–229.

Barnes, L., & Rudge, T. (2005). Virtual reality or real virtuality: The space of flows and nursing practice. *Nursing Inquiry, 12*(4), 306–315.

Bassendowski, S. L. (2005). NursingQuest: Supporting an analysis of nursing issues. *Journal of Nursing Education, 46*(2), 92–95.

Bell, S. (2003). Cyber-guest lecturers: Using Webcasts as a teaching tool. *TechTrends, 47*(4), 10–14.

Benner, P., Tanner, C., & Chelsa, C. (1997). The social fabric of nursing knowledge. *The American Journal of Nursing, 97*(7), 16BBB–16DDD.

Berg, J. A. (2005). Creating a professional poster presentation: Focus on nurse practitioners. *Journal of the American Academy of Nurse Practitioners, 17*(7), 245–249.

Bergren, M. D. (2000). Power up your presentation with PowerPoint. *Journal of School Nursing, 16*(4), 44–47.

Black, C. D., & Watties-Daniels, A. D. (2006). Cutting edge technology to enhance nursing classroom instruction at Coppin State University. *ABNF Journal, 17*(3), 103–106.

Bracke, P. J., & Dickstein, R. (2002). Web tutorials and scalable instruction: Testing the waters. *Reference Services Review, 30*(4), 330–338.

Carty, B., & Ong, I. (2006). The nursing curriculum in the information age. In V. Saba & K. McCormick (Eds.), *Essentials of nursing informatics* (4th ed., pp. 517–532). New York: McGraw-Hill.

Chase, D. (2007). Transformative sharing with instant messaging, Wikis, interactive maps, and Flickr. *Computers in Libraries, 27*(1), 7–56.

Clochesy, J. M. (2004). Hardware and software options. In J. Fitzpatrick & S. Montgomery (Eds.), *Internet for Nursing Research* (pp. 120–128). New York: Springer Publishing Company.

Cockrell, K., Caplow, J., & Donaldson, J. (2000). A context for learning: Collaborative groups in the problem-based learning environment. *Review of Higher Education, 23*(3), 347–363.

Colevins, H., Bond, D., & Clark, K. (2006). Nurse refresher students get a hand from handhelds. *Computers in Libraries,* 6–7, 46–48.

Costa, D. M. (2007). The collaborative fieldwork model. *OT Practice, 12*(1), 25–26.

Dede, C. (2005). Planning for neomillennial learning styles. *EDUCAUSE Quarterly, 28*(1) [Online]. Retrieved from http://www.educause.edu/apps/eq/eqm05/eqm0511.asp?bhcp=1

DeSantis, S. (2002). *Re-envisioning the pedagogical bridge: The new instructional designer.* Presented at the Pennsylvania Association for Educational Communications and Technology, Hershey, PA.

Dewald, N. H. (1999). Transporting good library instruction practices into the Web environment: An analysis of online tutorials. *Journal of Academic Librarianship, 25*(1), 26–32.

Dickerson, P. S. (2005). Evaluation: Part I. evaluating learning activities. *The Journal of Continuing Education in Nursing, 36,* 191–192.

EDUCAUSE Learning Initiative. (2006, June). *7 things you should know about … virtual worlds.* Retrieved November 13, 2007, from http://connect.educause.edu/Library/ELI/7ThingsYouShouldKnowAbout/39392?time=1209214921

Edwards, M. J. A., & Drury, R. M. (2000). Using computers in basic nursing education, continuing education, and patient education. In M. J. Ball, K. J. Hannah, S. K. Newbold, & J. V. Douglas (Eds.), *Nursing informatics: Where caring and technology meet* (pp. 49–68). New York: Springer.

Felder, R., & Prince, M. (2007). The case for inductive teaching. *Prism, 17*(2), 55.

Froman, R. D., Hall, A. W., Shah, A., Bernstein, J. M., & Galloway, R. Y. (2003). A methodology for supporting research and scholarship. *Nursing Outlook, 51*(2), 84–89.

Gabbard, R. B., Kaiser, A., & Kaunelis, D. (2007). Redesigning a library space for collaborative learning. *Computers in Libraries, 27*(5), 6–12.

Gagen, L., & Bowie, S. (2005). Effective mentoring: A case for training mentors for novice teachers. *Journal of Physical Education, Recreation & Dance, 76*(7), 40–45.

Garavalia, L. S. (2002). Selecting appropriate assessment methods: Asking the right questions. *American Journal of Pharmaceutical Education, 66*, 108–112.

Gillibrand, W. P., Burton, C., & Watkins, G. G. (2002). Clinical networks for nursing research. *International Nursing Review, 49*(3), 188–193.

Gordon, A. M. (2007). Sound off! The possibilities of podcasting. *Book Links*, 16–18.

Grant, M. J., & Brettle, A. J. (2006). Developing and evaluating an interactive information skills tutorial. *Health Information and Libraries Journal, 23*(2), 79–88.

Hebda, T., Czar, P., & Mascara, C. (2005). *Handbook of informatics for nurses & health care professionals* (3rd ed.). Upper Saddle River, New Jersey: Prentice Hall.

Hibbison, E. (2001). *Hybrid courses.* Retrieved November 19, 2007, from http://vccslitonline.cc.va.us/mrcte/many_media.htm

Johnson, D. W., & Johnson, R. T. (1990). *Learning together and alone: Cooperative, competitive and individualistic learning.* Boston: Allyn & Bacon.

Kramer, M. (1974). *Reality shock.* St. Louis, MO: Mosby.

Leasure, A., Davis, L., & Thievon, S. (2000). Comparison of student outcomes and preferences in a traditional vs. World Wide Web-based baccalaureate nursing research course. *Journal of Nursing Education*, (39), 149–154.

Maag, M. (2005). The potential use of "blogs" in nursing education. *CIN: Computers, Informatics, Nursing, 23*(1), 16–26.

McHugh, M. L. (2006). Computer hardware. In V. Saba & K. McCormick (Eds.), *Essentials of nursing informatics* (4th ed., pp. 517–532). New York: McGraw-Hill.

Menix, K. D. (2007). Evaluation of learning and program effectiveness. *Continuing Education in Nursing, 38*(5), 201–208.

Neary, M. (2000). Supporting students' learning and professional development through the process of continuous assessment and mentorship. *Nurse Education Today, 20*, 463–474.

Nicholl, H., & Tracey, C. (2007). Networking for nurses. *Nursing Management, 13*(9), 26–29.

Oblinger, D. G. (2005). Learners, learning, & technology: The EDUCAUSE learning initiative. *EDUCAUSE Review*, 66–75.

Pediatric Nursing Certification Board. (2007). *About recertification.* Retrieved November 2, 2007 from www.pncb.org/ptistore/control/certs/cpn/index

Peterson, T. (2007, November 19). *Here's the skinny: What you need to do to become and stay certified.* Retrieved November 19, 2007, from www.medscape.com/viewarticle/562945

Phillips, V. (1999). *Internet changing economics of higher education.* Retrieved November 2, 2007, from http://www.cnn.com/TECH/computing/9905/05/neted.idg/index.html

Pravikoff, D. S., & Levy, J. R. (2006). Computerized information resources. In V. Saba & K. McCormick (Eds.), *Essentials of nursing informatics* (4th ed., pp. 517–532). New York: McGraw-Hill.

Prensky, M. (2001). Digital natives, digital immigrants. *On The Horizon. 9*(5). Retrieved from www.marcprensky.com/writing/

Pusic, M. V., Pachev, G. S., & MacDonald, W. A. (2007). Embedding medical student computer tutorials into a busy emergency room department. *Academic Emergency Medicine, 14*(2), 138–148.

Redman, R., Lenburg, C. B., & Walker, P. H. (1999). Competency assessment: Methods for development and implementation in nursing education. *Online Journal of Nursing.* Retrieved November 2, 2007 from http://nursingworld.org/MainMenuCategories/ANAMarketplace/ANAPeriodicals/OJIN/TableofContents/Volume41999/No3Sep1999/InitialandContinuingCompetenceinEducationandPracticeCompetencyAssessmentMethodsforDeve.aspx

Ridley, R. T. (2007). Interactive teaching: A concept analysis. *Journal of Nursing Education, 46*(5), 206–209.

Riley, J. B. (1996). Educational applications. In V. K. Saba & K. A. McCormick (Eds.), *Essentials of computers for nurses* (2nd ed., pp. 527–573). New York: McGraw-Hill.

Shaffer, S. C., Lackey, S. P., & Bolling, G. W. (2006). Blogging as venue for nurse faculty development. *Nursing Education Perspectives, 27*(3), 126–128.

Schlomer, R. S., Anderson, M. A., & Shaw, R. (1997). Teaching strategies and knowledge retention. *Journal of Nursing Staff Development, 13*(5), 249–253.

Seropian, M. A., Brown, K., Gavilanes, J. S., & Driggers, B. (2004). Simulation: Not just a manikin. *Journal of Nursing Education, 43*(4), 164–170.

Skiba, D. J. (2007a). Do your students Wiki? *Nursing Education Perspectives, 26*(2), 120–121.

Skiba, D. J. (2007b). Nursing education 2.0: Second Life. *Nursing Education Perspectives, 28*(3), 156–157.

Sousa, D. A. (1995). *How the brain learns.* Reston, VA: National Association of Secondary School Principals.

Spillane, J. (2006). Virtual reality takes on patient safety. *Nursing Spectrum (New York/New Jersey Metro Edition), 18A*(7), 13.

Thackeray, R., Neiger, B. L., & Roe, K. M. (2005). Certified health education specialists' participation in professional associations: Implications for marketing and membership. *American Journal of Health Education, 36*(6), 337–344.

Turley, J. P. (2000). Nursing's future: Ubiquitous computing, virtual reality, and augmented reality. In M. J. Ball, K. J. Hannah, S. K. Newbold, & J. V. Douglas (Eds.), *Nursing informatics: Where caring and technology meet* (pp. 49–68). New York: Springer.

University of Colorado at Boulder, Office of Planning, Budget and Analysis. (2001). *Assessment methods used by academic departments and programs.* Retrieved November 17, 2007, from http://www.colorado.edu/pba/outcomes/ovview/mwithin.htm

Winfield, W., Mealy, M., & Scheibel, P. (1998). In Distance Learning '98. *Proceedings of the annual conference on distance teaching and learning.* Madison, WI.

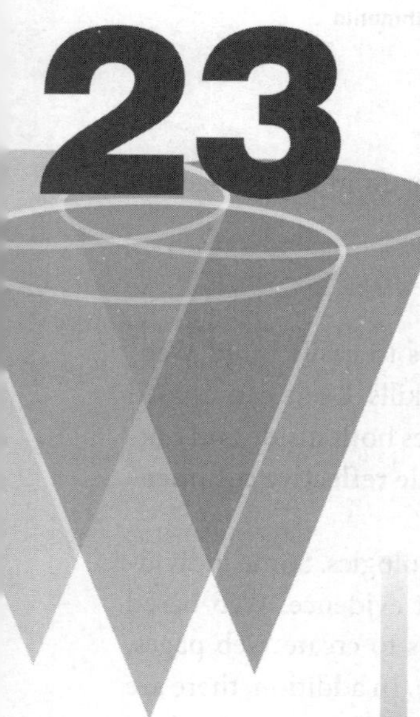

23 E-Portfolios: Processing and Dissemination of Professional Accomplishments

Glenn Johnson

Objectives

1. Describe an e-portfolio.
2. Distinguish between social networking and professional networking.
3. Examine the e-portfolio process.

Key Terms

E-portfolio
Evidence
Privacy
Professional networking
Reflective commentary
Social networking
Web publishing

INTRODUCTION

Web-based electronic portfolios (**e-portfolios**) have fast become a popular and powerful way for students in postsecondary educational programs to demonstrate not only what they know but also what they can do with what they know. The process of developing a meaningful e-portfolio is as important as the presentation of the final e-portfolio product. This process involves synthesizing and then purposefully presenting **evidence** of the learning and experiences that an individual has accumulated both inside and outside of the classroom. The purpose and the audience of a professional e-portfolio are also important. An e-portfolio might focus on what was learned in a single course, another might span an entire program of study, or in fact chronicle an entire career. The audience may also change. An e-portfolio may be required for review by faculty, might be used by advisors or mentors, or could be shared with prospective employers. Once completed, today's Internet-based technology infrastructure allows for convenient and efficient sharing of a variety of media types—how the e-portfolio is put together depends on the author's purpose and audience.

WHAT IS AN ELECTRONIC PORTFOLIO?

Today's information technology infrastructure allows users to easily build Web-based collections that include evidence of knowledge and skills. Users can upload artifacts that represent evidence of their learning experiences both inside and outside of the classroom. E-portfolios also allow users to include **reflective commentary** about their learning experiences.

E-portfolios can be built using a range of different technologies. Some individuals use PowerPoint presentations to capture and present evidence. Web-based e-portfolios are built using common **Web publishing** tools to create Web pages, which are then published on the Internet (Penn State, 2007). In addition, there are an increasing number of institutional e-portfolio systems that users can log into which allow them to upload, enter, and share information or evidence related to their experiences. Examples of such systems include PebblePad, Epsilen, ANGEL e-Portfolio, TaskStream, Livetext, iWebfolio, and Open Source Portfolio Initiative to mention a few (see resources list at the end of this chapter).

E-PORTFOLIOS IN POSTSECONDARY EDUCATION

As an instructional strategy, portfolios have been around for a long time. Instructionally, portfolios, whether electronic or paper based, require students to demonstrate or provide evidence that they have attained a specific learning outcome. For instance in the arts, portfolios have been used to demonstrate the depth and breadth of the work of an artist. While performance-based programs of study are more likely to be familiar with the concept of demonstrating what a student knows and can do, other areas of study have begun to adopt this method of assessment as well.

Portfolios can be particularly helpful in areas where higher-level thinking and analysis are essential. For instance, being a good doctor is more than being able to get high scores on exams. Doctors need to be able to collect information, analyze the information presented, relate it to past experience, apply related knowledge, and evaluate various options, and from this, present a diagnosis and a plan of action. In short, doctors need to be able to think critically and make informed decisions. In learning to become a doctor, portfolios can be used to capture, support, and improve this type of thinking as it develops.

Like the artist, the medical student can connect, share, and present cases and findings and include with this evidence the reflective commentary that serves to unveil how he or she arrived at a decision, what information or experiences were vital, and how his or her action plan evolved. However, from the variety of evidence that an individual might use to represent themselves, what should one select and how should this be shared?

SOCIAL NETWORKING VERSUS PROFESSIONAL NETWORKING

New opportunities to share information via social networks have grabbed the headlines. But to what degree does **social networking** serve the same purpose as an e-portfolio? How do online profiles differ from what is included in an e-portfolio?

Since their inception in 2004, the rise of social networking tools such as *Facebook* (http://www.facebook.com), *MySpace* (http://www.myspace.com), and many others has been phenomenal. In 2007, *Facebook* reported over 30 million users, over 40 billion page views every month, and is reportedly the top photo-sharing site on the Web (Locke, 2007). What makes these sites so attractive? Web-based applications such as *Facebook* allow users to connect and share information in ways that they had never been able to before. Users develop online profiles that contain information they select to share with others. Using simple online utilities, users easily connect and share their profile, communicating with friends over the Internet. Virtual groups of users with similar profiles are created connecting users with others who have similar interests.

Is the Web Changing How We Communicate?

The popularity of social networking applications is one indication of how new Web-based technologies are changing our communication preferences. Before the Internet, one-way broadcasts of information, i.e., information received from television and radio broadcasts, from a small number of major sources were the norm. As information technologies and the Internet have evolved, getting information from around our world from multiple channels and a variety of sources is becoming more common. Surfing today's Internet and using Web 2.0 tools involves entering a world of many sources all producing and sharing information among a range of contacts on every topic regardless of global location.

The Social Networking Dilemma

Whereas professional e-portfolios have a specific goal in mind, information use within a *Facebook* or *MySpace* profile may or may not target a specific purpose. For many, the social aspects of connecting with others is simply a fun thing to do. However, a social dilemma results from the openness required to make social networks fun—the accessibility of personal information about someone. Differentiating between what is fun personal information and professional personal information is easy for owners to delineate. For others, using what is published as an online representation of an individual, this differentiation may not be so clear cut. Photos and/or journal entries that may be viewed as seemingly innocent by one may be interpreted entirely differently by another audience. Biases and judgments that blur what for some might be a simple distinction naturally occur.

E-PORTFOLIO FOR PROFESSIONAL DEVELOPMENT

Using an e-portfolio to support **professional networking** involves a predetermined and focused purpose. The purpose may be to foster better communication between oneself and a mentor. Or the purpose may be to establish how what the nurse is doing fits into the goals of the institution or perhaps an institution for which the individual would like to work. A professional e-portfolio is evidence based and uses this evidence to make a case that highlights one's capacity to not only perform but also grow and develop professionally within one's chosen field.

THE E-PORTFOLIO PROCESS

The four steps involved in developing an e-portfolio are recursive in nature in that during the process one can backtrack to fill in missing pieces or reevaluate earlier decisions that were made. These four steps are: (1) collect, (2) select, (3) reflect, and (4) connect.

Collect

Evidence should demonstrate what a person knows, what she can do, or the values that she holds as being important. When it comes to developing e-portfolios, it is important to think of evidence in very broad terms. This evidence might include the results of what someone has learned in courses that he's taken, especially in terms of demonstrating a new skill or increased knowledge of a subject. More importantly, evidence can come from experiences that take place outside of the classroom. For instance, someone may have been involved in an internship or clinical observation where she had the opportunity to connect what she learned in the classroom with how this is applied in a real world setting. Not only is this experience valuable but it represents her understanding of how this knowledge can be applied, thus it enhances others' perception of the depth of what she knows.

Resumes are evidence documents. They are very important and every professional should have an updated copy handy. However, they only list an individual's experiences or accomplishments. E-portfolios, on the other hand, can go beyond the resume to emphasize personal attributes that are very important in the nursing profession. These attributes include, but are not limited to, interpersonal skills, leadership skills, appreciation of diversity, ability to work in a team, and self-sufficiency. These attributes are difficult if not impossible to feature in a resume. Using reflective commentary that accompanies evidence of an individual's involvement, these attributes and values can become the highlights of an e-portfolio.

Select

Everyone has his own unique pool of evidence from which to pull, and over time this evidence pool can get quite large. What will someone choose to feature and why? Putting together a professional e-portfolio requires that two intertwining questions related to purpose and audience be addressed.

What is the purpose? What is it that someone is attempting to gain by putting an e-portfolio together? Is the purpose related to personal development, i.e., feedback and advice about the professional direction that is being taken? Is the purpose to connect with colleagues? Or an individual may be interested in using her e-portfolio to find a job or gain admission into a graduate program. Each of these purposes addresses a different audience, which in turn informs the careful selection of what evidence to feature (Figure 23-1).

While an e-portfolio can link to everything that has been accomplished, this may not be the best strategy. Instead, it is essential that an individual consider his audience and establish a plan that will enable him to select the most appropriate pieces of evidence for his particular purpose and audience. A helpful way to start is to select the top five pieces of evidence that support his plan. Next, he should consider why he selected these pieces of evidence. What it is about each piece of evidence that makes it representative of who he is—what he knows, what he can do, and what he values as important.

FIGURE 23-1
Constructing a plan.

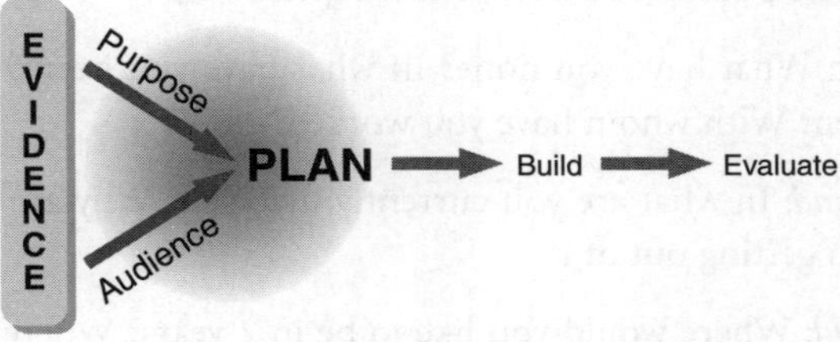

SOURCE: Penn State's e-Portfolio Initiative, 2007.

Reflect

Reflection and reflective commentary take an e-portfolio to the next level. This may be included in a single reflective statement or it can be attached to the evidence throughout an e-portfolio. Reflective comments should open up a window into why an individual thinks this evidence is important, the ways in which the individual values what she has learned or why she thinks it is important for her profession. For instance, she may present an experience where she was challenged to provide assistance. Describing this experience would be important; however, her reflective comments can extend this description—she can talk about the alternatives that she considered as the basis for how she made her decision to provide the type of assistance she provided and the manner in which she provided it. By itself, a description of this experience is good. With reflective comments, readers have a much more thorough perception of an individual's professional thinking.

Connect (Connections)/Feedback

The connection/feedback step is important to validate the assertions someone makes about what it is he knows, understands, or values. Individuals may choose to receive feedback from those who are close to them and from here reach out to others who may provide different perspectives. For instance, if one was thinking about using his e-portfolio as a part of applying for a position, he may want to start by getting feedback from friends and family first. He might share his e-portfolio with a mentor or faculty, raising the bar by getting professionally grounded feedback before he shares his e-portfolio with a prospective employer.

E-Portfolio Process—Summary Comments

With this process in mind, one might think about the process of developing a professional e-portfolio as boiling down to the telling of a rather simple story, a story that has three parts: looking back, looking around, and looking ahead. Think of your own evidence pool as you answer these questions:

Looking back: What have you done? In what have you been involved? Where have you been? With whom have you worked?

Looking around: In what are you currently involved? Why are you doing this? What are you getting out of it?

Looking ahead: Where would you like to be in 2 years? Where would you like to be in 5 years? Why do you feel this way? What makes you think this is a realistic goal?

CHALLENGES AND ISSUES: PRIVACY AND SECURITY

The ease and popularity that both Web-based social networking and professional e-portfolio tools bring to users also raises several challenges and issues. Never before has information been so accessible or personal. For this reason, issues related to **privacy** and security need to be addressed. What might be appropriate socially can be deadly in a professional context.

What Kind of Personal Information Should Be Available About Someone?

Is the information you find about yourself by searching the Internet for your own name unsettling? Give it a try and see what results! An e-portfolio is one place that an individual should have control over what personal information is included. How personal an individual wants this to be is up to the individual. What contact information should be included? Usually an e-mail address is all that would be required. Those creating an e-portfolio should look for mechanisms that will allow them to restrict access to certain pages they deem personal. When publishing in open Web space, users will likely have to engineer this themselves, whereas in larger online e-portfolio systems these capabilities are built in. In any case, users should get feedback from family, colleagues, or other professionals to help gauge whether an e-portfolio is or is not personal enough.

How Much Information Should Be Revealed?

Especially true in the medical profession, patient/client identity is critical. While one might write about an experience or relate an observation, this should be done in a manner that does not include any personal information about patients or clients. Including personal information is not only a violation of a patient's right to privacy, it demonstrates a lack of ethical judgment on the part of the e-portfolio maker!

SUMMARY—WHY CREATE AN E-PORTFOLIO?

While academic institutions may use e-portfolios for assessment of student learning, for the individual, e-portfolios are all about opportunity. This opportunity might be to support a working relationship with a mentor, network with other professionals, or to help represent certain qualities and characteristics to prospective employers. In any of these cases, having gone through the process of developing an e-portfolio requires critical examination of what qualities make an individual who she is and why these qualities are important to her and her profession. It is important for every professional to have a foundational understanding of where he is in his career trajectory and how this fits his long-term professional goals.

Practically speaking, e-portfolios are efficient. When introducing oneself in an e-mail message, a self-starting individual who has taken the initiative to develop and publish an e-portfolio can add this line to her message: "Here is a link to my e-portfolio." The recipient can click on this link, which automatically opens that individual's e-portfolio in a Web browser. Metaphorically, she has just walked into the recipient's office with information that features who she is, what she knows, what she can do, and what she values as important. She has just walked in with what can be a multimedia showcase of her qualities! The Internet is a very powerful communication medium, and individuals with professional e-portfolios can take advantage of this!

To find information about how e-portfolios are developed and used, visit Penn State University's e-portfolio support Web site at http://portfolio.psu.edu.

What the Future Holds

What I would like to leave you with is that the e-portfolio phenomena is not going to go away. There are significant initiatives underway both in the United States and in Europe. For example, the state of Minnesota allocates e-portfolio space to each of its citizens to "reach their career and education goals" (eFolio Minnesota, 2007, ¶ 1) The state of Indiana announced Indiana@Work, which provides free e-portfolio space to those who apply (Indiana@Work, 2004). In Europe, goals established at professional meetings include an e-portfolio for all European citizens by the year 2010 under the justification that, "In the context of a knowledge society, where being information literate is critical, the portfolio can provide an opportunity to demonstrate one's ability to collect, organize, interpret and reflect on documents and sources of information" (EIfEL, 2007, ¶ 1).

THOUGHT-PROVOKING Questions

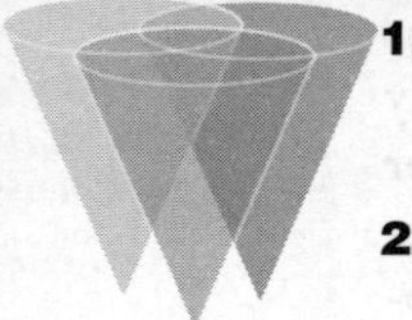

1. What would be the top five pieces of evidence that you would select to be featured in your own portfolio? Why did you select these pieces of evidence? What was it about them that made you think they would represent who you are?
2. Some institutions that require students to develop e-portfolios as a part of their program of study also may use this evidence of student learning to evaluate the program quality or generate evidence for accreditation reports. What do you think should be the driving purpose behind requiring electronic portfolios—professional development planning or institutional evaluation? What are the merits of each approach?

Web-based technologies will continue to evolve to find better ways to support an individual's ability to articulate personalized representations of who she is and what she is doing. The questions themselves have not changed. The ability to support this thinking process and the sharing of results with others through electronic portfolios will become more commonly available.

Resources

ANGEL e-Portfolio: http://www.angellearning.com/products/eportfolio/default.html

Epsilen: http://www.epsilen.com/Epsilen/Public/Home.aspx

Facebook: http://www.facebook.com

iWebfolio: http://www.iwebfolio.com

MySpace: http://www.myspace.com

Open Source Portfolio Initiative: http://www.osportfolio.org

PebblePAD: http://www.pebblepad.com

TaskStream: https://www.taskstream.com/pub

References

eFolio Minnesota. (2007). *Welcome.* Retrieved August 29, 2007, from http://www.efoliominnesota.com

European Institute for E-Learning (EIfEL). (2007). *Why do we need an ePortfolio?* Retrieved August 29, 2007, from http://www.eife-l.org/publications/eportfolio

Indiana@Work. (2004). *State launches new online career development, job search tool.* Retrieved August 29, 2007, from http://www.insideindianabusiness.com/newsitem.asp?id=12497

Locke, L. (2007, July 17). The future of Facebook. *Time.* Retrieved August 29, 2007, from http://www.time.com/time/business/article/0,8599,1644040,00.html

Penn State's e-Portfolio Initiative. (2007). Retrieved August 29, 2007, from http://portfolio.psu.edu

section

V Imagining the Future of Nursing Informatics

Nursing informatics is the synthesis of nursing science, information science, computer science, and cognitive science to manage and enhance the healthcare data, information, knowledge, and wisdom for the dual betterment of patient care and the nursing profession. After reading the first four sections of this book, you should have a good idea of the current state of the science of nursing informatics. This final section will help you think about the future. Since you have reflected on what is, this section will challenge you to think of what will or what could be. Envision your current practice setting and the NI applications that you use now. What will come next? What should come next?

As you are aware, the material within this book is placed within the context of the Foundation of Knowledge model (Figure V-1) to meet healthcare delivery systems', organizations', patients', and nurses' needs. We have attempted to capture this process in the Foundation of Knowledge model used as an organizing framework for this text. The first chapter, Nursing Science and the Foundation of Knowledge Model, provided a thorough overview of the Foundation of Knowledge model, thus providing a framework that embraces knowledge so that the readers can develop the wisdom necessary to apply what they have learned. Wisdom is the application of knowledge to an appropriate situation. In the practice of nursing science, we expect action and/or actions directed by wisdom. Wisdom uses knowledge and experience to heighten common sense and insight, allowing us to exercise sound judgment in practical matters. Wisdom is developed through knowledge, experience, insight, and reflection. Wisdom is sometimes thought of as the highest form of common sense resulting from accumulated knowledge or erudition (deep thorough learning) or enlightenment (education that results in understanding and the dissemination of knowl-

FIGURE V-1
Foundation of Knowledge model. (Designed by Alicia Mastrian.)

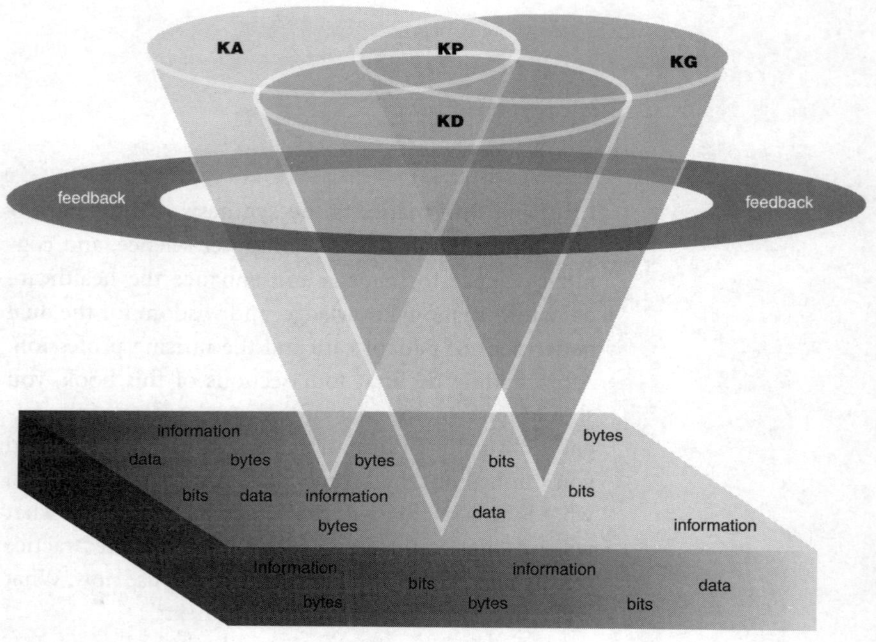

KA- Knowledge Acquisition
KD- Knowledge Dissemination
KG- Knowledge Generation
KP- Knowledge Processing

edge). Wisdom is the ability to apply valuable and viable knowledge, experience, understanding, and insight while being prudent and sensible. Knowledge and wisdom are not synonymous since knowledge abounds with others' thoughts and information while wisdom is focused on our own minds and the synthesis of our experience, insight, understanding, and knowledge.

Reflect on the model as you read through this final section. We challenge you to ask yourself, "How can I use my wisdom to help create the theories, tools, and knowledge of the future?"

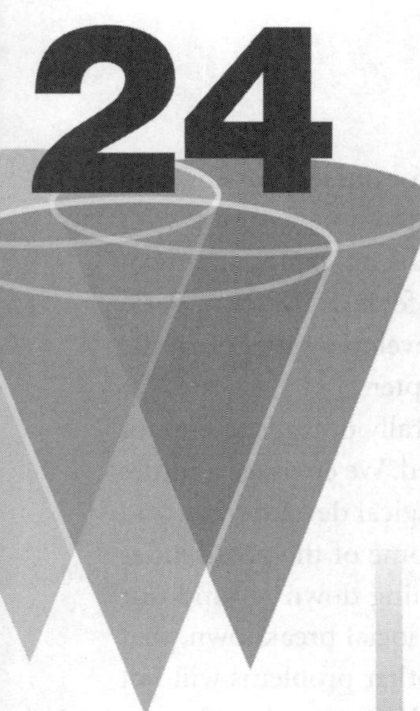

Emerging Technologies and the Generation of Knowledge

Peter J. Murray and W. Scott Erdley

Objectives

1. Outline the history of technology development and informatics applications.
2. Describe the state of the art technologies of today.
3. Predict the evolution of technology and its impact on knowledge generation in nursing.

Key Terms

Blogs
Change
Electronic data interchange
Emerging technologies
Folksonomies
Futurologists
Genomics
Half-life of knowledge
HealthVault
Information mediator
Lab-on-a-chip device
Mobile e-health (mobile health, m-health)
Nanotechnology
Podcasts
Relational databases
Really simple syndication (RSS)
Social bookmarking
Social networking
Tags/tag clouds
Transistor
Transparent technology
Ubiquitous

INTRODUCTION

"The future is here. It's just not evenly distributed . . ."
(William Gibson, novelist and visionary)

Anyone foolhardy enough to try to predict the future holds himself hostage to fortune as soon as the words are on the page—or in the case of many people's ways of writing today, as data have been saved to the hard drive, flash drive, Web page, or other storage medium. Many nursing colleagues have written about the future of nursing and about the challenges and changes that will either affect nursing or that nursing might influence. We do not, therefore, claim to be doing anything radically new in this chapter; in the best standing on the shoulders of giants tradition (especially in view of the increasing tendency of many to use tools such as Google Scholar for finding much of their literature), we use some of their works as a launch pad for our thoughts.

We have for several years been specifically working on projects and making conference presentations about some of the **emerging technologies** that are in both general, everyday use and in use and development within

Key Terms *Continued*
Ubiquitous health (u-health)
Virtual peers
Virtual worlds
Wearable computing
Web 2.0
Weblogs
Wikis

health care, and about what the future might hold for nurses, nursing, and health care more generally. We were also fortunate enough, along with nursing colleagues from around the world, to be able to explore many of these issues during the NI2006 Post Congress conference (Murray, Park, Erdley, & Kim, 2007), from which we draw and develop a number of the ideas and issues we present and discuss in this chapter.

In this chapter, we base our thoughts in a generally optimistic view of the future—one that some might say is unwarranted. We envisage a future that assumes a high degree of continuing technological development and general worldwide economic growth, and an absence of some of the possibilities that might bring much of our global infrastructure crashing down around our ears. We assume that there will not be widespread global social breakdown, that the predicted possible pandemics of avian influenza and other problems will not happen, or that catastrophic climate **change** will not produce as rapid effects as the worst prognostications suggest. However, we are aware that many of these things could happen, to some degree or other.

We do know that there is change coming, and that much of it is far enough advanced as to be virtually unavoidable. We know that the demographic changes that are occurring (changes to population age structures, increasing rates of dementia, crises in funding of retirement) will have a profound impact on all aspects of society, health, and care. We do not take the view that technology will solve all our future problems; some emerging technologies could create more problems than they solve. However, it is by having an awareness of likely and possible technological developments that we can assess what impact they might have on the ways in which we work and live, and whether the many issues can be addressed.

While not explicitly at each point addressing the four key areas of the Foundation of Knowledge model, we do, in the sections of this chapter, consider how emerging technologies may address the four areas of knowledge acquisition, knowledge processing, knowledge generation, and knowledge dissemination/feedback. We also do not focus explicitly on changes in health care and nursing technologies, but on the more general changes that might be adapted or adopted for use by nurses or within health care.

One of the most important features for nursing informatics in the future, and that will face health care in general, will be the vast amount of information that will be available to everyone. Knowledge is growing exponentially (Siemens, 2005), and in many disciplines its useful life span can be measured in months, with an ever-decreasing half-life (**half-life of knowledge** is the time span from when knowledge is gained to when it becomes obsolete). Many people think that we have information overload now; however, the present situation will be nothing compared to the future amount of data and information that we will be able to acquire, from new forms of patient monitoring, from advances in genomic medicine, and from the continuing explosion of knowledge generation and publishing, and we will need to be able to store and manipulate that data and information. Perhaps the key challenges for the future lie within identifying which emerging technologies will best provide the usable tools that nurses will need to manage the knowledge explosion.

LOOKING BACK FROM THE FUTURE

Visions of societies of the future, both utopias and dystopias, have been produced by many people. Sometimes they have been science fiction writers, while **futurologists** have used scenario planning to examine possible alternatives for the future and then examine how they might be achieved—or prevented—and the implications for society. This technique was used, in part, in the NI2006 Post Congress conference (Murray et al., 2007), but other useful scenarios that we can use to take a what-if look at possible emerging technologies also exist.

Eastel and Demosthenes (2005) postulated one such future that contains some interesting and already very plausible possibilities. We present some brief examples of the kinds of what-if thinking that might help us in exploring the implications of emerging technologies. What if, for example:

- "Googlezon" (formed from a merger of Google and Amazon) used fact-stripping robots to dynamically create personalized news stories for delivery to health information portal subscribers (patients, nurses, or family caregivers);
- personalized "genoming" (the sequencing of an individual's genome) was a routine procedure;
- biomedical research institutes had only executives and intellectual property lawyers as their permanent staff, with all the actual research outsourced and conducted under contract in India and China;
- "GoogleHealth" allowed individuals to store privately or publish their own health information, combining diverse information provided by patients, their own monitoring devices, and records supplied by hospitals, pathology and imaging services, and the general practitioner;
- GoogleHealth's search engines and **social networking** spaces allowed people to explore information held in 'virtual populations' of individuals who were genetically and behaviorally like themselves, so that they could see health trends in these populations that had real and direct meaning to their lives, and adopt the best practices of their "**virtual peers**," so as to derive the same health benefits.

In 2005, when this scenario was written, these were speculative ideas. However, in 2007, just 2 years later, we saw Nobel laureate James Watson—codiscoverer of the DNA double helix and father of the Human Genome Project—become the first human to receive the data that encompasses his personal genome sequence (Williams, 2007). Microsoft has launched its **HealthVault** online personal health record system, and rumors persist of similar developments from Google and others. Search engine technology, combined with the forms of open information-sharing and tools underpinning social networking Web sites (such as Facebook and MySpace), could rapidly support the sharing of health behavior information. The future will be upon us much more rapidly than many expect, and as nurse informaticians, we need to be at least aware of, if we are not directly involved in determining, the many new emerging technologies and their possibilities for use within our domains of interest and practice.

HISTORICAL OVERVIEW

There are several ways to view the explosive growth of information technologies and applications (Saba & Erdley, 2006; Sackett & Erdley, 2002). Regardless of perspective, the growth of information technologies follows a pathway leading from simple to complex. This path is long and twisted at times; detailed examination uncovers the significance of these developments. Initial generations of computers were analog devices focusing on military uses such as cryptography as well as weapons flight paths. Evolution proceeded from hardware to software for business administration and accounting tasks. The invention of **transistors** (solid-state semiconductors) resulted in the second generation of computers—digital devices much smaller and faster than analog computers. Silicon chips, smaller and more powerful than transistors, eventually replaced transistors, advancing the process of miniaturization. Future directions point to a shift towards advanced miniaturization (**nanotechnology**) for CPU and data storage capabilities as well as increased ubiquity of computational devices in general (discussed in, for example, Kurzweil, 2005, Chapter 2).

The pathway of computing history can be illustrated with eight time groupings, or demarcations, beginning with the pre-1800s; this schema is modeled on Sackett & Erdley's work (Sackett & Erdley, 2002). They are pre- to mid-1800s, later 1800s, 1900–1950s, 1960s, 1970s, 1980s, 1990s, and early 21st century.

Pre-1800 computing, in general, primarily represents human communication in its many forms (speech, oral history, hieroglyphics, and so forth) (Sackett & Erdley, 2002). Examples of some ancient tabulation devices include shells, rocks, and pieces of bone for adding or subtracting, thus creating a sum. The Chinese abacus, a counting device, emerged around 5000 BC. Other counting devices such as Napier's bones, and Pascal's arithmetic engine, became popular during the mid-1600s. Napier's bones, named for John Napier, are numbered white rods which, when laid side-by-side, allow a person to multiply numbers. Pascal's arithmetic engine, a gear and wheel device, was able to subtract and add numbers. In spite of the individual impact of these devices, continued growth and advancement of these devices was strongly influenced by the mobility of people and dispersion of ideas from the Old World to the New World (Sackett & Erdley, 2002).

The 1800s witnessed technological developments such as Babbage's difference engine in England (seen by many as the predecessor of the modern computer), as well as the invention of the telephone by Alexander Graham Bell. Bell's invention eventually provided the initial infrastructure on which computer connectivity began. From a software focus, a development of large significance was the first foray into standardized language. Dr. Peter M. Roget, a Scottish surgeon, is credited for this initial attempt at some sort of standardized nomenclature for the English language, which culminated in his *Roget's Thesaurus of English Words and Phrases,* based on synonyms, in 1852.

From the early 1900s through the 1950s, a number of hardware developments emerged with respect to computing. Examples include the Z1 and Colossus during World War II and then the Mark I, Electronic Numerical Integrator and Computer (ENIAC), and Universal Automatic Computer (UNIVAC), which emerged just after World War II. In health care, one of the first computers to be used was the IBM 704, which also was one of the first computers to use a number of the upcoming technologies such as magnetic core memory. The invention of transistors and their subsequent integration into computational devices also helped shape the future of computing.

Software growth was even more foundational during this time period. The idea of storing and running applications, a stored program concept, directly on and/or in the computer, was developed by Neumann. A key premise of this was a shift to a binary system from the traditional base 10. An extremely important hardware and software development was magnetic core memory by Charles Wang, which allowed applications to be stored without loss (software) as well as providing hardware advantages such as less energy and less heat production (Collen, 1995).

The next decade (1960s) saw a burst of activity and inventiveness, which provided important direction and substance to future computing needs. Transistor use in computers marked the end of first-generation computers and the beginning of the second generation. Kilby and Noyce's discovery that transistors could function as their own circuit boards greatly diminished the size and power requirements of computers and led to minicomputers (Collen, 1995). Noyce and his colleagues also developed the first integrated silicon chip, which eventually led to the use of very large-scale integration (VLSI) chips in the late 1960s (Collen, 1995). These integrated circuits demarcated second-generation computers (Blum, 1986; Saba & McCormick, 1986). Noyce went on to found Intel in the late 1960s, which grew into one of the world's leading manufacturers of computational and other chips.

Software application growth exploded during this decade, too. The Health Evaluation through Logical Processing (HELP) system was developed at the Latter Day Saints/LDS Hospital in Salt Lake City, Utah, in the late 1950s and early 1960s (Warner, Olmsted, & Rutherford, 1972). In 1962, Clark and Molnar of Massachusetts Institute of Technology (MIT) developed LINC (a laboratory-specific application) (Collen, 1995). The National Library of Medicine committed to computerization when they placed its journal collection, *Medlars/Medline,* onto a computer in 1963 (Collen, 1995). PLATO, from the late 1960s, was one of the first computer-based education programs. In health care, a number of landmark applications appeared, including the Technicon Medical Information System (TMIS) initiated in 1965; the problem-oriented medical record (POMR) and problem-oriented medical information systems (PROMIS) in the 1960s; and the computer-stored ambulatory record (COSTAR), which was developed and implemented in the late 1960s and used the Massachusetts General Hospital utility multiprogramming system (MUMPS) (Barnett et al., 1979).

In the 1970s, the focus of information technology related to health shifted from hardware to software or applications (Boutros, 1993; Brandejs, 1976; Collen, 1995; Elioutina & Tarasov, 1995; Hannah, Ball, & Edwards, 1999; Mandil, Moidu, Korpela, Byass, & Forster, 1993). The invention and subsequent use of the silicon chip in 1975, leading to a rapid proliferation of personal computers based on this chip, denoted a worldwide revolution in computer hardware and subsequent software developments. Shortly after this development, Paul Allen and Bill Gates founded Microsoft Corporation, which was destined to create an operating system of eventual global importance.

Internationally, from Canada and the United Kingdom, we have examples of computerized information systems in nursing practice. King's College Hospital in London pioneered computerized nursing care plans; Ninewells Hospital in Scotland implemented a real-time system for nursing documentation, and York Central Hospital in Richmond Hills, Ontario implemented a computerized patient care system (Sackett & Erdley, 2002).

Also in the 1970s, in the United States, hospital information systems (HISs) began adding in care management and cost control functionality. Edgar F. Codd's work with **relational databases** provided the framework and underpinnings for growth in data collection, manipulation, and analysis (Haux, Knaup, & Schmucker, 1999). Examples of other U.S. HISs include Technicon at El Camino, California (a continuation of work from the mid-1960s) and PROMIS (Medical Center Hospital, Burlington, Vermont) (Collen, 1995). The Patient Care System (PCS), developed at Duke Medical Center, focused on nursing staffing. Refinement of the PROMIS continued during this decade. MYCIN, a program designed to identify bacteria and recommend antibiotics (so named because of the typical suffix of antibiotics at the time), made real inexact reasoning in medicine (Shortliffe & Buchanan, 1975).

The decade of the 1980s witnessed continued growth in both application and hardware arenas. The continuing evolution of the computer chip by Intel, along with subsequent manufacture of personal computer clones, overtook Apple Computer's proprietary personal computers. The shift in computer focus, from mainframe architecture to individual machines, signaled a shift of power to the user. Hardware and software growth became collaborative in use and purpose. The U.S. Defense Agency Research Projects Agency's (DARPA) network was developed to cope with communication in the event of an atomic war. The concept of something titled *ethernet* by Bob Metcalf defined a form of communication over wires, which, along with developments in communication protocols such as transmission control protocol/Internet protocol (TCP/IP), provided the framework for not only necessary communication but future collaborations, too (e.g., client–server architecture).

One of the more prominent software developments in the healthcare field in the early 1980s was Internist-1 (Miller, Pople, & Myers, 1982). This application sought to apply symbolic reasoning to develop computer-assisted diagnoses through modeling physician behavior as a decision-support aid (van Ginneken, 1999). Other examples following in Internist-1's footprint include QMR, Internist-1's direct successor; DxPlain, Iliad, and Meditel. A hospital information systems project, based on MUMPS, was initiated at Obafemi Awolowo University Teaching Hospital in Ile-Ife, Nigeria in 1988 (Daini, Makanjuola, & Ojo, 1993).

Technology applications "exploded" in the 1990s with the advent of increasingly sophisticated hardware, software, increased memory and speed, and the decreased cost of digital computer technology. From the development and use of the Internet to satellites, to wireless innovations, from mainframes to minicomputers to microcomputers to work stations to global networks, the amount of knowledge generated and the necessity for management of increasingly complex information systems was evident everywhere and especially noticeable in health care.

International examples of information systems included CARE Telematics Project, led by the World Health Organization regional office for Europe (Zollner,

1995) and OPADE: Optimization of Drug Prescription Using Advanced Informatics (de Zegher et al., 1995), a joint venture between individuals from Belgium, France, Italy, Sweden, and the United Kingdom. TELENURSING was a European Commission-funded project

> … to promote standardized and formalized clinical nursing care data based on uniform definitions of data items with the purpose of developing countable and comparable nursing minimum data sets as a means of communicating nursing care information electronically between clinical setting, health care sectors nationally and European-wide and a means of producing Euro-Nursing Health statistics on people's need for nursing care. (Mortensen & Nielsen, 1995, p. 115)

South America has begun several healthcare initiatives (Stammer, 2000) including, for example, swipe cards to validate patient identity and eligibility at public health centers.

As the healthcare market has become increasingly complex, so has healthcare software. The number of software applications for health care numbers in the thousands, with what seems to be a program for any and all purposes. Figures quoted range from approximately 300 to over 500 vendors or more. In the last years of the 1990s, healthcare informatics was swept up by both the Internet and the lure of the World Wide Web (www). The increased popularity of **electronic data interchange** (EDI), with its ability to reduce human errors, altered the financial aspect of health care forever. Carrying through to the early 21st century, this trend has continued with a call for electronic health records for all U.S. citizens (Bush, 2004). Regionalism and interoperability have become the buzzwords for healthcare informatics in the United States and increasingly abroad. Denmark has provided a health portal for its citizens and health providers, which is accessible for all and any healthcare concerns ranging from scheduling an appointment to reviewing laboratory results (The Danish eHealth Portal, 2008). Second-generation Web applications (**Web 2.0**) are increasing in popularity for both health care and the population in general, in the United States and worldwide. Thus knowledge and information continue to evolve from specific uses by individuals to growth, evolution, and application by the population. This shift will continue to impact the role of providers as well as health care in general.

This shift of information access, acquisition, and interpretation, for both provider and patient, may result in overload in terms of content and comprehension. Managing this overload will increasingly consume both providers and patients. How this issue will be managed is of great concern, whether by an increased use of technology or a regression away from technology.

SOME TECHNOLOGIES WE HAVE TODAY

In many countries, not just the United States, much of the most recent focus of technology use in nursing and health care has been aimed at improving patient safety (reducing medication errors, etc.), as described by Oren, Shaffer, & Guglielmo (2003), among others. They point out, however, that there are few studies providing evidence for the impact of introducing these technologies on error reduction and the reducing of adverse events. This perhaps reflects two interacting sets of issues—first, that priorities for use of technologies often change with changing political drivers; and second, that many technologies are changing so rapidly that, by the time they are evaluated in large-scale, controlled trial environments, a new generation of devices and applications has succeeded them. Patient safety issues are a strong driver to using technology today, and will probably continue to be so as long as the politicians see benefit from such a focus, but as other priorities, often political, emerge, the focus will shift. We are already beginning to see some of this changing focus with the emerging discussions on personal health records.

However, many nurses often see technology as a hindrance or a barrier, rather than something that provides real benefit within their practice. Murray et al. (2007), for example, state that "Much technology currently gets in the way of care, and there is a need for increasingly **transparent technology** [boldface added], which will need to function in the background; if you talk about the technology, it is not transparent" (p. 18). This may be for a wide variety of reasons, but is often related to lack of consultation with end users in technology application to care processes. The true potential of technology to support nursing and health care will only come when it is both **ubiquitous** (everywhere) and transparent. The point has been made by Weaver et al. (2007), who say that "small, inexpensive, unobtrusive" (p. 80) devices will facilitate future monitoring of patients and data collection, while Kirovski, Oliver, Sinclair, and Tan (2007) suggest that the current generation of wearable physiological sensors are obtrusive and so meet resistance from users. If they are to gain widespread acceptance, they will need to provide for little or no change in the user's daily routine, with transparency being the key to widespread adoption (Kirovski et al.)

Even the most cursory examination of the proceedings of any recent health or nursing informatics conference will demonstrate the plethora of ways in which nurses are currently using a wide range of technologies to support and advance their practice. We are also beginning to see adoption of the kinds of near-transparent and ubiquitous technologies just discussed. Taking examples from just two recent events by way of illustration; from the NI2006 International Congress on Nursing Informatics (Park, Murray, & Delaney, 2006), we can find examples from around the world of the folowing:

- Computerized decision support systems to prevent unnecessary visits to health care facilities in South Africa (Horner, Hanmer, & Mbananga, 2006)
- Wireless speech recognition and touchscreen triage support systems in emergency departments in Taiwan (Chang et al., 2006)
- Nurse-managed telehealth services in United Kingdom dermatology clinics (Lawton & Timmons, 2006)
- Use of open-source software for development of Web-based nursing informatics education in Germany (Schrader, 2006)
- Nurse-led development of a personal health record system in the United States (Lee, Delaney, & Moorhead, 2006)
- Demonstrated uses of wireless biomedical sensors for invasive monitoring in Norway (Øyri, Balasingham, & Hogetveit, 2006)

From the 2007 Summer Institute in Nursing Informatics at the University of Maryland school of nursing, we can find examples of:

- Critical care telemedicine and virtual nurses teleconsultation systems
- Using wireless point-of-care applications
- Internet-accessible patient portals providing online access to healthcare professionals and information

Two recent reports, focusing on nursing and technology, have also summarized some of the practical ways in which nurses are involved in using technologies. The report of the February 2007 Technology Informatics Guiding Education Reform (TIGER) Initiative summit (TIGER, 2007) set out a 3-year action plan toward achieving a 10-year vision to enable practicing nurses and nursing students to fully engage in the unfolding digital era of health care, so enabling nurses to use information technology (IT) seamlessly to provide safer, higher quality patient care. Among the examples of current use cited were Web-based patient health records, such as the U.S. Department of Veterans Affairs' MyHealtheVet (http://www.myhealth.va.gov), which patients can access from anywhere, and which empowers them in making their own decisions about their health.

The 2004 report on technology's role is addressing the nursing crisis in Maryland (Technology Workgroup, Maryland Statewide Commission on the Crisis in Nursing, 2004) while noting that technology was not the solution to issues, but it could be a facilitator, demonstrated by pockets of innovation, including:

- The use of wearable, hands-free communication badges (Vocera, 2007)
- Bar-coded medication administration schemes that have demonstrated reductions in error rates

- Use of intranets for providing current and consistent protocol and procedure information

However, in addition to the technologies available, there are changes occurring in the ways in which these technologies facilitate interaction, in particular through the emergence of a wide range of what are termed Web 2.0 applications. Web 2.0 has many definitions and descriptions. O'Reilly (2005) first described it extensively, and many more recent descriptions still focus on interaction, the development of online communities and support for collaboration and sharing as being the key elements. Among the technologies that are seen as contributing to Web 2.0 are **blogs (weblogs)**, **wikis**, **podcasts**, **really simple syndication (RSS)** feeds and other methods of providing many-to-many publication and communication. Social networking and social educational applications (Anderson, 2005), which facilitate interaction and collaboration, are also a central component of Web 2.0 (Murray & Maag, 2006).

Web 2.0 technologies allow for the possibility of increased participation among formal and informal online communities of users. As such, they are disruptive technologies that have the potential to transform the ways in which knowledge is generated and shared. We do not have space within this chapter to explore at length the emerging tools and technologies generally labeled Web 2.0, nor to provide detailed discussion of their potential implications. However, they will undoubtedly have profound impacts on the ways in which data, knowledge, and information (and perhaps even wisdom) are generated, and so it is worth using a few paragraphs to summarize some emerging ways in which they are being used within nursing and health care.

Maag (2006) has described the use of podcasts of lecture materials with nursing students (the term *podcast* originated as an amalgam of *broadcasting* and Apple's proprietary *iPod* MP3 music player, although podcasts can be played on any computer or MP3 player). While much argument still exists of whether podcasts will provide long-term benefits and changes to ways in which people learn, there is some evidence that they can enhance the learning experience and engage learners. Maag (2005) is among those who have explored the potential use of blogs within nurse education, and she cites examples of small-scale evaluations within other educational contexts, for teaching and research purposes. She concludes that health professionals' writing, reading, and communication skills can be enhanced through the use of blogs, and that blogs also facilitate collaborative and information-gathering skills. Other practical examples support the use of blogs within formal education (e.g., Godwin-Jones, 2003; Martindale & Wiley, 2004) for professional development, sharing information, interacting as part of a learning community, and building an open knowledge base. In addition, they have been used for encouraging informal knowledge sharing and professional development around health and nursing informatics conferences (Murray & Ward, 2004). The emergence of **social bookmarking**, **tags** and **tag clouds**, and **folksonomies** are providing opportunities for the exploration of new ways of linking, ordering, and searching information, based in large part on popularity of its use among a community. These tools have implications for the ways in which health and nursing informatics are classified.

WHAT WILL AFFECT THE FUTURE? SOME VIEWS

Several of our nursing informatics colleagues have concluded their books by looking to the future and imagining scenarios for the life and work of the 21st century nurse. McCormick (2001), writing a possible scenario for 2020, envisaged the nurse using voice recognition to interact with her computer (portable, of course) and with components of the hospital systems, telehealth applications for physiological monitoring, use of genetic screening information in treatment decisions, and smart cards for storing a form of electronic health record. We've passed more than one third of the time from then until 2020, and we see many of these applications becoming almost routine, and the growth of networks (especially the Internet) mean that we have already moved beyond some of the ideas in our development of ways of working.

Ball (2005) also advocates the use of technology, including wireless networks and PDAs, to reduce the time spent on documentation (and so potentially increase the time available for direct patient care). She also sees technology supporting new roles, such as an Internet guide to assist patients in accessing appropriate educational resources. McCormick et al. (2007), in discussing American Medical Informatics Association Nursing Informatics Work Group's white paper on how the nursing informatics profession needs to set new directions, identified many areas that will impact the nature of nursing and of health care in the future, although many of these were nontechnological.

Some of the Issues from NI2006

In mid-2006, following the NI2006 International Congress on Nursing Informatics in Seoul, Korea (Park et al., 2006), a group of nurse informaticians from around the world participated in an intensive workshop-based exploration of possible futures and the implications for nursing and nursing informatics. Some of the issues that they identified are worth exploring. It was acknowledged that nursing and nursing informatics would—and would have to—change. Among the new roles for nurses, arising out of current developments was that of

information mediator, but the implications of this were, again, the need for technology to support immediate access to up-to-date knowledge anywhere and anytime.

Many of the issues that were explored were not, in fact, technological, nor related to IT. Discussions explored the many demographic changes that we know or can predict are likely to occur (e.g., growing and aging populations, changes in population structure, especially the numbers of productive working-age members able to contribute tax and other revenues to support healthcare systems, growing proportions of populations living in urban areas) (DCDC, 2007). Possible trends in healthcare provision and delivery as health policies and priorities change (e.g., moves toward less costly preventive or interventional measures, growing use of telehealth) and the impact these and other changes might have on the nature of nursing were also discussed.

Among the key issues that emerged from the discussions that are important for the international nursing informatics community to explore in coming years were:

- The development of the concept, and a possible model, of u-nursing (ubiquitous nursing), which, as well as having implications for the practice of nursing, also has profound implications for all aspects of the education and continuing professional development of nurses (Øyri et al., 2007)
- The role of the nurse changing to become more of a knowledge professional, working in partnership with the patients and their other caregivers
- The continuing growth of patient informatics, perhaps as a growth and evolution of the current concept of consumer health informatics, and with the increasing centrality of the patient as the controlling force in the whole enterprise
- The vast impact that **genomics** will have on all aspects of life, and in particular health care (Turley, Murray, Saranto, Ehnfors, & Seomun, 2007)

Such discussions of technologies as emerged were often focused on the interaction with these other changes. Among the issues discussed were nanotechnology, remote (e.g., wireless) monitoring of vital signs, wearable monitoring and treatment devices, ubiquitous access to computer networks, lifelong personal and electronic health records, and treatments, not only preventive and interventional, but also predictive of likely development of diseases, based in genetic medicine (Øyri et al., 2007).

Nanotechnology and its specific applications within medicine and health care (nanomedicine), open up many possibilities, including the development of minute biomedical devices, the size of molecules, that could provide drug delivery systems, precise targeting of therapies (e.g., delivery of drugs or radiation sources to individual cancer cells), or even nanorobots to undertake surgical procedures on cells. These types of technology are currently still in development stages. One project is the **lab-on-a-chip device** for undertaking comprehensive blood analyses (Schmidt, 2007). As nurses and informaticians, we need to consider what, if any, would be the nursing or informatics role in such interventions. As Loescher & Merkle (2005) point out in relation to other emerging technologies, without knowledge of genomic technologies, reasons for their use, and the possible implications of genetic diagnosis and genomic-based treatments, nurses will be increasingly unable to provide the quality of care needed and demanded by patients. The same applies to all new and emerging technologies that may impact on or become integral parts of the delivery of health care, in whatever setting.

While we are tending to focus on the technologies and can only summarize discussion of the issues, the technologies cannot be divorced from or considered in isolation from wider societal issues and the handling of increasingly large and complex volumes of data; readers are directed to the Post Congress Conference proceedings for more detailed discussion (Murray et al., 2007).

Among the issues explicitly identified and implicitly emerging from the NI2006 discussions was that the amount of data available about all aspects of health care will increase tremendously. Genomics, proteomics, and the plethora of related -omics, many of which are often gathered in the general field of bioinformatics, will produce many challenges for the nature of health care, and for all forms of health informatics. As Martin-Sanchez et al. (2004) have suggested, there will be many technological challenges, but also wider ethical and other issues to be addressed. They point out that, while new genetic and proteomic data provide the possibility of developing new therapies and of implementing new preventive measures, it is important to be able to deal with the large amounts of data generated. The new knowledge available and the new technologies will blur the distinctions between clinical and molecular information, while increased amounts of knowledge will lead to a greater need for genetic counseling as an even more important part of clinical, hands-on care. Martin-Sanchez et al. see a place for culture brokers—i.e., people who can translate between science and clinical care and between science and the self-caring citizen. As Turley et al. (2007) also point out:

> from the genome information, we can determine the disease risks of a given patient, the drug allergies of that patient and to some extent the optimal drug treatments for individual patients. These all fall clearly within the purview of nursing concerns and the science of nursing, and have implications for truly personalized care. (p. 56)

Other issues also emerge, such as the nature and amount of genomic data/information to be included in the electronic health record, and how long it must be held, as well as a set of issues around the impact of the changes and emerging technologies on education for all health professionals. The necessity of collecting, storing, and manipulating huge amounts of genomic data will have impacts on the technologies to be used. Grid technologies (unique configurations of distributed computing) are being explored as mechanisms for manipulating the data, but issues such as how the knowledge will be extracted from the data repositories and how it will be represented in usable form will present challenges for the development of new technologies (Kuhn, Wurst, Bott, & Guise, 2006).

If, as many of the participants in the NI2006 Post Congress Conference suggest, one of the major roles of the nurse (and nurse informaticians) of the future will be that of a clinical knowledge worker (Weaver et al., 2007), then they will need to be familiar with the many new tools and technologies that will develop to enable them to retrieve, use, manipulate, present, and share the new knowledge with patients and other health professionals. In the next section, we specifically explore some technologies and probable trends, but as new applications are being developed on a seemingly daily basis, we do not dwell on any in detail, but explore some of the trends.

SOME EMERGING TECHNOLOGIES AND OTHER ISSUES THAT WILL IMPACT NURSING AND HEALTH CARE

For many years we have had *e-health* for which Oh, Rizo, Enkin and Jadad (2005) have identified 51 unique published definitions. The definitions address not only health but also technology and commerce with a general tendency for health care to be viewed as a process rather than health as an outcome, and with technology seen both as a tool to enable a process/function/service and as a means to expand, to assist, or to enhance human activities rather than as a substitute for them. The European view of e-health, as developed by the Commission of the European Communities (2004), acknowledges the need for providing citizen-centered health-care systems, respecting the diversity of Europe's multicultural, multilingual health-care traditions. Examples of e-health developments include electronic health records, health portals, telemedicine and telehealth services, and wearable and portable monitoring systems.

More recently, we have seen the development of **m-health** (often termed *mobile e-health,* as opposed to simply *mobile health*), which, according to some (e.g., WHO, 2007) includes health-related uses of mobile technologies including mobile phones (and increasingly, Internet-enabled, wireless-connected smartphones), personal digital assistants (PDAs), tablet computers and subnotebook microcomputers, remote diagnostic and monitoring devices, and Global Positioning System (GPS)/geographic information system (GIS) mapping equipment.

M-health can therefore be described in terms of the application to healthcare systems and processes of network technologies and mobile communications and devices (Istepanian, Laxminarayan, & Pattichis, 2006). More recently, recognizing the increasing pervasiveness of technology in all aspects of our lives, including health care, we have had the emergence of the concept of *u-health.* **U-health** (or ubiquitous health or health care) is based in the concept of ubiquitous computing, which is considered a third wave of computing wherein technologies become increasingly invisible, becoming incorporated into our everyday use, and so fading into the background (Weiser, 1991). With true ubiquitous computing, which pervades all parts of the everyday environment, unobtrusively providing information and services, and with the very concept of the single device (computer) disappearing into the network (Bott, 2005), the real possibility of providing nurses and other healthcare professions with the information they need where and when they need it exists.

Øyri et al. (2007) have suggested that information and communications technologies will become ubiquitous within nursing, and that emerging technologies, including nanotechnology, wireless sensors, and minimally invasive technologies, will support not only health care, but also wellness management. They suggest a model for u-nursing that "will focus on the provision of nursing for anyone or any organization, anytime, anywhere, through any networks and any devices" (p. 32).

A TECHNOLOGY WISH LIST

There are doubtless many other technologies we could cover—and some readers will say that we should have covered. We have not addressed the prospects for robotics in delivering aspects of care, even though there are well-documented examples of robotic surgery and even robots for delivering nursing care. Similarly, we have not explored the possibilities of emerging **virtual worlds**, such as Second Life, and simulations, nor have we addressed many of the technologies, such as wearable devices, that are being used to provide remote monitoring of physiological parameters in care settings, including patients' own homes. These are certainly interesting and exciting developments, and we can only plead the excuse of lack of space in a printed text, and we urge readers to undertake their own explorations of these and other technologies.

In concluding our exploration, we present a short wish list for some new technologies that we would like to see emerge in the next few years. As with much of what we have discussed previously, the seeds of these developments are already present, and they may be with us sooner than we expect. Our technology wish list includes:

1. The kind of computer interface used in the film *Minority Report*—no mouse, no keyboard, just gesture-based interactions with virtual images projected into a vertical space at head height.
2. Ubiquity of computational devices to the extent that conversation and discussion of these devices will disappear from everyday social interactions.
3. The ability to access information when and where we want irrespective of modality—maximizing mobility and other personal resources. This may lead to cell phones becoming the main avenue of access for more than text messages, speech, and video clips. Knowledge acquisition and utilization will then become ubiquitous and pervasive; new work roles will emerge to cope with this new and different technology.

WHAT THE FUTURE HOLDS: SUMMARY

We know that the future will be different; however, it is likely that, in the foreseeable future, let us say the next 10–15 years, many of the changes that are likely to occur are already in development or will be extrapolations of current developments and trends. There is always, however, the possibility of new developments, or unexpected consequences, of the development of emerging technologies.

Within this chapter, we have touched briefly on some of the emerging technologies that are likely to have an effect on nursing, nurse informatics, and health care in the near future, and that might impact and interact with the Foundation of Knowledge model. We have probably not given some of the technologies as much coverage as hindsight will show that we ought to have; this is, in part, because some of the emerging technologies are evolving so rapidly that it is difficult to predict what might emerge within the next few months, let alone the next few years, and the impacts they will have. We have certainly not given as much coverage to the potential of Web 2.0, Web 3.0, and beyond as they are likely to deserve, again because the future evolution is difficult to predict. We have not touched on new interfaces with technology (such as Apple's iPhone), and have made little mention of the emergence of virtual worlds.

We can probably say, with a fair degree of certainty, that the implications of social networking technologies that are major elements of Web 2.0 will have significant impact on the amount of information and knowledge that is generated, and the ways in which it is used. We know that new healthcare technologies will develop, most likely based in genomic and nanotechnological sciences, and that they will lead to huge new volumes of data, with implications for what is captured and stored, for how long, and how it is used. We know that computing power and storage capabilities will lead to faster, smaller, more mobile, and more powerful devices with vastly greater capacities for storing data. Everyone will have the opportunity to be more connected, more readily, and more of the time, to many other people through the growth of wireless networks.

The major challenges for us all will be in finding the best tools and methods for managing, and making best use of, the information that will be available to us not only 24/7, but 60/60/24/7; i.e., every second of every day. For many of us, knowing what to keep up with, what is most relevant to our practice, our education, and our research will be a challenge. Nurse informaticians have a good track record in finding ways to use information and will need to rise to that challenge.

The potential to generate more health data, for example from new forms of physiological monitoring, or from the implications of the new -omics sciences will raise important new needs for storing that data, in both the short and long terms, and for generating from it the information and knowledge needed to support clinical practice, research, and education. The key words to describe the changes in the ways in which nursing and healthcare knowledge are acquired, processed, generated, and disseminated are smaller, more integrated, more mobile, more wearable, more connected, and ubiquitous.

Devices for capturing and storing data will become smaller, and the amount of data that can be stored within a device will increase. Devices the size of today's cell phones are likely, as smartphone technology evolves, to have all the functionality—and more—of today's desktop computers. We are already seeing the integration of more functions into today's cell phones and PDAs, and this trend is also likely to continue. Both of these trends make the information processing power available to nurses more mobile, enabling nurses to spend more time with patients and also develop new ways of interacting with patients and delivering care in a wide range of settings.

Of course, all this increased computing power in mobile devices is of little use if mobile communications are restricted. Access to information and use of information on the move will increase, as new forms of wireless communications are implemented, meaning that nurses are less restricted to particular physical spaces to interact with patients' records. And finally, while **wearable computing** may have more to offer in terms of capturing data from patients, there are many emerging tools that may mean the nurse will not be restricted to holding and handling physical devices, but may interact, through voice and other commands, with computing devices carried elsewhere on their persons. As nurses work in environments where they can be always connected to ubiquitous computing resources, they will no longer be able to say that they did not have access to the information they needed to undertake their roles. The challenge will be to find not only technological ways of dealing with the available information, but ways of using and prioritizing information, new ways of thinking, and new ways of interacting with information resources, so that they have the right information, at the right time, to do the right job, and are not overwhelmed with extraneous and irrelevant "noise." The technology is the easy part; the nontechnological issues will be the greater, and perhaps more urgent, challenge.

In this chapter, we explored some of the emerging technologies that are in both general use and in use and development within health care, and we discussed what the future might hold for nurses, nursing, and health care more generally. We do not take the view that technology will solve all our future problems; some emerging technologies could create more problems than they solve. However, it is by having an awareness of likely and possible technological developments that nurses can assess what impact they might have on the ways in which we work and live. While not explicitly at each point addressing the four key areas of the Foundation of Knowledge model, we considered how some of the emerging technologies may address the four areas of knowledge acquisition, knowledge processing, knowledge generation, and knowledge dissemination/feedback. We also did not focus explicitly on changes in health care and nursing technologies, but on the more general changes that might be adapted or adopted for use by nurses or within health care. **The most important thought we would like to leave you with is**, the key challenges for the future lie within identifying which emerging technologies will best provide the usable tools that nurses will need to manage the coming knowledge "explosion" as more information becomes available to support diagnosis, treatment, and care.

THOUGHT-PROVOKING Questions

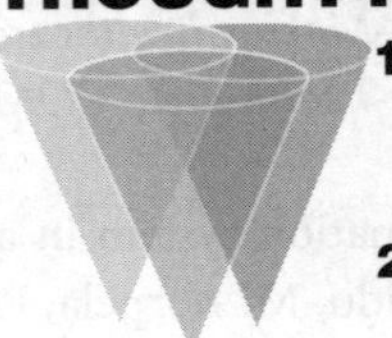

1. This chapter raises several important issues related to nursing knowledge, not the least of which might be the uniqueness of nursing knowledge. Is this uniqueness requisite for future care by nurses and/or nursing informatics specialists?
2. Given the future is relatively unpredictable, what might be said regarding what can be predicted and to what degree of certainty?

References

Anderson, T. (2005). *Distance learning—Social software's killer ap?* Retrieved November 13, 2007, from http://www.unisa.edu.au/odlaaconference/PPDF2s/13%20odlaa%20-%20Anderson.pdf

Ball, M. J. (2005, February). Nursing informatics of tomorrow. *Healthcare Informatics*, 74–75.

Barnett, G., Justice, N., Somand, M., Adams, J., Waxman, B., Beaman, P., et al. (1979). COSTAR—A computer-based medical information system for ambulatory care. In J. van Bemmel (Ed.), *Yearbook of Medical Informatics—The Promise of Medical Informatics* (pp. 262–273). New York: Schattauer.

Blum, B. (1986). *Clinical Information Systems.* New York: Springer-Verlag.

Bott, O. J. (2005). Ubiquitous health care systems: A new paradigm for medical informatics? In R. Haux & C. Kulikowski (Eds.), *IMIA Yearbook of Medical Informatics 2005: Ubiquitous Health Care Systems* (pp. 213–218). Stuttgart: Schattauer.

Boutros, S. (1993). Egyptian experience with microcomputers in monitoring and evaluating of health care programmes. In S. Mandil, K. Moidu, M. Korpela, P. Byass, & D. Forster (Eds.), *Health Informatics in Africa HELINA 93* (pp. 58–63). Amsterdam, Netherlands: EXCERPTA MEDICA.

Brandejs, J. (1976). *Health Informatics Canadian Experience.* New York: American Elsevier Publishing Company.

Bush, G. W. (2004). *President Bush touts benefits of health care information technology.* Retrieved December 7, 2007, from http://www.whitehouse.gov/news/releases/2004/04/20040427-5.html

Chang, P., Sheng, Y-H., Sang, Y-Y., Wang, D-W., Hsu, Y-S., & Hou, I-C. (2006). Developing and evaluating a wireless speech-and-touch-based interface for intelligent comprehensive triage support systems. In H-A. Park, P. J. Murray, & C. Delaney (Eds.), *Consumer-centered computer-supported care for healthy people. Proceedings of NI2006* (pp. 693–697). Amsterdam: IOS Press.

Collen, M. F. (1995). *A history of medical informatics in the United States: 1950–1990.* Indianapolis, IN: American Medical Informatics Association.

Commission of the European Communities. (2004). *E-Health–Making healthcare better for European citizens: An action plan for a European e-health area. COM (2004) 356 final.* Brussels, Belgium: Author.

Daini, O., Makanjuola, R., & Ojo, J. (1993). A hospital information system in a Nigerian university teaching hospital. In S. Mandil, K. Moidu, M. Korpela, P. Byass, & D. Forster (Eds.), *Health Informatics in Africa HELINA 93* (pp. 86–89). Amsterdam, Netherlands: EXCERPTA MEDICA.

The Danish eHealth Portal. (2008). Retrieved May 15, 2008, from http://www.sundhed.dk/wps/portal/_s.155/1922?_FOLDER_ID_=1023050919183419&_ARTIKELGRUPPE_ID_=1023050919180045

Development, Concepts and Doctrine Centre (DCDC). (2007). *The DCDC Global Strategic Trends Programme 2007–2036.* Swindon, UK: DCDC, Ministry of Defence. Retrieved November 13, 2007, from http://www.dcdc-strategictrends.org.uk/viewdoc.aspx?doc=1

deZegher, I., Venot, A., Milstein, C., Sene, B., deRosis, F., DeCarolis, B., et al. (1995). OPADE: optimization of drug prescription using advanced informatics in health informatics in health. In M. F. Laires, M. J. Ladeira, & J. P. Christensen, (Eds.), *The new communications age health care telematics for the 21st century* (pp. 251–259). Amsterdam, Netherlands: IOS Press.

Eastel, S., & Demosthenes, P. (2005, May 5). View from the future. *Bio-ITWorld.com.* Retrieved November 13, 2007, from http://cms.bio-itworld.com/issues/2005/May/future.html?page:int=-1

Elioutina, S., & Tarasov, V. (1995). Current state and perspectives of healthcare informatics in Russia. *International Journal of Bio-Medical Computing, 39,* 163–167.

Godwin-Jones, R. (2003, May). Emerging technologies. Blogs and wikis: environments for on-line collaboration. *Language Learning and Technology.* Retrieved November 13, 2007, from http://llt.msu.edu/vol7num2/pdf/emerging.pdf

Hannah, K., Ball, M., & Edwards, M. (1999). *Introduction to nursing informatics* (2nd ed.). New York: Springer-Verlag.

Haux, R., Knaup, P., & Schmucker, P. (1999). Commentary—Medical and health information systems; the boundaries are still fading. In A. McCray & J. van Bemmel (Eds.), *Yearbook of Medical Informatics 1999* (pp. 235–237). New York: Schattauer.

Horner, V., Hanmer L., & Mbananga, N. D. (2006). A consumer decision support system for common health ailments in South Africa. In H-A. Park, P. J. Murray, & C. Delaney (Eds.), *Consumer-centered computer-supported care for healthy people. Proceedings of NI2006* (p. 1027). Amsterdam: IOS Press.

Istepanian, R., Laxminarayan, S., & Pattichis, C. S. (Eds.). (2006). *M-Health: Emerging mobile health systems.* Berlin, Germany: Springer.

Kirovski, D., Oliver, N., Sinclair, M., & Tan, D. (2007). *Health-OS: A position paper.* Proceedings of the 1st ACM SIGMOBILE International Workshop. Retrieved November 13, 2007, from http://portal.acm.org/citation.cfm?id=1248077

Kuhn, K. A., Wurst, S. H. R., Bott, O. J., & Guise, D. A. (2006). Expanding the scope of health information systems: Challenges and developments. *IMIA Yearbook of medical informatics 2006.* Stuttgart, Germany: IMIA and Schattauer GmBH.

Kurzweil, R. (2005). *The singularity is near. When humans transcend biology.* London: Gerald Duckworth & Co. Ltd.

Lawton, S., & Timmons, S. (2006). The relationship between technology and changing professional roles in health care: A case study in teledermatology. In H-A. Park, P. J. Murray, & C. Delaney (Eds.), *Consumer-centered computer-supported care for healthy people. Proceedings of NI2006* (pp. 669–671). Amsterdam: IOS Press.

Lee, M., Delaney, C., & Moorhead, S. (2006). Building a personal health record from nursing perspective. In H-A. Park, P. J. Murray, & C. Delaney (Eds.), *Consumer-centered computer-supported care for healthy people. Proceedings of NI2006* (pp. 25–29). Amsterdam: IOS Press.

Loescher, L. J., & Merkle, C. J. (2005, June). The interface of genomic technologies and nursing. *Journal of Nursing Scholarship, 37*(2), 111–119.

Maag, M. (2005, January 1). The potential use of 'blogs' in nursing education. *CIN: Computers, Informatics, Nursing, 23*(1), 16–24.

Maag, M. (2006, January/February). Podcasting and MP3 players: Emerging education technologies. *CIN: Computers, Informatics, Nursing, 24*(1), 9–13.

Mandil, S., Moidu, K., Korpela, M., Byass, P., & Forster, D. (Eds.). (1993). *Health informatics in Africa HELINA93.* Amsterdam, Netherlands: EXCERPTA MEDICA.

Martin-Sanchez, F., Iakovidis, I., Norager, F., Maojo, V., de Groen, P., Vander Lei, J., et al. (2004, February). Synergy between medical informatics and bioinformatics: Facilitating genomic medicine for future health care. *Journal of Biomedical Informatics, 37*(1), 30–42.

Martindale, T., & Wiley, D. A. (2004). *An introduction to teaching with weblogs.* Retrieved November 13, 2007, from http://teachable.org/papers/2004_blogs_in_teaching.pdf

McCormick, K. A. (2001). Future directions. In V. K. Saba & K. A. McCormick (Eds.), *Essentials of computers for nurses: Informatics for the new millennium* (3rd ed., pp. 519–527). New York: McGraw-Hill.

McCormick, K. A., Delaney, C. J., Brennan P. F., Effken, J. A., Kendrick, K., Murphy, J., et al. (2007). Guideposts to the future—An agenda for nursing informatics. *Journal of the American Medical Informatics Association, 14*(1), 19–24.

Miller, R., Pople, H., & Myers, J. (1982). INTERNIST-1: An experimental computer-based diagnostic consultant for general internal medicine. *New England Journal of Medicine, 307,* 468–476.

Mortensen, R., & Nielsen, G. (1995). Telenursing. In M. F. Laires, M. J. Ladeira, & J. P. Christensen, (Eds.), *Health in the new communications age health care telematics for the 21st century* (pp. 115–126). Amsterdam, Netherlands: IOS Press.

Murray, P. J., & Maag, M. (2006). *Towards health informatics 2.0: Blogs, podcasts and Web 2.0 applications in nursing and health informatics education and professional collaboration: A discussion paper.* Retrieved November 13, 2007, from http://www.hi-blogs.info/media/publications/murraymaaghi20%20july06.rtf

Murray, P. J., Park, H-A., Erdley, W. S., & Kim, J. (Eds.). (2007). *Nursing informatics 2020: Towards defining our own future. Proceedings of NI2006 Post Congress Conference.* Amsterdam: IOS Press.

Murray, P. J., & Ward, R. (2004, October). Engaging in healthcare informatics—Let's use the technology. *BJHC&IM, 21*(10), 14.

Oh, H., Rizo, C., Enkin, M., & Jadad, A. (2005). What is ehealth (3): A systematic review of published definitions. *Journal of Medical Internet Research, 7*(1), e1. Retrieved November 13, 2007, from http://www.jmir.org/2005/1/e1

Oren, E., Shaffer, E. R., & Guglielmo, B. J. (2003). Impact of emerging technologies on medication errors and adverse drug events. *American Journal of Health-System Pharmacy, 60*(14), 1447–1458.

O'Reilly, T. (2005). *What is Web 2.0: Design patterns and business models for the next generation of software.* Retrieved June 6, 2008, from http://oreilly.com/pub/a/oreilly/tim/news/2005/09/30/what-is-web-20.html

Øyri, K., Balasingham, H., & Hogetveit, J. O. (2006). Implementation of wireless technology in advanced clinical practice. In H-A. Park, P. J. Murray, & C. Delaney (Eds.), *Consumer-centered computer-supported care for healthy people. Proceedings of NI2006* (pp. 730–733). Amsterdam: IOS Press.

Øyri, K., Newbold, S., Park, H-A., Honey, M., Coenen, A., Ensio, A. et al. (2007). Technology developments applied to healthcare/nursing. In P. J. Murray, H-A. Park, W. S. Erdley, & J. Kim (Eds.), *Nursing informatics 2020: Towards defining our own future. Proceedings of NI2006 Post Congress Conference* (pp. 21–37). Amsterdam: IOS Press.

Park, H-A., Murray, P., & Delaney, C. (2006). *Consumer-centered computer-supported care for healthy people. Proceedings of NI2006.* Amsterdam: IOS Press.

Saba, V. K., & Erdley, W. S. (2006). Historical perspectives of nursing and the computer. In V. K. Saba & K. A. McCormick (Eds.), *Essentials of nursing informatics* (4th ed., pp. 9–28). New York: McGraw-Hill.

Saba, V. K., & McCormick, K. A. (1986). *Essentials of computers for nurses.* Philadelphia: J. B. Lippincott Company.

Sackett, K. M., & Erdley, W. S. (2002). The history of health care informatics. In S. P. Englebardt & R. Nelson (Eds.), *Health care informatics: An interdisciplinary approach* (pp. 453–457). St. Louis, MO: Mosby.

Salata, O. V. (2004). Applications of nanoparticles in biology and medicine. *Journal of Nanobiotechnology,* 2. Retrieved December 9, 2007, from http://www.jnanobiotechnology.com/content/2/1/3

Schmidt, K. F. (2007). *Nanofrontiers: Visions for the future of nanotechnology. Project on Emerging Nanotechnologies* 6. Woodrow Wilson International Center for Scholars. Retrieved December 9, 2007, from http://www.nanotechproject.org/file_download/181

Schrader, U. (2006). Managing a lecture in nursing informatics in a blended learning format—A bottom-up approach to implement an open-source Web-based learning management system. In H-A. Park, P. J. Murray, & C. Delaney (Eds.), *Consumer-centered computer-supported care for healthy people. Proceedings of NI2006* (pp. 559–562). Amsterdam: IOS Press.

Shortliffe, E., & Buchanan, B. (1975). A model of inexact reasoning in medicine. *Math Biosci, 23,* 351–379.

Siemens, G. (2005). *Connectivism. A learning theory for the digital age.* Retrieved December 9, 2007, from http://www.constructict.com/blog/wp-content/themes/kiwi/featurepics/WBLEAlan/LinkedDocuments/ConnectivismLearningintheDigitalAge.doc

Stammer, L. (2000, August). Brazil & its neighbors. *Healthcare Informatics,* 26–36.

Technology Workgroup, Maryland Statewide Commission on the Crisis in Nursing (2004). *Technology's role in addressing Maryland's nursing shortage: Innovations & examples.* Retrieved December 9, 2007, from http://maryland.nursetech.com/F/NT/MD/NursingInnovations2004.pdf

TIGER. (2007). *The TIGER Initiative: Evidence and informatics transforming nursing: 3-year action steps toward a 10-year vision.* Retrieved December 9. 2007, from https://www.tigersummit.com/uploads/TIGERInitiative_Report2007_bw.pdf

Turley, J. P., Murray, P. J., Saranto, K., Ehnfors, M., & Seomun, G-A. (2007). What if nurses get what they have always sought: Totally personalized care? Trends affecting nursing informatics. In P. J. Murray, H-A. Park, W. S. Erdley, & J. Kim (Eds.), *Nursing informatics 2020: Towards defining our own future. Proceedings of NI2006 Post Congress Conference* (pp. 55–72). Amsterdam: IOS Press.

Vocera. (2007). *Vocera communications badge: Wearable instant voice communication.* Retrieved December 9, 2007, from http://www.vocera.com/downloads/voc_sys_datasheet_1206.pdf

Warner, H., Olmsted, C., & Rutherford, B. (1972). HELP—A program for medical decision-making. *Computers and Biomedical Research, 5*(1), 65–74.

Weaver, C., Kennedy, R., Erdley, W. S., Kim, J., Chang, P., Schrader, U. et al. (2007). Health care in 2020. In P. J. Murray, H-A. Park, W. S. Erdley, & J. Kim (Eds.), *Nursing informatics 2020: Towards defining our own future. Proceedings of NI2006 Post Congress Conference* (pp. 73–83). Amsterdam: IOS Press.

Weiser, M. (1991, September). The computer for the twenty-first century. *Scientific American,* 94–104.

Williams, L. (2007, May 31). *Nobel laureate James Watson receives personal genome in ceremony at Baylor College of Medicine.* Retrieved December 9, 2007, from http://www.bcm.edu/news/packages/watson_genome.cfm

World Health Organization (WHO). (2007, April 19). *WHO brainstorming session on mhealth.* Med-e-Tel Conference, Luxembourg, Luxembourg. Retrieved June 6, 2008, from http://www.medetel.lu/download/2007/parallel_sessions/abstract/0418/WHO_m-HEALTH_Brainstorm_Notes.pdf

Zollner, H. (1995). The CARE telematics project. In M. F. Laires, M. J. Ladeira, & J. P. Christensen, (Eds.), *Health in the new communications age, health care telematics for the 21st century* (pp. 279–289). Amsterdam: IOS Press.

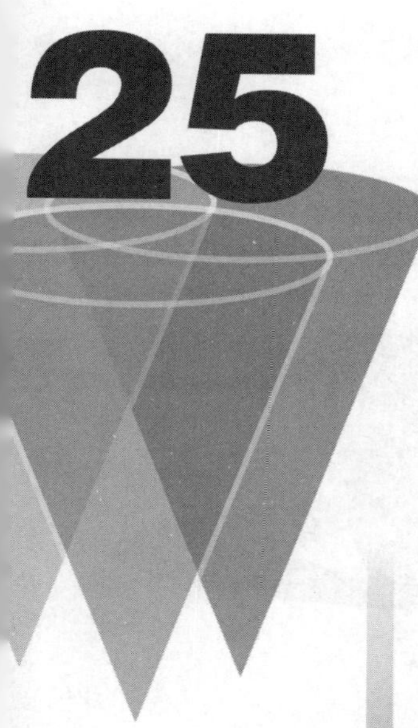

Nursing Informatics and the Foundation of Knowledge

Dee McGonigle and Kathleen Mastrian

Objectives

1. Assess nursing knowledge.
2. Explore the contribution of nursing informatics to the foundation of knowledge.

Key Terms

Comprehensive Health Enhancement Support System (CHESS)
Codify
Data
Data-centric
Information
Information technology (IT)
Knowledge
Knowledge acquisition
Knowledge-centric
Knowledge dissemination
Knowledge generation
Knowledge management system (KMS)
Knowledge repositories
Knowledge worker
Nursing informatics (NI)

INTRODUCTION

Throughout this book you have learned about many facets of **nursing informatics (NI)** and the interfacing of nurse **knowledge workers** and technology. The Foundation of Knowledge model (Figure 25-1) has provided a framework for examining the dynamic interrelationships between data, **information**, and **knowledge** used to meet healthcare delivery systems', organizations', patients', and nurses', needs.

At its base, the model has bits, bytes (computer terms for chunks of information), data, and information in a random representation. Growing out of the base are separate cones of light that expand as they reflect upward and represent **knowledge acquisition, knowledge generation**, and **knowledge dissemination.** At the intersection of the cones and forming a new cone is knowledge processing. Encircling and cutting through the knowledge cones is feedback, which acts on and may transform any or all aspects of knowledge represented by the cones. Now imagine the model as a dynamic figure with the cones of light and the feedback rotating and interacting rather than remaining static. In other words knowledge acquisition, knowledge generation, knowledge dissemination, knowledge processing, and feedback are constantly evolving for us as nurse scientists. The transparent effect of the cones is deliberate

FIGURE 25-1
Foundation of Knowledge model. (Designed by Alicia Mastrian.)

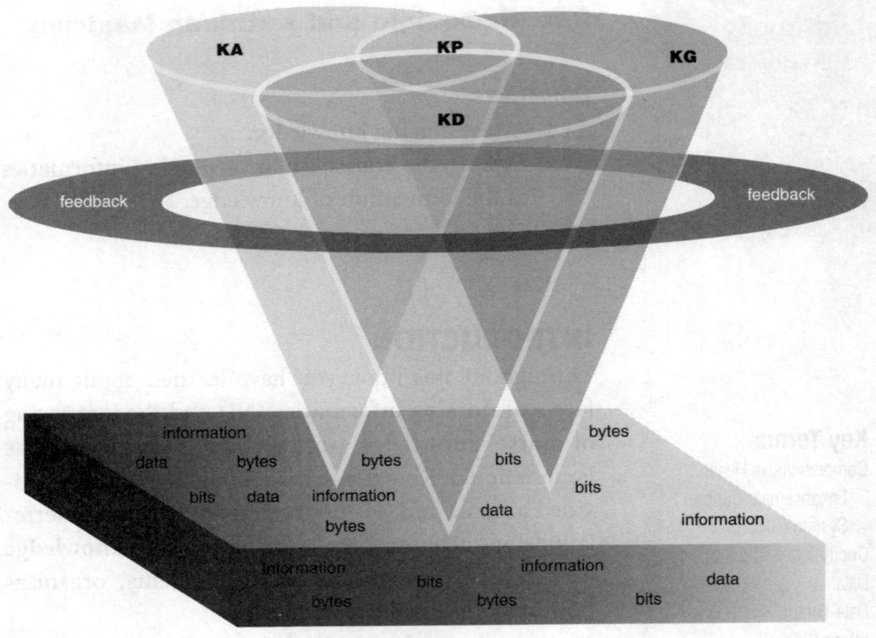

and is intended to suggest that as knowledge grows and expands its use becomes more transparent—that is, we use it without even being consciously aware of what aspect of knowledge we are using at any given moment during our practice.

If you are an experienced nurse, think back to when you were a novice. Did you feel like all you had in your head were bits of data and information that did not form any type of cohesive whole? As the model depicts, the processing of knowledge begins a bit later (imagine a time line applied vertically) with early experiences on the bottom and expertise growing as the processing of knowledge kicks in. Early on in our education as nurses, we focus our conscious attention mainly on knowledge acquisition and depend on our instructors and others to process, generate, and disseminate knowledge. As we become more comfortable with the science of nursing, we begin to take over some of the other knowledge functions. However, in order to keep up with the explosion of information in nursing and health care, we must continue to rely on the knowledge generation and dissemination of others. In this sense, we are committed to lifelong learning and the use of knowledge in the practice of nursing science.

As nurse knowledge workers, information is our primary resource, and when we deal with information it is done in overlapping phases. We are acquiring, processing or assimilating and retaining, and using this information to generate and disseminate knowledge. However, it is not a sequential phasing; instead, we are constantly gleaning data and information from our environment and massaging it into our knowledge bases so that we can apply and share (disseminate) what we know.

Knowledge is thought of as either explicit or tacit. Explicit knowledge is the knowledge that we can convey in letters, words, and numbers. This can be exchanged or shared in the form of data, manuals, product specifications, principles, policies, theories, and the like. Nurses can disseminate and share this knowledge publicly or on the record and scientifically or methodically. A nursing model or theory that is well developed and easily explained and understood would be an example of explicit knowledge. Tacit knowledge, on the other hand, is individualized and highly personal or private, including your values or emotions. This type of knowledge is difficult to convey, transmit, or share with others since it is your own insights or slant on things, perceptions, intuitions, sense, hunches, or gut feelings. Tacit knowledge reflects our skills and beliefs, and that is why we find it difficult to explain or communicate to others. Lake (2005) states:

> From close examination of and reflection on the literature it is possible to infer nursing prioritisation of the patient need for care as it is initially taught to nursing students and is then developed in practice and influenced by practice setting. The process of nursing prioritisation of the patient need for care involves discretionary judgment and ongoing assessment throughout and between unfolding patient situations. It is best understood from studies addressing clinical decision-making in nursing through the interpretive paradigm and in the plain language descriptions of nurse decision-making. The principles of such decision-making are discussed only in very general terms and the rationale remains the tacit knowledge of nursing (p. 152).

How we learn as nursing students and practicing nurses is therefore directly affected by our practice experiences within our own personal frame of reference. The quality of our clinical decision making is directly related to our experience and knowledge. Knowledge is situational. We use explicit and tacit knowledge to conduct our assessments, diagnoses, intervention implementation, and evaluation of our nursing actions for each individual patient in our care. **Knowledge management systems (KMSs)** must blend these knowledge needs and provide knowledge bases as well as decision support systems in order to inform our clinical decision making. We each process and assimilate knowledge in our own unique way influenced by our own unique perspectives.

According to Gent (2007), there are three types of knowledge workers—knowledge consumers, knowledge brokers, and knowledge generators. This breakdown of knowledge workers is not mutually exclusive but instead we transition between them as situations and our experience, education, and knowledge change. Knowledge consumers are mainly users of knowledge who do not have the expertise to provide the knowledge they need for themselves. Novice nurses can be thought of as knowledge consumers who use the knowledge of experienced nurses or who search information systems for the knowledge necessary to apply to their practice. As responsible knowledge consumers, they must also question and challenge what is known to help them learn and understand. Their questioning and challenging will facilitate critical thinking and the development of new knowledge. Knowledge brokers know where to find information and knowledge, they generate some knowledge but are mainly known for their ability to find what is needed. More experienced nurses and nursing students become knowledge brokers out of necessity, needing to know. Knowledge generators are the "primary sources of new knowledge" (Gent, ¶ 2). These are our nursing researchers and nursing experts—the people who know. They are able to answer our questions, craft theories, find solutions to nursing problems or concerns, and innovate practice.

The healthcare industry, the nursing profession, and our patients all benefit as we develop nursing intelligence and intellectual capital by gaining insight into nursing science and its enactment, practice. Nursing informatics applications of databases, knowledge management systems, and repositories where this knowledge can be analyzed and reused facilitates this process, enabling dissemination and reuse of knowledge.

In order to be able to enhance the acquisition, processing, generation, dissemination, and reuse of nursing knowledge, we must **codify** or be able to articulate our knowledge structures so that they can be captured within the KMSs. According to Markus (2001):

> Synthesis of evidence from a wide variety of sources suggests four distinct types of knowledge reuse situations according to the knowledge reuser and the purpose of knowledge reuse. The types involve shared work producers, who produce knowledge they later reuse; shared work practitioners, who reuse each other's knowledge contributions; expertise-seeking novices; and

> secondary knowledge miners. Each type of knowledge reuser has different requirements for knowledge repositories. (¶ 1)

Markus refers to the **knowledge repositories** as "organizational memory systems" (2001, ¶ 1). These memory systems gained popularity for help desk personnel who could access and reuse knowledge of solutions to similar problems on which clients seek help. Health care is an arena that could use the KMSs or knowledge repositories. Hsia, Lin, Wu, and Tsai (2006) recognize that nurses are "knowledge intensive" (¶ 4) professionals who are "required to take new nursing knowledge and experience that can be acquired through various net-enabled applications or the Internet. Nursing professionals are being asked to do more with less in such contexts, while their nursing care responsibilities have increased" (¶ 4). The **information technology** [boldface added] capabilities are expanding to develop and support a "**knowledge-centric** [boldface added] view rather than simply a **data-centric** view [boldface added]" (Hsia et al., ¶ 4). Nurse knowledge workers must be able to access, use, and share these new informatics tools since "a well-designed IT-based knowledge management system (KMS) has become an ever more central force in improving the quality of care in competitive e-health environments" (Hsia et al., ¶ 4). Capturing the explicit and tacit forms of knowledge will be paramount to truly harness nursing knowledge. As knowledge repositories evolve to enhance sharing and repurposing of knowledge, nurses will be able to easily access, process, evaluate, reuse, generate, and disseminate knowledge.

This book uses the Foundation of Knowledge model reflecting that knowledge is power, and for that reason, nurses focus on information as a key resource. The application of the model was described in each section of the book to help you understand and appreciate the foundation of knowledge in NI. All of the various nursing roles—practice, administration, education, research, informatics—involve the science of nursing. Nurses are knowledge workers, working with information and generating information and knowledge as a product. We are knowledge acquirers, providing convenient and efficient means of capturing and storing knowledge. We are knowledge users, individuals or groups who benefit from valuable, viable knowledge. Nurses are knowledge engineers, designing, developing, implementing and maintaining knowledge. We are knowledge managers, capturing and processing collective expertise and distributing it where it can create the largest benefit. We are knowledge developers or generators, changing and evolving knowledge based on the tasks at hand and information available.

Nursing science is dependent on knowledge generation, and NI should facilitate all aspects of nursing especially in the generation of knowledge and translational research where we attempt to bridge the gap between what we know (research) and what we do (practice). Swan, Lang, and McGinley (2004) describe NI and a common nursing language as an important vehicle to access stores of clinical information that can be used as the basis for research and to help answer the question, "What do nurses do?" "Embedding nursing language within informatics structures is essential to make the work of nurses visible and articulate evidence about the quality and value of nursing in the care of patients, groups, and populations" (¶ 27). In this text, we have established that NI is a vital tool for clinical decision making, especially when we are able to demonstrate how nurses structure and process information. An important direction for the future is to study the impact of NI on nursing science. For example, Goossen (2000) suggests the need for further study of nursing decision making and the need to model this process. He also suggests that we need to focus on the evaluation of technology systems themselves and the human–technology interface.

Nursing informatics can also be used to facilitate nursing administration and managerial studies of the work of nursing. We have previously described numerous opportunities for **data** mining in NI. Goossen (2000) suggests two approaches to data mining. The first approach involves a general search looking for repeated instances or patterns without preconceived notions about what will be found. Findings from the eyes wide open look at the database may suggest patterns that warrant more structured data mining, consistent with Goossen's second approach. Some of the larger healthcare systems store all of the clinical information from all of the affiliated hospitals and clinics in a central data warehouse. General data scans and analyses looking for patterns may suggest a trend toward better outcomes for patients with congestive heart failure in one of the affiliate hospitals. This identification of such a trend clearly begs for further analyses. A nurse researcher or administrator could ask, "What are the factors contributing to these better outcomes and how can they be put into practice across the system?" Other research studies might focus on assessing the effectiveness of strategic planning and organizational goal setting or studying work flow and communication processes in an organization. Poissant, Pereira, Tamblyn, and Kawasumi (2005) present the results of a systematic literature review on the time efficiency impacts of electronic health records in the clinical setting. There are numerous other examples of research aimed at advancing the state of the science of NI. Bakken (2006) provides one of the most comprehensive overviews of the effects of NI on patient safety. In her opening remarks, she writes, "The health information technologies deployed as part of the national framework must support nursing practice in a manner that enables prevention of medical errors and the promotion of patient safety and contributes to the development of practice-based nursing knowledge as well as best practices for patient safety"

(¶ 1). Shaw and colleagues (2006) summarize 15 years of research on the **Comprehensive Health Enhancement Support System (CHESS)**, a computer-based system designed to help underserved breast cancer patients manage their disease. A study of comparing routine instruction with computer-assisted video instruction about home exercise and the effects on compliance with the regimen and patient satisfaction is yet another example of research opportunities related to NI (Lysack, Dama, Neufeld, & Andreassi, 2005). As a final example, Hering, Harvan, D'Angelo, and Jasinski (2005) studied the effects of a specially designed Web page related to surgical teaching on patient acquisition of information and overall satisfaction with the surgical experience. We invite you to read each of these studies in more detail.

We hope that we have convinced you that in order for a profession to evolve, knowledge must be dynamically generated, disseminated, and assimilated. This dynamic interplay means that as knowledge is generated, disseminated, and assimilated, new questions about the impact of NI that will help new knowledge to be generated and assimilated and so on will arise. The assimilation of new knowledge in a profession is a multifaceted approach of individual perception, challenges, and collective thought applied to the practice of nursing. As nurses, we challenge what is known, and we want to acquire, process, generate, and disseminate knowledge.

SUMMARY

What we would like to leave you with is the same challenge that we have set for the entire text: become informatics savvy and ask yourself the following questions:

- How can I apply the knowledge I gain from my practice setting to benefit my patients and enhance my practice?
- How can I help my colleagues and patients understand and use the current technology that is available?
- How can I use my wisdom to help create the theories, tools, and knowledge of the future?

As a result of reading this book, you should have a deeper understanding of knowledge and informatics and the power they have to inform the science of nursing. We hope that you also gained valuable insights into the core principles of NI and the NI practice specialty. The future is exciting. The previous chapter in this section was an excellent insight into what will/can be. This chapter should motivate you to continue to learn more and perhaps delve into the science of NI in a nursing research role. We invite you to become active participants in molding the future of both nursing and informatics sciences.

References

Bakken, S. (2006). Informatics for patient safety: A nursing research perspective. *Annual Review of Nursing Research, 24,* 219–254. Retrieved January 27, 2008, from ProQuest Nursing & Allied Health Source database (Document ID: 1106698271).

Gent, A. (2007). *Three types of knowledge workers.* Retrieved January 26, 2008, from http://incrediblydull.blogspot.com/2007/10/three-types-of-knowledge-workers.html

Goossen, W. (2000). Nursing informatics research. *Nurse Researcher, 8*(2), 42. Retrieved January 27, 2008, from ProQuest Nursing & Allied Health Source database (Document ID: 67258628).

Hering, K., Harvan, J., D'Angelo, M., & Jasinski, D. (2005). The use of a computer Website prior to scheduled surgery (a pilot study): Impact on patient information, acquisition, anxiety level, and overall satisfaction with anesthesia care. *AANA Journal, 73*(1), 29–33. Retrieved January 2, 2008, from ProQuest Nursing & Allied Health Source database (Document ID: 795995771).

Hsia, T., Lin, L., Wu, J., & Tsai, H. (2006). A framework for designing nursing knowledge management systems. *Interdisciplinary Journal of Information, Knowledge and Management.* Retrieved January 26, 2008, from http://www.ijikm.org/Volume1/IJIKMv1p013-022_Hsia02.pdf

Lake, S. (2005). *Nursing prioritization of the patient need for care: Tacit knowledge of clinical decision making in nursing.* Retrieved January 26, 2008, from http://researcharchive.vuw.ac.nz/bitstream/10063/22/6/thesis.pdf

Lysack, C., Dama, M., Neufeld, S., & Andreassi, E. (2005). Compliance and satisfaction with home exercise: A comparison of computer-assisted video instruction and routine rehabilitation practice. *Journal of Allied Health, 34*(2), 76–82. Retrieved January 2, 2008, from ProQuest Nursing & Allied Health Source database (Document ID: 855324561).

Markus, M. (2001). Toward a theory of knowledge reuse: Types of knowledge reuse situations and factors in reuse success. *Journal of Management Information Systems, 18*(1), 57–94. Retrieved January 26, 2008, from http://jmis.bentley.edu/articles/v18_n1_p57/index.html

Poissant, L., Pereira, J., Tamblyn, R., & Kawasumi, Y. (2005). The impact of electronic health records on time efficiency of physicians and nurses: A systematic review. *Journal of the American Medical Informatics Association, 12*(5), 505–516. Retrieved January 21, 2008, from ProQuest Nursing & Allied Health Source database (Document ID: 908812431).

Shaw, B., Gustafson, D., Hawkins, R., McTavish, F., McDowell, H., Pingree, S., et al. (2006). How underserved breast cancer patients use and benefit from ehealth programs: Implications for closing the digital divide. *American Behavioral Scientist, 49*(6), 823–834. Retrieved January 2, 2008, from ABI/INFORM Global database. (Document ID: 974889131).

Swan, B., Lang, N., & McGinley, A. (2004). Access to quality health care: Links between evidence, nursing language, and informatics. *Nursing Economics, 22*(6), 325–332. Retrieved January 27, 2008, from Health Module database (Document ID: 768191851).

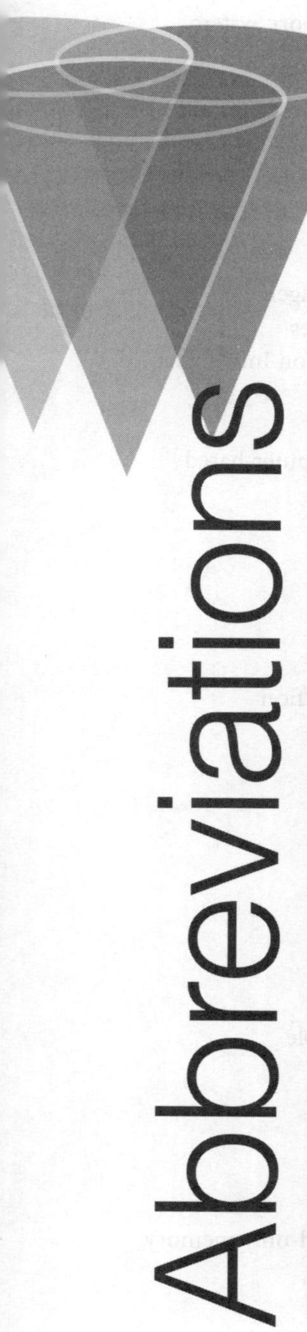

Abbreviations

ABC	Alternative billing codes
ADT	Admission, discharge, and transfer system
AHRQ	Agency for Healthcare Research and Quality
AI	Artificial intelligence
ALA	American Library Association
Alt	Alternate key on the computer keyboard
ALU	Arithmetic logic unit
ANA	American Nurses Association
ANGEL	A New Global Environment for Learning
ANSI	American National Standards Institute
API	Application programming interface
b	Bit
B	Byte
BIOS	Basic input/output system
bit/s or bps	Bits per second
BMP	Bitmap image
BRFSS	Behavioral risk factor surveillance system
CAI	Computer assisted instruction
CBIS	Computer-based information system
CCC	Clinical care classification
CD	Compact disc
CDC	Centers for Disease Control and Prevention
CD-R	Compact disc recordable
CD-ROM	Compact disc-read only memory
CD-RW	Compact disc recordable and rewritable
CDS/CDSS	Clinical decision support/clinical decision support system

CHESS	Comprehensive Health Enhancement Support System
CHF	Congestive heart failure
CHI	Consolidated health informatics
CI	Cognitive informatics
CINAHL	Cumulative Index to Nursing & Allied Health Literature
CIO	Chief information officer
CIS	Clinical information systems
CMIS	Case management information system
CMS	Course management system; content management system; Centers for Medicare and Medicaid Services
CNPII	Committee for Nursing Practice Information Infrastructure
COPD	Chronic obstructive pulmonary disease
CPGs	Clinical practice guidelines
CPOE	Computerized physician order entry; computer-based provider order entry
CPU	Central processing unit
CRA	Community risk assessment
CRT	Cathode ray tube
CSS	Cascading style sheets
CTA	Cognitive task analysis
CTO	Chief technical officer; chief technology officer
Ctrl	Control key on the computer keyboard
CWA	Cognitive work analysis
DBMS	Database management system
DHR	Digital health record
DRAM	Dynamic random access memory
DSS	Decision support system
DVD	Digital versatile disc; digital video disc
DVD-R	Digital video disc-recordable
DVD-RW	Digital video disc-recordable and rewritable
DW	Data warehouse
EB	Exabyte
EBP	Evidence-based practice
EDI	Electronic data interchange
EEPROM	Electronically erasable programmable read-only memory
EHR	Electronic health record
EMR	Electronic medical record

EPROM	Erasable programmable read-only memory
ERD	Entity relationship diagram
ERIC	Education Resources Information Center
ESC	Escape key
ESLI	Ethical, social, and legal implications
F key	Function key on the computer keyboard
FHIE	Federal Health Information Exchange
FPROM	Field programmable read only memory
FPU	Floating point unit
GB	Gigabyte
GHz	Gigahertz
GLBA	Gramm-Leach-Bliley Act
GUI	Graphical user interface
HCI	Human–computer interaction
HCT	Human–computer technology
HHA	Home health agency
HIE	Health information exchange
HIPAA	Health Insurance Portability and Accountability Act
HIT	Health information technology
HL7	Health Level 7
HMO	Health maintenance organization
HTI	Human–technology interaction
HTML	Hypertext markup language
ICNP	International classification of nursing practice
IDE	Integrated drive electronics
IEEE	Institute of Electrical and Electronics Engineers
IHIE	Indiana Health Information Exchange
IM	Instant message
IN	Informatics nurse
INS	Informatics nurse specialist
I/O	Input/output
IP	Internet protocol
IS	Information system
ISO	International Organization for Standardization
IT	Information technology

KB	Kilobyte
KMS	Knowledge management system
LAN	Local area network
LCD	Liquid crystal display
LOINC	Logical Observation Identifiers Names and Codes
LOS	Length of stay
LTC	Long-term care
MAN	Metropolitan area network
MB	Megabyte
MCIS	Managed care information system
MHDC	Massachusetts Health Data Consortium
MHz	Megahertz
Modem	Modulator-demodulator
Moodle	Modular Object-Oriented Dynamic Learning Environment
MP3	MPEG-1 Audio Layer-3
MPEG	Moving Picture Experts Group
MPI	Master patient index
MRI	Magnetic resonance imaging
NANDA-I	North American Nursing Diagnosis Association-International
NCPHI	National Center for Public Health Informatics
NGC	National Guideline Clearinghouse
NGI	Next-generation Internet
NHII	National Health Information Infrastructure
NHIN	National Health Information Network
NI	Nursing informatics
NIC	Nursing Intervention Classification; network interface cards
NIDSEC	Nursing Information and Data Set Evaluation Center
NIS	Nursing information system
NLS	National language support
NMDS	Nursing minimum data set
NMMDS	Nursing management minimum data set
NOC	Nursing outcome classification
NPI	National provider identifier
OASIS	Outcomes and assessment information set
OS	Operating system

OSI	Open systems interconnection
OWL	Web ontology language
PACS	Picture archiving and communication system
PADS	Planned accelerated discharge protocols
PB	Petabyte
PBL	Problem-based learning
PC	Personal computer
PCA	Patient-controlled analgesia
PCI	Peripheral component interconnection
PCIS	Patient care information system
PDA	Personal data assistant; personal digital assistant
PERS	Personal emergency response system
PHI	Protected health information; public health informatics
PHR	Personal health record
PNDS	Perioperative nursing data set
POSIX	Portable operating system interface for UNIX
PPS	Prospective payment system
PROM	Programmable read-only memory
PrtSc or Prnt Scrn	Print screen key
PS/2	Personal system/2
PT/INR	Prothrombin time/international normalized ratio
QA	Quality assurance
RAM	Random access memory
RATS	Readiness assessment tests
RDBMS	Relational database management system
RDF	Resource description framework
RFID	Radio frequency identification
RHIO	Regional health information organization
RIS	Radiology information system
ROM	Read-only memory
RSS	Really simple syndication
RSVP	Rapid Syndromic Validation Project
RU	Research utilization
SCSI	Small computer system interface
SDO	Standards developing organization
SDRAM	Synchronous dynamic random access memory

SGML	Standard generalized markup language
SNOMED CT	Systematic Nomenclature of Medical Clinical Terms
SOX	Sarbanes-Oxley Act
SPRC	Suicide Prevention Resource Center
TB	Terabyte
TCP	Transmission control protocol
URL	Uniform resource locator
USB	Universal serial bus
VNA	Visiting Nurse Association
VoIP	Voice-over-Internet protocol
VR	Virtual reality
W3C	World Wide Web Consortium
WAN	Wide area network
WWW	World Wide Web
XML	Extensible markup language
YB	Yottabyte
YRBSS	Youth Risk Behavior Surveillance System
ZB	Zettabye

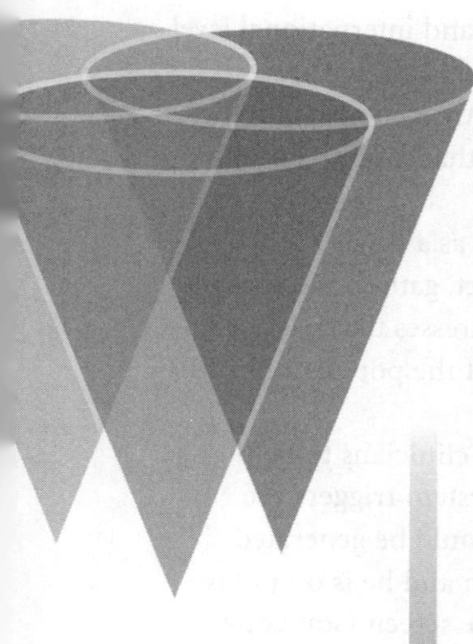

Glossary

Acceptable use A corporate policy that defines the types of activities that are acceptable on the corporate computer network, identifies the activities that are not acceptable, and the consequences for violations.

Accessibility Ease of accessing the information and knowledge needed to deliver care or manage a health service; the extent to which a system is usable by as many users as possible.

Acquisition The act of acquiring, to locate and hold. We acquire data and information.

Acuity system System that calculates the nursing care requirements for individual patients based on severity of illness, specialized equipment and technology needed, and intensity of nursing interventions; determines the amount of daily nursing care needed for each patient in a nursing unit.

Administrative processes The electronically performed functions of a healthcare agency including such items as billing, scheduling appointments and procedures, and insurance claim processing.

Admission, discharge, and transfer (ADT) system System that provides the backbone structure for the other types of clinical and business systems (Hassett & Thede, 2003); it contains the groundwork for the other types of healthcare information systems since it includes the patient's name, medical record number, visit or account number and demographic information such as age, sex, home address, and contact information. They are the central source for collecting this type of patient information and communicating it to the other types of healthcare information systems including clinical and business systems.

Advocate To act in the patients' best interest; to act and/or speak on our patients' behalf; to make the healthcare delivery system responsive to our patients' needs.

Advocate/policy developer A nurse informatics specialist who is key to developing the infrastructure of health policy. Policy development on a local, national, and international level is an integral part of this role.

Agency for Healthcare Research and Quality (AHRQ) An agency within the Department of Health and Human Services (DHHS), that supports health services research initiatives.

Aggregate data Any types of data that can be referenced as a single entity, but that also consist of more than one piece of data. Collect, gather, and report data that is related and kept together in a way that addresses that relationship; for example the population of a state is an aggregate of the populations of its cities, counties, and regions.

Alerts Warnings or additional information provided to clinicians to help with decision making; the action of the clinician or system triggers the generation of an alert. An example of when an alert could be generated would be if the patient's serum potassium level is high and he is on potassium chloride, the system would alert the nurse on the screen (soft copy alert) with or without audio and/or by a printed (hard copy alert) warning; also known as triggers.

Alternatives Choice between two or more options.

American Library Association (ALA) U.S.-based organization that promotes libraries and library education internationally.

American National Standards Institute (ANSI) An organization dedicated to promoting consensus on norms and guidelines related to the assessment of health agencies.

A New Global Environment for Learning (ANGEL) A course management system designed to support classroom learning in academic settings.

Analysis Separating a whole into its elements or component parts. Examination of a concept or phenomena, its elements, and their relations.

Antiprinciplism Theory that emerged with the expansive technological changes and the tremendous rise in ethical dilemmas accompanying these changes. Opponents of principlism include those who claim that its principles do not represent a theoretical approach and those who claim that its principles are too far removed from the concrete particularities of everyday human existence; the principles are too conceptual, intangible, or abstract, or disregard or do not take into account a person's psychological factors, personality, life history, sexual orientation, religious, ethnic, and cultural background.

Antivirus software A computer program that is designed to recognize and neutralize computer viruses, malicious codes that replicate over and over and eventually take over the computer's memory and interfere with normal functioning.

Application Refers to the implementation software of a computer system. This software allows users to complete tasks such as word processing, developing presentations, and managing data.

Archetype Broad or general, idealized model of an object or concept from which similar instances are derived, copied, patterned, or emulated. Original model after which other similar things are patterned. First form from which varieties arise or imitations are made.

Arithmetic logic unit (ALU) Essential building block of the central processing unit (CPU) that digitally performs arithmetic and logical functions.

Artificial intelligence (AI) The field that deals with the conception, development, and implementation of informatics tools based on intelligent technologies. This field attempts to capture the complex processes of human thought and intelligence.

Asynchronous That which is not synchronous. Not in real time, or does not occur or exist at the same time, having the same period or time frame. Learning anywhere and anytime using Internet and World Wide Web software tools (course management systems, e-mail, electronic bulletin boards, Web pages, etc.) as the principal delivery mechanisms for instruction.

Attribute Quality or characteristic; field or element of an entity in a database.

Audiopod Utility to download podcasts.

Authentication Processes to serve to authenticate or prove who is accessing the system.

Autonomy Right of individual to choose for herself/himself.

Avatar Image on the Internet that represents the user in virtual communities or other interactions on the Internet; 3-dimensional or 2-dimensional image representing one user on the Internet.

Behavioral Risk Factor Surveillance System (BRFSS) An assessment system initially designed to collect information on the movement of mentally impaired persons from state-operated facilities into community settings. The assessments have been expanded to include other populations and are designed to determine the effectiveness of programs in meeting healthcare needs of at-risk populations.

Beneficence Actions performed that contribute to the welfare of others.

Binary system System used by computers. A numeric system using two symbols: 0 and 1.

Bioethics The study and formulation of healthcare ethics. Bioethics takes on relevant ethical problems experienced by healthcare providers in the provision of care to individuals and groups.

Bioinformatics The application of computer science, information science, and cognitive science principles to biological systems, especially in the human genome field of study.

Biometrics Study of processes or means to uniquely recognizing individual users (humans) based upon one or more intrinsic physical or behavioral attributes or characteristics. Authentication devices that recognize thumb prints, retinal patterns, or facial patterns are available. Depending on the level of security needed, organizations will commonly use a combination of these types of authentication.

BIOS Basic input/output systems, binary input/output systems, basic integrated operating system, or built-in operating system that resides or is embedded on a chip that recognizes and controls the computer's devices.

Bioterrorism The use of pathogens or other potentially harmful biologic agents to sicken or kill members of a targeted population. Informatics database applications are used to track strategic indicators, such as emergency room visits, disease case reports, frequency and type of lab testing ordered by physicians and/or nurse practitioners, missed work, and over-the-counter medication purchases, that may indicate an outbreak that can be attributed to bioterrorism.

Bit (b) Unit of measurement that holds one binary digit, 0 or 1. The smallest possible chunk of data memory used in computer processing, exhibited as either 1 or 0, making up the binary system of the computer.

Blended A term used to describe a program format in which students take courses both face to face and online. A program of study that combines face-to-face courses and online courses.

Blog Interactive, online weblog. Typically a combination of what is happening on the Web as well as what is happening in the blogger's or the creator's life. A blog is as unique as the blogger or person creating it. Thought of as a diary and guide.

Blogger Someone who creates and maintains a blog. A person who blogs.

Borrowed theory Theories borrowed or made use of from other disciplines; as nursing began to evolve, theories from other disciplines such as psychology, sociology, etc., were adopted to try to empirically describe, explain, or predict nursing phenomena. As nursing theories continue to be developed, nurses are now questioning whether or not these borrowed theories were sufficient or satisfactory in their relation to the nursing phenomena they were used to describe, explain, or predict.

Brain The central information processing unit of humans. An organ that controls the central nervous system, is responsible for cognition and the interpretation, processing, and reaction to sensory input.

Browser Software used to locate and display Web pages. Also known as a Web browser or Internet browser.

Building block Basic element or part of nursing informatics such as information science, computer science, cognitive science, and nursing science.

Bus Subsystem that transfers data between a computer's internal components or between computers.

Byte (B) Unit of memory equal to eight bits or eight informational storage units and represents one keystroke; e.g., any push of a key on a keyboard such as pressing the space bar, a lower case a or an upper case T, for example; a chunk of memory that consists of eight bits, and is considered to be the best way to indicate computer memory or storage capacity.

Cache memory Smaller and faster memory storage used by the central processing unit (CPU) to store copies of frequently used data in main memory.

Call centers Registered nurse-staffed facilities at which nurses typically act as case managers for callers or perform patient triage.

Care ethics An ethical approach to solving moral dilemmas encountered in health care that is based on relationships and a caring attitude toward others.

Care plan A set of guidelines that outline the course of treatment and the recommended interventions that will achieve optimal results.

Case management information system (CMIS) Computer programs and information management tools that interact to support and facilitate the practice of case managers.

Case study An account of a nursing informatics activity, event, or problem containing some of the background and complexities actually encountered by a nurse. The case is used to enhance one's learning about nursing informatics principles, practices, and trends. Each case describes a series of events that reflect the nursing informatics episode as it actually occurred.

Casuist approach Approach to ethical decision making that grew out of the concern for more concrete methods of examining ethical dilemmas. Casuistry is a case-based ethical reasoning method that analyzes the facts of a case in a sound, logical, and ordered or structured manner. The facts are compared to the decisions arising out of consensus in previous paradigmatic or model cases.

Centers for Disease Control and Prevention (CDC) An agency of the United States Department of Health and Human Services that works to protect public health and safety related to disease control and prevention.

Centers for Medicare and Medicaid Services (CMS) The largest health insurer in the United States, particularly for home healthcare services, and for the elderly, for healthcare services.

Central processing unit (CPU) Processors that execute computer programs, thought of as the brains, controlling the functioning of the computer; the computer component that actually executes, calculates, and processes the binary computer code instigated by the operating system and other applications on the computer. It serves as the command center that directs the actions of all other components of the computer, and manages both incoming and outgoing data.

Central stations Multifunctional telehealthcare platforms for receiving, retrieving, and/or displaying patients' vital signs and other information transmitted from telecommunications-ready medical devices.

Certification System that validates that a nurse possesses certain skills and knowledge or is competent to complete a task. Competence and skill level determined by or based on an external review, assessment, examination, or education.

Change A transition to something different.

Chat Real-time electronic communications; users type what they want to say, and it is displayed on the screens of all participants in the same chat. Internet relay chat (IRC) is the Internet protocol for chat.

Chief information officer (CIO) Person involved with the information technology infrastructure of an organization. This role is sometimes called chief knowledge officer.

Chief technology officer or chief technical officer (CTO) Person focused on organizationally based scientific and technical issues and responsible for technological research and development as part of the organization's products and services.

Chronic disease Range of long-term diseases, such as congestive heart failure, diabetes, and respiratory ailments.

Clinical analytics Process of analysis by which clinical data is used to help make decisions and develop predictive analytics.

Clinical database A collection of related patient records stored in a computer system using software that permits a person or program to query the data in order to extract needed patient information.

Clinical decision support (CDS) A computer-based program designed to assist clinicians in making clinical decisions by filtering or integrating vast amounts of information, and providing suggestions for clinical intervention. May also be called a clinical decision support system (CDSS).

Clinical documentation system Array or collection of applications and functionality; amalgamation of systems, medical equipment, and technologies working together that are committed or dedicated to collecting, storing, and manipulating healthcare data and information and providing secure access to interdisciplinary clinicians navigating the continuum of client care. Designed to collect patient data in real time to enhance care by providing data at the clinician's fingertips and enabling decision making where it needs to occur—at the bedside. Also known as clinical information system (CIS).

Clinical guidelines That which provides a guide to decisions and criteria for specific practice areas.

Clinical information system (CIS) Array or collection of applications and functionality; amalgamation of systems, medical equipment, and technologies working together that are committed or dedicated to collecting, storing, and manipulating healthcare data and information and providing secure access to interdisciplinary clinicians navigating the continuum of client care. Designed to collect patient data in real time to enhance care by providing data at the clinician's fingertips and enabling decision making where it needs to occur—at the bedside. Also known as clinical documentation system.

Clinical outcomes Patient's results and consequences from clinical interventions.

Clinical practice council Group that uses the information generated by the clinical information systems (CIS) to design clinical education programs. Also called nursing practice council.

Clinical practice guidelines (CPGs) Informal or formal rules or guiding principles that a healthcare provider uses when determining diagnostic tests and treatment strategies for individual patients. In the electronic health record they are included in a variety of ways such as prompts, pop-ups, and text messages.

Coded terminology Nursing terminologies that are given a specific and standardized designation so that they can be easily entered into computerized nursing documentation systems, searched for, and easily retrieved.

Codify To classify, reduce to code, or articulate.

Cognitive That which uses one's capacity to think. Process of cognition is important to generate knowledge. Conscious intellectual or mental activity such as thinking, reasoning, and remembering, it includes imagination or the ability to imagine and the ability to learn.

Cognitive activity Any process or task (activity) that involves the capacity to think, reason, imagine, and learn.

Cognitive informatics (CI) Field of study made up of the disciplines of neuroscience, linguistics, artificial intelligence and psychology. The multidisciplinary study of cognition and information sciences, which investigates human information processing mechanisms and processes and their engineering applications in computing.

Cognitive science The interdisciplinary field that studies the mind, intelligence, and behavior from an information processing perspective.

Cognitive task analysis (CTA) Examination of the nature of a task by breaking it down into its component parts and identifying the performers' thought processes.

Cognitive walkthrough A technique used to evaluate a computer interface or a software program by breaking down and explaining the steps that a user will take to accomplish a task.

Cognitive work analysis (CWA) A multifaceted analytic procedure developed specifically for the analysis of complex, high-technology work domains.

Collaboration The sharing of ideas and experiences for the purposes of mutual understanding and learning.

Column Field or attribute of an entity in a database.

Communication science Area of concentration or discipline that studies human communication.

Communication software Technology programs used to transmit messages via e-mail, telephonically, paging, broadcast such as MP3, Internet such as instant messaging, voice-over-Internet protocol (VoIP), or lists, etc.

Communication system Collection of individual communications networks and transmission systems. In health care, it includes call light systems, wireless phones, pagers, e-mail, instant messaging and any other devices or networks that clinicians use to communicate with patients, families, other professionals, and internal and external resources.

Communications hub A device that captures and assists in the transmission of information from peripheral equipment. A processor organizes the data, appropriately encrypts it to assure confidentiality, and transmits it to appropriate decision makers. Data can be transmitted via traditional phone lines, the Internet, or over wireless networks. Typically the hub will be a small box, to which peripheral equipment is connected.

Community risk assessment (CRA) A comprehensive examination of a community to identify factors that potentially affect the health of the members of that community. Often used in public health program planning.

Compact disc read-only memory (CD-ROM) Disc that can hold approximately 700 megabytes of data accessible by a computer.

Compact disc-recordable (CD-R) Compact disc that can be used once for recording.

Compact disc-rewritable (CD-RW) Compact disc that can be recorded onto many times.

Compatibility The ability to work with each other or other devices or systems; e.g., software that is compatible with a computer.

Comprehensive health enhancement support system (CHESS) A computer-based system designed to help underserved breast cancer patients manage their disease.

Computer A machine that stores and executes programs; a machine with peripheral hardware and software to carry out selected programming.

Computer assisted instruction (CAI) Any instruction that is aided by the use of a computer.

Computer-based That which uses the computer to interact; the computer is the base tool.

Computer-based information system (CBIS) Combinations of hardware, software and telecommunications networks that people build and use to collect, create, and distribute useful data, typically in organizational settings.

Computer science Branch of engineering (application of science) that studies the theoretical foundations of information and computation and their implementation and application in computer systems. The study of storage/memory, conversion and transformation, and transfer or transmission of information in machines—that is computers—through both algorithms and practical implementation problems. Algorithms are detailed unambiguous action sequences in the design, efficiency, and application, and practical implementation problems deal with the software and hardware.

Computerized physician order entry systems (CPOE) A system that automates the way that orders have traditionally been initiated for patients. Clinicians place orders within these systems instead of using traditional handwritten transcription onto paper. These systems provide major safeguards by ensuring that physician orders are legible and complete, thereby providing a level of patient safety that was historically missing with paper-based orders. These systems provide decision support and automated alert functionality that was previously unavailable with paper-based orders.

Conceptual framework Framework used in research to chart feasible courses of action or to present a desired approach to a study or analysis. Framework built from a set of concepts that are related to a proposed or existing system of methods, behaviors, functions, relationships, and objects. A relational model. A formal way of thinking or conceptualizing about a phenomenon, process, or system under study.

Conferencing software Electronic communications system or software that supports and facilitates two or more people meeting for discussion. One of the high-end systems offers telepresence (creates a life-like experience allowing people to feel as if they were present in person—it would be as though the nurse were physically there with the patient—so people can work, learn, and play in person over the Internet or have an effect at a remote location).

Confidentiality All personal information that must be safeguarded by ensuring that access is limited to only those who are authorized.

Connectivity Ability to hook up to the electronic resources necessary to meet the user's needs. The ability to use computer networks to link to people and resources. The unbiased transmission or transport of Internet protocol packets between two end points.

Consequences Outcomes or products resulting from our decision choices.

Consolidated health informatics (CHI) A collaborative effort to adopt health information interoperability standards, particularly health vocabulary and messaging standards, for implementation in federal government systems.

Consultant A person hired to provide expert advice, opinions, and recommendations based on his or her area of expertise.

Context of care The setting, services, patient, environment, and professional and social interactions surrounding the delivery of patient interventions.

Continuing education Coursework or training completed postbaccalaureate, often for the purpose of recertification.

Continuous learner One who gleans lessons or learns from success as well as failures, or who constantly searches for information to add to one's knowledge base.

Copyright A legal term used by many governments around the world that gives the inventor or designer of an original product sole or exclusive rights for a limited time; the same laws that cover physical books, artwork, and other creative material are still applicable in the digital world.

Core business system System that enhances administrative tasks within healthcare organizations. Unlike clinical information systems whose aim is to provide direct patient care, these systems support the management of health care within an organization. These systems provide the framework for reimbursement, support of best practices, quality control, and resource allocation. There are four common core business systems: (1) admission, discharge and transfer (ADT), (2) financial, (3) acuity, and (4) scheduling systems.

Core sciences The branches of study and knowledge that form the foundation of nursing informatics, including nursing, computer, and information sciences. Some, including the editors of this text, believe that cognitive science should also be included in the list of NI foundational sciences.

Courage The strength to face difficulty.

Course management system (CMS) Software system designed for both faculty and students that supports educational episodes including tools for grading, learner assessment, content presentation/interaction, and communication. These systems provide for the support of learning activities throughout course delivery; proprietary examples include ANGEL, Blackboard, WebCT, Learning Space, and eCollege.

Creativity software Programs that support and facilitate innovation and creativity (intellectual process relating to the creation or generation of new ideas, concepts, or new relationships between currently existing ideas or concepts); allow users to focus or concentrate more on creating new things in our digital age and less on the mechanics or workings of how they are created or developed.

Cumulative Index to Nursing and Allied Health Literature (CINAHL) A comprehensive nursing and allied health literature database.

Data Raw fact that lacks meaning.

Data-centric Data is the central focus.

Data dictionary Software that contains a listing of the tables and their details including field names, validation settings, and data types.

Data file A collection of related records.

Data gatherer One involved in the direct procurement of raw facts (data). Raw fact (data) collector.

Data mart Collection of data focusing on a specific topic or organizational unit or department created to facilitate management personnel making strategic business decisions; could be as small as one database or larger such as a compilation of databases; generally smaller than a data warehouse.

Data mining A process of utilizing software to sort through data in order to discover patterns and ascertain or establish relationships. This process may help to discover or uncover previously unidentified relationships among the data in a database.

Data warehouse (DW) An extremely large database or repository that stores all of an organization's or institution's data and makes this data available for data mining. A combination of an institution's many different databases that provides management personnel flexible access to the data.

Database A collection of related records stored in a computer system using software that permits a person or program to query the data in order to extract needed information; may consist of one or more related data files or tables.

Database management system (DBMS) Software program/s and the hardware used to create and manage data.

Decision making Output of cognition. Outcome of our intellectual processing.

Decision support Recommendations for interventions based on computerized care protocols. The decision support recommendations may include such items as additional screenings, medication interactions, or drug and dosage monitoring.

Decision support/outcomes manager Person charged with reviewing the effects of interventions suggested by the computerized decision support system.

Decision support system (DSS) Computer applications designed to facilitate human decision-making processes. Usually DSSs are rule-based, using a specified knowledge base and a set of rules to analyze data and information and provide recommendations typically through the use of a knowledge base and rules to make recommendations to users.

Degradation Loss of quality; e.g., in telecommunications, it is the loss of quality in the electronic signal.

Desktop Computer's interface that resembles the top of one's desk, where one keeps things one wants to access quickly, such as paper clips, pens, paper, etc. On the computer's desktop, one can customize the look and feel to have easy access to the programs, folders, and files on the hard drive that one uses the most.

Digital divide The gap between those who have and those who do not have access to online information.

Digital health record (DHR) An electronic record of patient assessments that are collected over time, typically by a telemonitoring device. For example, daily assessments of weight and blood pressure can be captured electronically and graphically displayed to allow for the detection of subtle trends.

Digital pen Actual writing implement that can also digitally capture handwriting or drawings. It is battery operated and generally comes with a universal serial bus (USB) cradle that permits uploading captured materials to one's desktop, laptop, or palmtop computer. The user can use it as a ballpoint pen and write on regular paper just as he would with a normal pen, or he can capture it digitally after writing on digital paper.

Digital video disc-recordable (DVD-R) Disc on which a user can record once.

Digital video disc-recordable and rewritable (DVD-RW) Disc on which a user can record many times.

Digital video disc or digital versatile disc (DVD) Optical disc storage format that can generally hold or store more than six times the amount of data that a CD can.

Dissemination A thoughtful, intentional, goal-oriented communication of specific, useful information or knowledge.

Distance education Education provided from a remote location.

Document To capture and save information for later use.

Documentation Communication in the form of written or typed text, audio, video, graphics, photographs, pictures or any blending of these means used to describe some characteristics or elements of an object, system, or practice; for example, nursing documentation generates information about a patient (individual, family, group, community, populations) that describes the care and/or services that have been provided and allows for the communication necessary between nurses and other healthcare providers.

Domain name Series of alphanumeric characters that forms part of the Internet address or URL, such as psu.edu which denotes Penn State's address.

Drill-down Means of viewing data warehouse information by going down to lower levels of the database to focus on information that is pertinent to her/his needs at the moment.

Duty One's feeling of being bound or obligated to carry out specific tasks or roles based on one's rank or position.

Dynamic random access memory (DRAM) Type of RAM chip requiring less space to store the same amount on a similar SRAM (static RAM) chip; however, DRAM requires more power than SRAM since DRAM needs to keep its charge by constantly refreshing.

E-brochure Electronic brochure. Patient education material that is typically tied to an agency Web site, and may include such information as descriptions of diseases and their management, medication information, or where to get assistance with a healthcare issue.

E-health Healthcare initiatives and practice supported by electronic or digital media. The most typical use is in patient and family education where information is communicated electronically.

E-learning Electronic learning or learning that is facilitated by electronic means such as computers and the Internet. E-learning, online, and Web-based education has caused a significant shift in student–teacher relationships in nursing education.

E-mail Electronic mail. To compose, send, receive, and store messages in electronic communication systems.

E-mail client Program that manages e-mail functions.

E-portfolio Personalized collections of evidence from coursework, experiences outside of the classroom, and reflective commentary related to this evidence that can be shared with others electronically; categorized electronic presentation of one's skills, education, and examples of work and/or career achievements.

Educational Resources Information Center (ERIC) A comprehensive educational resources database. An international database of educational literature.

Educator Sage, leader, and/or guide who assists in the process or practice of learning.

eHealth Initiative Initiative developed to address the growing need for managing health information and to promote technology as a means of improving health information exchange, health literacy, and healthcare delivery.

Electronic communication Any exchange of information that is transmitted electronically.

Electronic data interchange (EDI) Specific set of standards for exchanging information between/among computers (computer to computer).

Electronic health record (EHR) A computer-based data warehouse or repository of information regarding the health status of a client, replacing the former paper-based medical record; it is the systematic documentation of a client's health status and health care in a secured digital format, meaning that it can be processed, stored, transmitted, and accessed by authorized interdisciplinary professionals for the purpose of supporting efficient, high quality health care across the client's healthcare continuum. Also known as electronic medical record (EMR).

Electronic mailing list Automatic mailing list server such as LISTSERV that sends an e-mail that is addressed to the list to everyone who has subscribed to the list automatically. Similar to an electronic bulletin board or news forum.

Electronic medical record (EMR) See electronic health record (EHR).

Electronically erasable programmable read-only memory (EEPROM) A non-volatile storage chip used in computers and other devices to store small amounts of volatile data, e.g., calibration tables or device configuration.

Emerging technologies New technology that is likely to impact health care in a significant way such as nanotechnology or biotechnology.

Empiricism That knowledge which is derived from our experiences or senses.

Empowerment Promoting self-actualization. Achieve power or control one's own life.

Entity Represents a table, and each field within the table becomes an attribute of that entity. The database developer must critically think about the attributes for each specific entity. For example, the entity disease might have the attributes of chronic disease, acute disease, or communicable disease. The name of the entity, disease, would imply that the entity is about diseases. The fields or attributes would be chronic, acute, or communicable.

Entity relationship diagram (ERD) Diagram that specifies the relationship among the entities in the database. Sometimes the implied relationships are apparent based on the entities' definitions; however, all relationships should be specified as to how they relate to one another. There are typically three relationships, one to one, one to many, and many to many.

Entrepreneur One who assumes the risks of beginning an enterprise or business and accepts responsibility for organizing and managing the organization.

Enumerative approach Nursing terminology in which words or phrases are represented in a list or a simple hierarchy; gives an explicit and exhaustive listing of all the objects that fall under the concept or term in question.

Epidemiology The study of identifying things that come upon the people. Incidence, prevalence, and control of disease. Case finding.

Epistemology Study of the nature and origin of knowledge; what it means to know.

Erasable programmable read-only memory (EPROM) Type of computer memory chip that retains its data when its power supply is switched off, and can be erased with ultraviolet light.

Ergonomics In the United States, this term is used to describe the physical characteristics of equipment, for example, the optimal fit of a scissors to a human hand. In Europe, the term is synonymous with human factors. It is the interaction of humans with physical attributes of equipment or the interaction of humans and the arrangement of equipment in the work environment.

Ethical decision making The process of making informed choices about ethical dilemmas based on a set of standards differentiating right from wrong. The decision making reflects an understanding of the principles and standards of ethical decision making, as well as philosophical approaches to ethical decision making. Requires a systematic framework for addressing the complex and often controversial moral questions.

Ethical dilemma A difficult choice or issue that requires the application of standards or principles to solve. Issues that challenge us ethically.

Ethical, social, and legal implications (ESLI) Consideration and understanding of the ethical, social or legal connections or aspects of an issue that relates to a moral question of right and wrong.

Ethicist Expert in the arbitrary, ambiguous, and ungrounded judgments of other people. Ethicists know that they make the best decision they can based on the situation and stakeholders at hand.

Ethics A process of systematically examining varying viewpoints related to moral questions of right and wrong.

Eudaemonistic A system of ethical evaluation that involves consideration of what actions lead to being an excellent and happy person.

Evidence Artifacts, productions, attestations, or other examples that demonstrate what an individual's knowledge, skills, or valued attributes are.

Evidence-based practice (EBP) Nursing practice that is informed by research generated evidence of best practices.

Exabyte (EB) One quintillion bytes of computer memory.

Execute To carry out software's or a program's instructions.

Expert system A type of decision support system that implements the knowledge of one or more human experts.

Extensibility System design feature that allows for future expansion without the need for changes to the basic infrastructure.

Extensible markup language (XML) Computer language that began as a simplified subset of standard generalized markup language (SGML). Its major purpose is to facilitate the exchange of structured data across different information systems, especially via the Internet. It is considered an extensible language since it permits its users to define their own elements allowing customization to enable purpose-specific development.

Face-to-face Most widely used teaching method among nurse educators where teacher and learners meet together in one location at the same time.

Fair use Doctrine that permits the limited use of original works without copyright holder's permission; an example would be quoting or citing an author in a scholarly manuscript.

Federal Health Information Exchange (FHIE) A federal information technology (IT) healthcare initiative that enables the secure electronic one-way exchange of patient medical information from the Department of Defense's legacy health information system, the Composite Health Care System (CHCS), for all separated service members to Veterans Affairs' (VA) VistA Computerized Patient Record System (CPRS). The point of care in veterans affairs.

Feedback Input in the form of opinions about or reactions to something such as shared knowledge. In an information system, feedback refers to information from the system that is used to make modifications in the input, processing actions, or outputs.

Fidelity Right to what has been promised.

Field Column or attribute of an entity in a database.

Field study Study in which end users evaluate a prototype in the actual work setting prior to its general release. Also called field test, alpha test, or beta test.

Financial system System used to manage the expenses and revenue for providing health care. The finance, auditing, and accounting departments within an organization most commonly use financial systems. These systems determine the direction for maintenance and growth for a given facility. Financial systems often interface to share information with materials management, staffing, and billing systems to balance the financial impact of these resources within an organization. These systems report the fiscal outcomes in order to track them against the organizational goals of an institution. Financial systems are one of the major decision-making factors as healthcare institutions prepare their fiscal budgets. These systems often play a pivotal role in determining the strategic direction for an organization.

Firewall A common tool used by organizations to protect their corporate networks when they are attached to the Internet. A firewall can be either hardware or software or a combination of both. A firewall examines all incoming messages or traffic to the network. The firewall can be set up to only allow messages from known senders into the corporate network. Firewalls can also be set up to look at outgoing information from the corporate network.

FireWire Apple Computer's version of a high performance serial bus used to connect devices to a computer.

Firmware Hardware and software programs or data written onto ROM, PROM, and EPROM.

Flash drive Small, removable storage device.

Flash memory Special type of EEPROM that can be erased and reprogrammed in blocks instead of one byte at a time. Many modern PCs have their BIOS stored on a flash memory chip so that it can easily be updated if necessary.

Folksonomies Organization and classification of online content by users; derived from folk and taxonomy. Users tag information with key words to make it easier to index and search vast amounts of information.

Foundation of Knowledge model Model that proposes that humans are organic information systems constantly acquiring, processing, and generating information or knowledge in both their professional and personal lives. The organizing framework of this text.

Futurologist Guru who is a forward thinker and looks to the future.

Genomics The extensive study of the genetic make-up of an organism, especially the sequencing, mapping and interactions of the individual components of the gene.

Gigabyte (GB) Unit of measure used to express bytes of data storage and capability in computer systems; 1 gigabyte equals 1,000 megabytes.

Gigahertz (GHz) Unit of measure used to express speed and power of some components such as the microprocessor; 1 gigahertz or GHz is equal to 1,000 megahertz.

Good Favorable outcome in ethics.

Gramm-Leach-Bliley Act (GLBA) Federal legislation in the United States to control how financial institutions handle the private information they collect from individuals.

Graphical user interface (GUI) Software that provides a user-friendly desktop metaphor interface that is made up of the input and output devices as well as icons that represent files, programs, actions, and processes.

Graphics card A board that plugs into a personal computer to give it display capabilities.

Grey gap A term used to reflect the age disparities in computer connectivity; there are fewer persons over age 65 who use computer technology than those in younger age groups.

Gulf of evaluation The gap between knowing one's intention (goal) and knowing the effects of one's actions.

Gulf of execution The gap between knowing what one wants to have happen (the goal) and knowing what to do to bring it about (the means to achieve the goal).

Hacker Computer savvy individual most commonly thought of as a malicious person who hacks or breaks through security to steal or alter data and information, but it can also be computer aficionados who band together in clubs and organizations or who use their skills as a hobby.

Half-life of knowledge The time span from when knowledge is gained to when it becomes obsolete.

Hard disk Magnetic disk that stores electronic data.

Hard drive Permanent data storage area that holds the data, information, documents, and programs saved on the computer, even when the computer is shut off. The actual physical body of the computer and its components.

Hardware Physical or tangible parts of the computer. Computer parts that one can touch and that are involved in the performance or function of the computer, such as the keyboard and monitor.

Harm Physical or mental injury or damage. Unfavorable outcome in ethics.

Health information exchange (HIE) Organization that prepares and organizes people and resources to manage healthcare information electronically across organizations within a community or region.

Health Information Portability and Accountability Act (HIPAA) Law signed by President Bill Clinton in 1996 addressing the need for standards to regulate and safeguard health information and making provisions for health insurance coverage for employed persons who change jobs.

Health Level 7 (HL7) An accredited standards-developing organization that is committed to developing standard terminologies for information technology that support interoperability of healthcare information management systems.

Health literacy The acquisition of knowledge that promotes the ability to understand and to manage one's health.

HealthVault Microsoft's online personal health record system.

Heuristic evaluation An evaluation in which a small number of evaluators (often experts in relevant fields such as human factors or cognitive engineering) evaluate the degree to which the interface design complies with recognized usability principles (the "heuristics").

High-fidelity A high level of realism generated by the equipment used in simulations.

Home health agency (HHA) Organization that delivers part-time and intermittent skilled services including nursing and other therapeutic services in the patient's home.

Home health care Alternate site for healthcare services typically focusing on posthospital discharge patient needs.

Home telehealth care Home healthcare clinical and educational services provided via telecommunications-ready tools.

HONcode One of the two most common symbols that power users look for to identify trusted health sites.

Human–computer interaction (HCI) The study of how people use computers and software applications and the ways that computers influence people.

Human–computer interface The hardware and software through which the user interacts with the computer.

Human–technology interaction (HTI) How users interact with technology. The study of that interaction.

Human–technology interface The hardware and software through which the user interacts with any technology (e.g., computers, patient monitors, telephone, etc.).

Hybrid That which defines individual courses in which instruction is delivered using multiple formats such as online, face to face, print-based, or audio or videoconference such as PicTel.

Hypertext Clickable words that allow users to access another document at a remote location.

Indiana Health Information Exchange (IHIE) Collaborative effort among institutions in Indiana to provide high quality patient care and enhance safety and efficiency.

Industrial Age Late 18th and early 19th centuries when there were major changes in manufacturing, farming, and transportation; inventions and innovations led these changes.

Informatics A specialty that integrates the specialty's science, computer science, cognitive science, and information science to manage and communicate data, information, knowledge, and wisdom in a specialty's practice.

Informatics innovator Process of making enhancements or improvements and creative, novel, and inventive solutions in the informatics specialty.

Informatics nurse (IN) A nurse with specialized skills, knowledge, and competencies in informatics. An RN with an interest or experience working in an informatics field. A generalist in the field of informatics in nursing.

Informatics nurse specialist (INS) An RN with formal, graduate education in the field of informatics or a related field and is considered a specialist in the field of nursing informatics.

Informatics solution A generic term used to describe the product an informatics nurse specialist recommends after identifying and analyzing an issue. Informatics solutions may encompass technology and nontechnology products such as information systems, new applications, nursing vocabulary, or informatics curricula.

Information Data that are interpreted, organized, or structured. Data that is processed using knowledge or data made functional through the application of knowledge.

Information Age Period at the end of the 20th century, when information was easily accessible using computers, networks, and the Internet.

Information literacy Recognizing when information is needed and having the ability to locate, evaluate, and effectively use the needed information. An intellectual framework for finding, understanding, evaluating, and using information.

Information mediator New nursing role arising out of the need for technology to support immediate access to up-to-date knowledge anywhere and anytime.

Information science The science of information, studying the application and usage of information and knowledge in organizations and the interfacings or interaction between people, organizations, and information systems. An extensive, interdisciplinary science that integrates features from cognitive science, communication science, computer science, library science, and social sciences.

Information system (IS) The manual and/or automated components of a system of users or people, recorded data, and actions used to process the data into information for a user, group of users, or an organization.

Information technology (IT) Use of hardware, software, services, and supporting infrastructure to manage and deliver information using voice, data, and video or the use of technologies from computing, electronics, and telecommunications to process and distribute information in digital and other forms. Anything related to computing technology, such as networking, hardware, software, the Internet, or the people who work with these technologies. Many hospitals have IT departments for managing the computers, networks, and other technical areas of the healthcare industry.

Information user The person who accesses and makes use of information made available to her/him.

Informatique French term that refers to the computer milieu.

Infrastructure Structural elements that provide the framework supporting a system. In the case of information technology, infrastructure refers to the architecture of the computer system, its operating system and various other systems that are fundamental to its operation.

Input Data and information entered into a computer system.

Input devices Hardware and software used to enter data and information into a computer.

Input/output system (I/O) (Pronounced "eye-oh.") The term I/O is used to describe any program, operation or device that transfers data to or from a computer and to or from a peripheral device.

Instant message (IM) Form of real-time communication between two or more people based on typed text conveyed via computers connected over a network.

Integrated drive electronics (IDE) Technology where the drive controller is located on the drive itself instead of being a separate controller connected to the motherboard.

Integrity Quality and accuracy. Employees need to have confidence that the information they are reading is in fact true. To accomplish this, organizations need clear policies to clarify how data is actually inputted, who has the authorization to change such data and to track how and when data are in fact changed.

Intelligence Mental ability to think logically, reason, prepare, ideate, assess alternative solutions to problems, problem solve by choosing a proposed solution, think abstractly, comprehend and grasp ideas, understand and use language, and learn.

Interdisciplinary knowledge team A team composed of members of various disciplines in a healthcare organization who each contribute their unique knowledge to the team in problem-solving or management situations.

Interface Mechanism or a system used by separate things to interact. For example, if one wants to change a CD in a CD player, one could use a remote; one is not related to the CD player but can interact with it using the remote control. Therefore, the remote control becomes the interface that enables that person to tell the CD player which CD to play.

International Organization for Standardization (ISO) An international network supporting collaboration among the standards developing agencies of numerous countries for the development of consistent standards in a multitude of industries to support a global economy. ISO is best known in the technology industries for the ISO 9000 standards.

Internet A worldwide system of computer networks whose connectivity promotes worldwide communications via computers.

Internet2 A nonprofit consortium which develops and deploys advanced network applications and technologies, for education and high-speed data transfer purposes. Led by 212 universities, it is also known as University Corporation for Advanced Internet Development.

Internet browser Software used to locate and display Web pages. Also known as Web browser or browser.

Intranet A computer network contained within an enterprise and which has restricted access. Has the look and feel of the Internet, often providing links to the Internet. The purpose varies, but can include employee and departmental directories, policies and procedures, internal and external resources, schedules, and updates on programs and business. The benefits are browsing capabilities and the ability to maintain contact information and phone numbers in a central location, with easy dissemination.

Intrusion detection devices Both hardware and software that allow an organization to monitor who is using the network and what files that user has accessed.

Intrusion detection system Method of security that uses both hardware and software detection devices as a system that can be set up to monitor a single computer or an entire network. Corporations must diligently monitor for unauthorized access of their networks.

Intuition A way of acquiring knowledge that cannot be obtained by inference, deduction, observation, reason, analysis, or experience.

Iowa model A model that facilitates the translation of research evidence into clinical practice. Also known as the Iowa model of evidence based practice.

iPod The name given to a family of portable MP3 players from Apple Computer.

Jump drive Small, removable storage device.

Justice Fairness. Treatment of everyone in the same way.

Key field Within each database record, one of the fields is identified as the primary key or key field. This primary key contains a code, name, number, or other bit of information that acts as a unique identifier for that record. In a healthcare system, for example, a patient is assigned a patient number or ID that is unique for that patient.

Keyboard Set of keys resembling an actual typewriter that permits the user to input data into a computer.

Know-do gap Situation that exists because solutions to global health problems exist but are not implemented in a timely fashion because of the lack of access to important health information. The Internet connections in developing countries are widely scattered and may not be efficient/sufficient for viewing healthcare information.

Knowledge The awareness and understanding of a set of information and ways that information can be made useful to support a specific task or arrive at a decision; abounds with others' thoughts and information. Information that is synthesized so that relationships are identified and formalized. Understanding that comes through a process of interaction or experience with the world around us. Information that has judgment applied to it or meaning extracted from it. Processed information that helps to clarify or explain some portion of our environment or world that we can use as a basis for action or upon which we can act. Internal process of thinking or cognition. External process of testing, senses, observation, and interacting.

Knowledge acquisition The act of acquiring or getting knowledge.

Knowledge brokers People who know where to find information and knowledge. They generate some knowledge but are mainly known for their ability to find what is needed. More experienced nurses and nursing students become knowledge brokers out of necessity—needing to know.

Knowledge builder Person who examines, interprets, and compares clinical data and trends with an eye toward improving clinical practice based on the available evidence.

Knowledge-centric Knowledge is the central focus.

Knowledge dissemination Distribution and sharing of knowledge.

Knowledge exchange The product of collaboration when sharing an understanding of information promotes learning to make better decisions in the future.

Knowledge generation Creating new knowledge by changing and evolving knowledge based on one's experience, education, and input from others.

Knowledge management system (KMS) A repository of information that contains the latest collective expertise based on experience and research. The knowledge is typically stored in a computerized system that promotes easy access for use.

Knowledge processing The activity or process of gathering or collecting, perceiving, analyzing, synthesizing, saving or storing, manipulating, conveying, and transmitting knowledge.

Knowledge repositories Collections of information made available to an organization's workers to support and inform their work.

Knowledge user Individuals or groups who benefit from valuable, viable knowledge.

Knowledge workers Those who work with information and generate information and knowledge as a product.

Lab-on-a-chip device A nanotechnology device designed to perform blood analyses.

Laboratory information system Report on blood, body fluid, and tissue samples along with biological specimens that are collected at the bedside and received in a central laboratory. These systems provide clinicians with reference ranges for tests indicating high, low, or normal values in order to make care decisions. Often the laboratory system provides result information directing clinicians toward the next course of action within a treatment regimen.

Laptop Portable battery-powered computer also known as a notebook that the user can take with him or her.

Legacy system Old computer systems or programs that are not replaced because the institution does not want to expend the resources; they can cause problems especially in interfacing with newer systems.

Liberty The independence from controlling influences.

Library science An interdisciplinary science that integrates law, applied science, and the humanities, to study issues and topics related to libraries (collection, organization, preservation, archiving, and dissemination of information resources).

Local area network (LAN) Organizationally based network; joined together locally.

Logic A system of thinking that uses principles of inference and reasoned ideas to govern action.

Long-term care facility A healthcare institution designed to support the needs of those who need ongoing care, especially the aged.

Longevity Usability beyond the immediate clinical encounter. Long-term value.

Main memory Computer's internal memory.

Mainframe Extremely high-performance computer that is smaller than supercomputer, used for high-volume, processor-intensive computing. Computers used by some large businesses and/or for scientific processing purposes.

Malicious code Software that includes spyware, viruses, worms, and Trojan horses.

Malicious insider An insider or employee who sabotages or adds malicious codes or hacks into systems to cause damage or to steal data and information.

Mask Method that a proxy server uses to protect the identity of a corporation's employees while surfing the World Wide Web. The proxy server keeps track of which employees are using which masks and directs the traffic appropriately.

Massachusetts Health Data Consortium (MHDC) A consortium of regional healthcare organizations that collects data, publishes comparative information, supports and promotes electronic standards, educates, and researches.

Medical informatics A specialty that integrates medical science, computer science, cognitive science, and information science to manage and communicate data, information, knowledge, and wisdom in medical practice.

Medication management devices Range of telecommunications-ready medication devices to remind or otherwise alert patients to medication compliance needs.

MEDLINE A database that contains more than 10 million records, maintained and produced by the National Library of Medicine.

Megabyte (MB) Unit of measure used to express the amount of data storage and capability in computer systems; 1 megabyte equals 1,000 kilobytes.

Megahertz (MHz) Unit of measure used to express the speed and power of some components such as the microprocessor.

Memory Data stored in digital format; generally refers to random access memory (RAM).

Meta-analysis A form of systematic review that uses statistical methods to combine the results of several research studies.

Microprocessor Chip that integrates the processor onto one circuit, incorporating the functions of the central processing unit (CPU) and continues to evolve processing capacity.

Mind The brain's conscious processing; encompasses thought processes, memory, imagination and creativity, emotions, perceptions, and inner drive or will.

Mobile e-health (mobile health, m-health) Health-related uses of mobile technologies including mobile phones (and increasingly, Internet-enabled, wireless-connected smartphones), personal digital assistants (PDAs), tablet computers and, sub-notebook microcomputers, remote diagnostic and monitoring devices, and Global Positioning System (GPS)/geographic information system (GIS) mapping equipment.

Model of terminology use A domain content model that is optimized for the management of particular entities within an informational and/or operational context.

Modem Hardware that allows a user to send and receive information over the phone or cable lines, for example, with a computer. It enables Internet connectivity via a telephone line or cable connection through network adaptors situated within the computer apparatus.

Monitor Computer display that allows the user to view text and graphic images.

Moral dilemma Situation for which there is no clear evidence that one of several alternatives is morally right or wrong.

Moral rights Ethical privileges.

Morals Social conventions about right and wrong human conduct that are socially constructed and tacitly agreed upon as good or right.

Motherboard A key foundational computer component. All other components are connected to it in some way (either via local sockets, attached directly to it, or connected via cables). The essential structures of the motherboard include the major chipset, super I/O chip, BIOS, read-only memory (ROM), bus communications pathways, and a variety of sockets that allow components to plug into it.

Mouse A small device that one can roll along or scroll to control the movement of the pointer or cursor on a display and click to search for and/or execute features.

MP3 aggregator A program that can facilitate the process of finding, subscribing to, and downloading podcasts. A commonly known aggregator is Apple Computer's iTunes, which is a free program available as a download from apple.com. Using a program such as iTunes gives one the ability to search for podcasts based on many criteria including category, author, or title. iTunes provides access to audio downloads, which may be either songs or podcasts.

MPEG-1 Audio Layer-3 (MP3) Digital or electronic audio programming format.

Multimedia A computer-based technology that incorporates traditional forms of communication to create a seamless and interactive learning environment.

Multispatial Relating to the need for educators in the age of technology to account for both physical and virtual spaces and their relationship to the learning process.

Nanotechnology Microscopic technology on the order of one billionth of a meter.

National Center for Public Health Informatics (NCPHI) Center created in 2005 by the Centers for Disease Control and Prevention (CDC) to provide leadership in the field of public health informatics.

National Guideline Clearinghouse (NGC) A comprehensive database of clinical practice guidelines developed as a result of research. The NGC Web site allows users to browse for the clinical guidelines, view abstracts and full-text links, download full-text clinical guidelines to personal digital assistive (PDA) devices, obtain technical reports, and compare guidelines.

National Health Information Infrastructure (NHII) An initiative set forth to improve the effectiveness, efficiency, and overall quality of health and health care in the United States. A comprehensive knowledge-based network of interoperable systems of clinical, public health, and personal health information that would improve decision making by making health information available when and where it is needed. The set of technologies, standards, applications, systems, values, and laws that support all facets of individual health, health care, and public health. The NHII is voluntary and not a centralized database of medical records or a government regulation.

Nationwide Health Information Network (NHIN) An agency of Health and Human Services charged with the development of a safe, secure, interoperable health information infrastructure.

National provider identifier (NPI) A standard 10-position unique identifier (code) mandated by HIPAA legislation and designed to replace previous provider identifiers.

Negligence A departure from the standard of due care, prudent reasonable care, toward others, including intentionally posing risks that are unreasonable as well as unintentionally, but carelessly, imposing risks.

Net generation Students used to surfing the Web and interacting online.

Network Connection of computers that can be local and/or organizationally based, joined together into a local area network (LAN), on a wider area scope (such as a city or district) using a metropolitan area network (MAN), or from an even greater distance (e.g., a whole country or continent or the Internet in general) using a wide area network (WAN) configuration.

Network security Refers to the specific precautions taken to ensure that the integrity of a network is safe from unauthorized entry and that the data and information stored on the network are only accessible by authorized users.

Neuroscience The study of the nervous system.

New England Health EDI Network (NEHEN) An example of an implementation model for building regional health information organizations that are functional, sustainable, and growing while reducing administrative costs.

Next-Generation Internet (NGI) A government project to develop new, faster technologies to enhance research and communication.

Nicomachean Vocabulary of technical terms used in a particular field, subject, science, or art. Terminology.

Nonmaleficence Doing no harm.

Nonsynchronous That which is not in real time or does not occur or exist at the same time, having the same period or time frame. Occurring anywhere and anytime using Internet and World Wide Web software tools (course management systems, e-mail, electronic bulletin boards, Web pages, etc.) as the principal delivery mechanisms.

Nursing informatics (NI) A specialty that integrates nursing science, computer science, and information science to manage and communicate data, information, knowledge, and wisdom in nursing practice.

Nursing informatics competencies A set of essential skills related to informatics deemed appropriate for various levels of nursing practice.

Nursing knowledge A body of facts accumulated over time from experience, education, and research that are used to make nursing decisions.

Nursing science The ethical application of knowledge acquired through education, research, and practice to provide services and interventions to patients in order to maintain, enhance, or restore their health; to advocate for health, and to acquire, process, generate, and disseminate nursing knowledge to advance the nursing profession.

Nursing terminology Body of the terms used in nursing. Terminology for nursing.

Nursing theory Concepts, propositions, and definitions that represent a methodical viewpoint and provide a framework for organizing and standardizing nursing actions.

Office suite Software that is generally distributed together with a consistent user interface that is designed for knowledge workers and clerical personnel. These software packages can interact with each other to enhance productivity and ease of use.

Online Something accomplished while connected to or using a computer.

Ontological approach Theory that considers ontology development (domain analysis) and its mapping to object models (specification of infrastructure). Based on enumerating all concepts used in a domain and in providing their formal definitions according to suitable formalisms (usually logic based).

Ontology Study of that which is compositional in nature and a partial representation of the entities within a domain and the relationships that hold between them. An explicit specification of a conceptualization.

Open Access Initiative A worldwide movement to make a library of knowledge available to anyone with Internet access.

Open source software (OSS) Computer software where the source code is made available for use and/or modification without charge. The developers share code in the hopes that the software will evolve as others modify and improve upon the base.

Open systems interconnection (OSI) A model of standardization for communications in a network developed to insure that various programs would work efficiently with one another.

Operating system (OS) The most important software on any computer. It is the very first program to load on computer start-up and is fundamental for the operation of all other software as well as the computer's hardware.

Order entry management A program that allows a clinician to enter medication and other care orders directly into a computer including laboratory, microbiology, pathology, radiology, nursing, medicine, supply orders, ancillary services, and consults.

Order entry system A system that automates the way that orders have traditionally been initiated for patients. Clinicians place orders within these systems instead of using traditional handwritten transcription onto paper. They provide major safeguards by ensuring that physician orders are legible and complete, thereby providing a level of patient safety that was historically missing with paper-based orders. These systems provide decision support and automated alert functionality that was previously unavailable with paper-based orders.

Outcome Changes, results, and/or impacts from inputting and processing.

Output Changes that exit a system and that can activate or modify processing.

Palmtop or palm computer Miniature or small computer that fits in the palm of the hand.

Parallel port Interface for connecting an external device that is capable of receiving more than one bit at a time.

Password A code established by the user to identify her/him when she/he enters the system. Most organizations today enforce a strong password policy. Strong password policies include using combinations of letters, numbers, and special characters such as plus (+) signs and ampersands (&). Policies typically include the enforcement of changing passwords every 30 or 60 days.

Patient care information system (PCIS) Patient-centered information systems focused on collecting data and disseminating information related to direct care. Several of these systems have become mainstream types of systems used in health care. The four systems most commonly found include (1) clinical documentation systems, (2) pharmacy information systems, (3) laboratory information systems, and (4) radiology information systems.

Patient care support system System of components that make up each of the specialty disciplines within health care and their associated patient care information systems. The four systems most commonly found include (1) clinical documentation systems, (2) pharmacy information systems, (3) laboratory information systems, and (4) radiology information systems.

Patient-centered Change from a focus on illness/healthcare professional to a focus on the patient/person with patients becoming active participants in their own healthcare initiatives. Patients as active participants receive services designed to meet their individual needs and preferences, under the guidance and counsel of their healthcare professionals. Data, observations, interventions, and outcomes focused on direct patient care.

Patient outcomes Measurable effects resulting from best practice treatment interventions that improve/stabilize the course of health over time.

Patient informed consent Document that a patient signs to agree to treatment. Document that a home healthcare patient signs to agree to receive telehealthcare services in addition to conventional home health care.

Patient support The total array of tools and software that can be used to provide information and assistance to help meet the healthcare needs of consumers.

Payor organization Those organizations that contract with healthcare agencies and service providers to attempt to manage healthcare costs.

Perception The process of acquiring knowledge about our environment or situation by obtaining, interpreting, selecting, and organizing sensory information from seeing, hearing, touching, tasting, and smelling. Sensory experience foundational to formulating knowledge.

Performance improvement Enhancing or improving performance. Quality indicators.

Performance improvement analyst Person who analyzes performance improvement initiatives. Person who is intimately involved in the design of the system used by nursing.

Peripheral biometric (medical) devices Range of telecommunications-ready measurement devices, such as blood pressure cuffs and blood glucose meters, that typically use the household telephone jack to transmit patient data to a central server location.

Peripheral component interconnection (PCI) Mechanism for attaching peripheral devices to a motherboard that can be via computer bus, expansion slots, or integrated circuits.

Peripheral devices Devices with a digital readout typically used in home telehealth and whose output is capable of being captured by computer. Generally this equipment is self-administrated by the patient or family caregiver. Examples of the most commonly used peripheral devices include: a weight scale, blood pressure monitor, pulse oximeter, thermometer, glucometer, spirometer, prothrombin/international normalized ratio (PT/INR) meter, digital camera (to capture images of wounds), and a personal digital assistant-based or telephonic self-reporting device.

Personal computer (PC) Computer made for individual use or directly used by an end user.

Personal digital assistant (PDA) A handheld device, miniature or small computer or palmtop that uses a pen for inputting instead of a keyboard. Also called a handheld computer. Also known as personal digital assistive.

Personal emergency response systems (PERS) Signaling devices for patients to access emergency and other care needs.

Petabyte (PB) A unit of information or computer storage equal to one quadrillion bytes, or 1,000 terabytes.

Pharmacy information system Information system that facilitates the ordering, managing, and dispensing of medications for a facility. It also commonly incorporates allergies and height and weight information for effective medication management; streamline the order entry, dispensing, verification, and authorization process for medication administration while they often interface with clinical documentation and order entry systems so that clinicians can order and document the administration of medications and prescriptions to patients while having the benefits of decision support alerting and interaction checking.

Picture archiving and communication system (PACS) Systems that are designed to collect, store, and distribute medical images such as computed tomography (CT) scans, magnetic resonance imaging (MRI) and X-rays; replace traditional hard copy films with digital media that is easy to store, retrieve, and present to clinicians. These systems may also be stand-alone systems, separate from the main radiology system, or they can be integrated with radiology information systems (RIS) and computer information systems (CIS). The benefit of PACS systems is their ability to assist in diagnosing and storing vital patient care support data.

Plug and play What a user can do to add new devices to a computer easily without having to manually install and reconfigure the computer to accept the device.

Podcast A digital media file or collection of related files that are distributed over the Internet using syndication or subscription feeds for playback on portable media players such as MP3 players, laptops, and personal computers. Subscribe using RSS feeds. Online media delivery. Enhanced podcasts contain slides and pictures. Vodcasts contain videos.

Population health management A term adopted by healthcare management companies to express their goal of achieving optimum health outcomes at a reasonable cost. The management process involves data collection and trend analyses that are used to predict clinical outcomes.

Port Interface between a computer and other devices or other computers.

Portability Ability to be transported easily. For example, users can easily take handheld computers wherever they go.

Portable operating system interface for UNIX (POSIX) A uniform set of standards adopted by the Institute of Electrical and Electronics Engineers (IEEE) and the International Organization for Standardization (ISO) that define an interface between programs and operating systems. The standardization ensures that software can be easily ported to other POSIX-compliant operating systems.

Portals Tools for organizing information from Web pages into simple menus on one's desktop. Also, multifunctional telehealthcare platforms for receiving, retrieving, and/or displaying patients' vital signs and other information transmitted from telecommunications-ready medical devices.

Portfolio A collection of evidence used to demonstrate knowledge and skill achievement. A nursing portfolio provides the opportunity for a student to document a variety of sometimes unquantifiable skills, such as creativity, communication, and critical thinking.

Presentation Act of presenting or showing; typically uses presentation software in a slide show format. The most commonly used presentation software in the United States is Microsoft PowerPoint.

Primary key A field within a record also known as the key field. This field contains a code, name, number, or other bit of information that acts as a unique identifier for that record. In a healthcare system, for example, a patient is assigned a patient number or ID that is unique for that patient.

Principlism A foundation for ethical decision making. Principles were expansive enough to be shared by all rational individuals, regardless of their background and individual beliefs.

Privacy An important issue related to personal information, about the owner or about other individuals, that is included for sharing with others electronically and the mechanisms that restrict access to this personal information.

Problem-based Typically refers to a type of student-centered instructional strategy where students collaboratively solve problems and reflect on their experiences.

Problem solving Cognitive process of critically thinking through a problem or issue to determine a course of action.

Processing Acting on something by taking it through established procedures in order to convert it from one form to another. Examples include: information is processed data, and we process a credit application to get a loan.

Product developer One who designs, creates, and builds a product; for example, a computer program, network, and/or system. One who employs productivity software to create a product.

Productivity software Programs or software that help us compose, create, or develop. An example is the Microsoft Office suite of productivity tools, which offers word processing, spreadsheet, database, presentation, and Web tools to help us complete our tasks both professionally and personally.

Professional development Acquisition of skills required for maintaining a specific career path or to general skills offered through continuing education, including the more general skills area of personal development. It can be seen as training to keep current with changing technology and practices in a profession or in the concept of lifelong learning.

Professional networking Connecting with other professionals in a field with a predetermined and focused purpose as well as an identified target audience in mind.

Programmable read-only memory (PROM) Form of digital memory where the setting of each bit is locked on a chip by a fuse or antifuse. Such PROMs are used to store programs permanently, and thus are useful in applications where the programming needs to be permanent. The device cannot be erased, therefore it must be replaced if changes are deemed necessary in the system.

Project manager Responsible for the success of a project by managing the planning and enactment of the project.

Protected health information (PHI) Any and all information about a person's health that is tied to any type of personal identification.

Proxy server Hardware security tool to help protect an organization against security breaches.

PSYCHINFO A comprehensive database in the field of education and psychology.

Psychology The field that studies the mind and behavior.

Public health The science of protecting the well-being of communities and the population through education, research, intervention, and prevention.

Public health informatics (PHI) An aspect of informatics focused on the promotion of health and disease prevention in populations and communities.

Public health interventions Actions taken to promote and secure the well-being of a population or a community.

Publishing The process of production and dissemination of information.

Qualitative study A type of research design that focuses on the human experience of a phenomenon using words, concepts, language, and meanings rather than numbers to capture the essence of the subject under study. Subjective study.

Quality assurance (QA) The systematic process of assessing and testing to verify that a product or service being developed or used is meeting its specified requirements; focuses on discovering and correcting defects before they become part of the final product.

Quantitative study Research that looks at the what, where, and when to provide understanding of phenomena based on quantifying data and using statistical measures; depending on the research, can ascertain cause and effect relationships. Objective study.

Query A form of questioning. A request for information; an example would be a database query.

QWERTY Name given to the typical computer keyboard layout, derived from the six letters in the first row below the numeric or number row.

Radio frequency identification (RFID) chip ID chip that stores the information for retrieval.

Radiology information system (RIS) Information system designed to schedule, report, and store information as it relates to diagnostic radiology procedures. One common feature found in most radiology systems is a picture archiving and communication system (PACS). The benefit of RIS and PACS systems is their ability to assist in diagnosing complex cases and storing vital patient care support data.

Random access memory (RAM) Volatile, temporary storage system that allows the processor to access program codes and data while working on a task. RAM is lost once the system is rebooted, shut off, or loses power.

Rapid Syndromic Validation Project (RSVP) System where local healthcare professionals report cases such as influenza. Data is analyzed centrally and the resulting information is shared with appropriate local authorities in an attempt to identify outbreaks early and prevent the spread of contagious diseases.

Rationalism An ethical position that contends that knowledge is derived from deductive reasoning and not from the senses.

RDF site summary Resource description framework site summary. See really simple syndication.

Read-only memory (ROM) Essential permanent or semipermanent, nonvolatile memory that stores saved data and is critical in the working of the computer's operating system and other activities. ROM is primarily stored in the motherboard but may also be available through the graphics card, other expansion cards, and peripherals.

Real environment data Refers to patient data collected in the home during telehealth monitoring. This data is typically more reflective of the true patient situation because it is collected in the "real" environment and not the "artificial" environment of a healthcare agency.

Real time Human time; occurs live with users or learners interacting at the same time.

Real-time telehealth Live interactions between two or more clinicians, usually performed with videoconferencing equipment.

Really simple syndication (RSS) A form of Web feed formats used to publish frequently updated content in podcasts, blog entries, or even news headlines. Subscribers receive update notices whenever new content is added or a site is updated. Also known as RDF site summary (RSS 1.0 and RSS 0.90) and rich site summary (RSS 0.91).

Reasoning Way of thinking, calculating, interpreting, or introspectively rethinking or critically thinking through an issue; reflective thought to reason or think through one's ideas and alternatives.

Record Row in a relational database representing one patient, for example. Also called a tuple. Group of related fields in a database. To record or capture audio and video using specific devices.

Reflective commentary Narrative comments that focus on why an individual thinks specific evidence is important, the ways in which he values what he has learned, or why he thinks it is important for his profession.

Regional health information exchange See Regional health information organization.

Regional health information organization (RHIO) A regional network of healthcare organizations and providers who exchange information related to the health of the population. The goal is to work together without duplication to provide cost effective health care and promote community well-being.

Relational database A collection of related records stored in a computer system using tables that can be related to one another and the data extracted in a variety of ways to gain needed information without having to reorganize the tables.

Relational database management system (RDBMS) A system that manages data using the relational model. A relational database could link a patient's table to a treatment table, for example, by a common field such as the patient ID number field.

Reporting The act of using of documents or information system outputs to convey information to stakeholders.

Reports Documents that contain data or information based on a query or investigation designed to yield customized content in relation to a situation and a user, group of users, or an organization; designed to inform, reports may include recommendations or suggestions based on programming and other embedded parameters.

Repository Central place where data are collected, stored, and maintained. Central location for multiple databases or files that can be distributed over a network or directly accessible to the user. Location for files and databases so that the data can be reused, analyzed, explored, or repurposed.

Research utilization (RU) The process of moving new understandings generated in research into practice.

Research validity A conclusion that can be drawn about the conduct of the research based on an analysis of the research design and methods (internal validity) and the applicability of the findings to the general population (external validity).

Results management An approach to evaluating the outcomes of a process to determine if the process was useful or valuable.

Reusability The extent to which software or other work-related artifacts can be used in more than one computing program or software system.

Rights Privileges; include the right to privacy, confidentiality, etc.

Risk assessment Determination of risk or danger, such as assessing for risk factors related to heart disease.

Role playing Situation that allows students to try on real-life scenarios by filling either prescripted or ad-libbed roles (doctor, nurse, patient, clinician, etc.) without the fear or pressure of putting another's life at risk while trying to determine the best course of action or find a solution to a fictitious patient's health issue.

Row A record in a database.

Sarbanes-Oxley Act (SOX) Legislation that was put in place to protect shareholders as well as the public from deceptive accounting practices in organizations.

Scenario Mock description of a situation or series of events.

Scheduling system A system designed to track resources within a facility while managing the frequency and distribution of those resources. For example, resource-scheduling systems provide information about operating room utilization, or availability of intensive care unit beds and regular nursing unit beds.

Second Life A proprietary virtual reality tool that allows users to create virtual communities.

Secure information Information that is protected from error, unauthorized access, and other threats that can compromise its integrity and safety.

Security Protection from danger or loss. In informatics, one must protect against unauthorized access, malicious damage, and incidental and accidental damage and enforce secure behavior and maintain security of computing, data, applications, information, and networks.

Security breach Any security violation.

Self-control Self-discipline. Strength of will.

Sensor and activity monitoring systems Systems for tracking activities of daily living of seniors and other at-risk individuals in their places of residence. Additional applications are sensors' use in detecting anomalies or problems such as faucets and stoves left turned on.

Serial port An interface for connecting an external device that is capable of receiving only one bit at a time, such as a mouse, a modem, and some printers.

Shoulder surfing Watching over someone's back as she is working. This is still a major way that confidentiality is compromised.

Simulation That which mimics reality, a real situation, or process by representing that reality's key characteristics or behaviors. Generally, a computer-generated imitation of an authentic or real situation that can be used for educational purposes. In nursing, simulation mannequins resembling human beings are common.

Situational awareness The ability to detect, integrate, and understand critical information that leads to an overall understanding of a problem or situation.

Small computer system interface (SCSI) Set of standards for physically connecting and transferring data between computers and peripheral devices. The SCSI standards define commands, protocols, and electrical and optical interfaces. Standardization among commercial products help to ensure that devices will interface with many different systems.

Smartphone A cell phone that has limited personal digital assistant capabilities. Smartphones have limited personal computer functionality; they have an operating system and facilitate the use of e-mail and other applications.

Social bookmarking Saving bookmarks or Internet URLs to a public Web site instead of on the user's private computer. The purpose is to share and grow the list of Web sites related to a specific topic. As users add bookmarks they also typically add keyword tags that aid in search and organization processes.

Social engineering The manipulation of a relationship based on one's position in an organization. For example, someone attempting to access a network may pretend to be an employee from the corporate information technology office who then simply asks for an employee's digital ID and password. A second example of social engineering is a hacker impersonating a federal government agent. After talking an employee into revealing network information, the hacker basically has an open door to enter the corporate network.

Social networking Subscribing to and utilizing Web-based applications for the purpose of sharing personal information with others.

Social sciences Collection of academic/scientific fields or disciplines concerned with the study of the human aspects of our world/environment.

Software Anything that can be stored electronically; it is divided into two types—system (software that includes the operating system and other software necessary for the computer to function) and application (software that allows users to complete specific tasks, e.g., word processors, spreadsheet software, presentation software, database managers, and media players).

Sound card A computer expansion card that facilitates the input and output of audio signals to/from a computer under control of computer programs. Also known as an audio card.

Spreadsheet Text and numbers located in cells on a grid and the software necessary to process formulas and other computations such as creating graphs and charts.

Spyware A program that may contain malicious code that may attack or attempt to "take over" a computer. Spyware may also be nonmalicious in intent and monitor the user's behavior in an attempt to gain information about the user for targeted advertising.

Staff development The process of providing opportunities for professional growth and skills development. Computer information systems are frequently used to assist with the ongoing education and development of nursing staff members since the medium can embed the prompts, information, and related questions in the nursing documentation system with a link to an appropriate clinical protocol.

Stakeholder An individual or group with the responsibility for completing a project, influencing the overall design, and is most impacted by success or failure of the system implementation.

Standard Benchmark. Criterion. Rule. Norm. Principle.

Standard generalized markup language (SGML) Metalanguage, markup language for documents. Extensible markup language (XML) began as a simplified subset of SGML.

Standardized nursing terminology A body of terms used in nursing that is in some ways approved by an appropriate authority or by general consent.

Standardized plan of care That which presents clinicians with treatment protocols to maximize their outcomes and support best practices.

Standards developing organization (SDO) Guidelines, standards, and rules to help healthcare entities collect, store, manipulate, dispose of, and exchange secure protected health information. Many SDOs are working to help develop standards. HIPAA guarantees the security and privacy of health information and curtails healthcare fraud and abuse while enforcing standards for health information.

Static medium Something that cannot be updated; for example, a print-based brochure may be outdated almost as soon as it is printed.

Store-and-forward telehealth transmission Application of telehealth care, in which images and other clinical data are captured and transmitted to specialist clinicians.

Suicide Prevention Community Assessment Tool Risk assessment method that addresses general community information, prevention networks, and the demographics of the target population as well as community assets and risk factors.

Summaries Condensed versions of the original designed to highlight the major points.

Supercomputer Fastest computer; designed to run special applications that require numerous calculations.

Surveillance The act of watching for trends in health-related data for early detection of health threats.

Surveillance data systems A networked computer system designed to use health-related data trends to predict the probability of an outbreak of a contagious or infectious disease, or to detect morbidity and mortality trends in a geographic area as a precursor to public health planning or response.

Synchronous Real time or occurring at the same time, having the same period or time frame. Learning anywhere and anytime in real time using any real time delivery modalities such as traditional face-to-face, Internet, and World Wide Web software tools (course management systems, chat, e-mail, electronic bulletin boards, audio-video communication tools, etc.).

Synchronous dynamic random access memory (SDRAM) Most common type of dynamic random access memory found in personal computers.

Syndromic surveillance A specialized system of data collection to detect trends in the incidence and severity of a specific disease or health-related syndrome and plan the public health response.

Synthesis Combining parts of existing material or ideas into a new entity or concept.

Table A collection of related records in a database.

Tags/tag clouds A collection of keywords (tags) that describe the contents of Web sites related to a topic of interest that are then organized by importance using differing colors and font sizes and styles (cloud). Many tag clouds are navigable; that is, the tags are hyperlinks to Web pages.

Task analysis Analytic technique that focuses on how a task must be accomplished, including detailed descriptions of task-related activities, task characteristics and complexity, and the environmental conditions required for a person to perform a given task.

Technologist Person skilled in the use of technology.

Technology Method by which people use knowledge and tools. Knowledge used to solve problems, control and adapt to our environment, and extend human potential. Generally people use technology to refer to machines or devices such as computers and the infrastructure that supports them. A simplistic example, examining cell phones and planes—they are technologies that are tangible—one can see and touch them but cannot see and touch the vast infrastructures supporting them such as the wireless communications between the device (cell phone) and the cell towers nor can one see and touch the electronic guidance used by the device (plane) to navigate the skies.

Telecommunications Broadcasting or transmitting signals over a distance from one person to another person or from one location to another location for the purpose of communication.

Telehealth Telecommunication technologies used to deliver health-related services or to connect patients and healthcare providers to maximize patients' health status. A relatively new term in our medical/nursing vocabulary, referring to a wide range of health services that are delivered by telecommunications-ready tools such as the telephone, videophone, and computer.

Telehealth care Health services delivered by telecommunications-ready tools, usually supervised by a nurse or other clinician.

Telehealth hardware Equipment that captures objective vital signs data. Some systems use interactive self-reporting devices to capture subjective information on how a patient feels as well. The values obtained from the patient are then collected and transmitted by a communication hub. Peripheral devices used in home telehealth can include any item with a digital readout. Generally this equipment is self-administrated by the patient or family caregiver.

Telehealth software Computer programs designed to collect and interpret health data gathered remotely via a telehealth communications system.

Telemedicine Health services delivered by telecommunications-ready tools supervised or directed by a physician.

Telemonitoring Remote measurement of patients' vital signs and other necessary data.

Telenursing Health services delivered by telecommunications-ready tools supervised or directed by a nurse.

Telepathology Use of telecommunications technology to facilitate the transmission and transfer of pathology data for the purposes of diagnosis, education, and research. Transmission and exchange of image-rich pathology data between remote locations.

Telephony Telephone monitoring of patients at their residences by off-site telenurses.

Teleradiology Use of telecommunications technology to electronically transmit and exchange radiographic patient images with the consultative text or radiologist reports from one location to another.

Terabyte (TB) A measurement term for data storage capacity. The value of a terabyte is 1,024 gigabytes.

Term At its simplest level, a word or phrase used to describe something concrete, e.g., leg, or abstract, e.g., plan.

Terminology Vocabulary of technical terms used in a particular field, subject, science, or art; concerned with the collection, description, processing, and presentation of terms belonging to specialized areas of usage of one or more languages; nomenclature.

Thick or fat client A computer connected to a network designed primarily for data processing and not communications or storage.

Thin client A computer that conveys input and output from the user to the server and back, but does no processing.

Throughput The amount of work a computer can do in a given time period; a measure of computer performance that can be used for system comparison.

Thumb drive Small removable storage device.

TIGER initiative Group called the Technology Informatics Guiding Education Reform—or TIGER—team. This is a team of nursing leaders who developed a vision for utilizing information technology to transform nursing practice.

Touch screen The display used as an input device for interacting with or relating to the display's materials or content. The user can touch or press on the designated display area to respond, execute, or request information or output.

Transistor Solid-state semiconductors that resulted in the second generation of computers. Digital devices much smaller and faster than analog computers.

Translational research Research that is conducted with a vision toward transforming clinical nursing practice (translating into practice).

Transparent Done without conscious thought.

Transparent technology Technology that is not visible or recognizable by the user, therefore allowing the user to focus on the function or output and not the challenges of the technology itself.

Transput Input and output activities collectively.

Trend General movement—a line of development. Process of getting others to emulate one's actions.

Trending Process of collecting and analyzing patient data that is collected over time via telehealth technology. Trending analysis provides a more accurate picture of health status than the analysis of episodic data collected during an agency visit.

Triage Process of assessing patients who are ill or injured and determining the need for intervention based on the severity of the health issue. Some software programs used in telehealth monitoring systems provide this function by comparing actual data with a preset standard and then alerting clinicians that an intervention is necessary.

Trojan horse Malicious code capable of replicating within a computer that is hidden in data or a program that appears to be safe.

Trust-e One of the two most common symbols that power users look for to identify trusted health sites.

Truth Fact. Certainty. Sincere action, character, and fidelity.

Tutorial Learning materials available to the learner, who must then be self-directed to study the specific topical area presented.

Ubiquitous Existing or being everywhere at the same time; widespread.

Ubiquitous health (u-health) The concept of health care that is so present in one's daily life that it seems invisible or in the background.

Ubiquity State of being everywhere at once (or seeming to be everywhere at once). Presence in many places especially simultaneously. With changing models of healthcare delivery, information and knowledge should be available anywhere.

Uncertainty Ambiguity. Insecurity. Vagueness.

Universal serial bus (USB) That which connects to a myriad of plug-in devices, such as portable Flash drives, digital cameras, MP3 players, graphics tablets, light pens, and so on using a plug and play connection without rebooting the computer.

Usability The ease with which people can use an interface to achieve a particular goal. Issues of human performance during computer interactions for specific tasks within a particular context.

User friendly Programs and peripherals that make it easy to interact or use computers. Design of a program to enhance the ease with which the user can utilize and maximize the productivity from computer programs.

User interface Mechanisms or systems used by users to interact with programs.

Values Relative worth of an object or action such as aesthetic beauty or ethical value.

Veracity Right to truth.

Video adapter card A board or card that is inserted or plugged into a computer to provide display capabilities.

Videopod Self-contained system with a video transmitter.

Virtual memory The use of hard disk space temporarily when the user is running many programs simultaneously. This temporary use frees up RAM to allow programs to run simultaneously and seamlessly.

Virtual peers Virtual populations of individuals who are genetically and behaviorally alike.

Virtual reality (VR) Technology that simulates reality in a virtual medium.

Virtual world World that exists in cyberspace where people can establish avatars, purchase land, and interact with others. Emerging virtual worlds such as Second Life are changing the meaning of social networking.

Virtue Certain ideals toward which we should strive that provide for the full development of our humanity. Attitudes or character traits that enable us to be and to act in ways that develop our highest potential; examples are honesty, courage, compassion, generosity, fidelity, integrity, fairness, self-control, and prudence. Like habits, they become a characteristic of a person. The virtuous person is the ethical person.

Virtue ethics Theory that suggests that individuals use power to bring about human benefit. One must consider the needs of others and the responsibility to meet those needs.

Virus Malicious code that attaches to an existing program and executes its harmful script when opened.

Visiting Nurse Association (VNA) A nonprofit home healthcare agency.

Voice recognition A type of software that allows the user to input data or to navigate the Web using voice commands. Voice interactivity should help to reduce the disparity associated with those who have limited keyboard or mousing skills.

Wearable computing Devices that one can don or put on as one would other articles of clothing or watches, jewelry, etc. Wearable devices are being used to provide remote monitoring of physiological parameters in care settings, including patients' own homes.

Web 2.0 Developing tools for social networking. The implications of the social networking technologies that are major elements of Web 2.0 will have significant impact on the amount of information and knowledge that is generated, and the ways in which it is used.

Web-based Originating from the World Wide Web.

Web enhanced That which uses the World Wide Web to enhance or promote functions or tasks such as effective learning and skill acquisition.

Web publishing The design and development of Web pages that include links to digital files that are all uploaded to Web servers so that these files are accessible to others via Web browsers.

Web quest A search of the World Wide Web for information.

Web servers Multifunctional telehealthcare platforms for receiving, retrieving, and/or displaying patients' vital signs and other information transmitted from telecommunications-ready medical devices.

Webcast Media distributed over the Internet as a broadcast; uses streaming media technology to facilitate downloading and participation. It could be distributed in real time, live, or recorded for asynchronous interaction.

Weblog A Web site that contains the contributions of single or multiple users about a particular topic or issue. Similar in nature to a threaded discussion board or a personal diary, weblogs or blogs can provide insight into the perceptions of the contributors about the topic.

Wi-Fi Wireless technology brand owned by Wi-Fi Alliance, which is used to improve the interoperability of wireless networking devices.

Wiki Server software that allows users to create, edit, and link Web page content from any Web browser. Server software that supports hyperlinks. The simplest online database; used to develop collaborative Web sites.

Wisdom Knowledge applied in a practical way or translated into actions; uses knowledge and experience to heighten common sense and insight to exercise sound judgment in practical matters. Sometimes thought of as the highest form of common sense resulting from accumulated knowledge or erudition (deep, thorough learning) or enlightenment (education that results in understanding and the dissemination of knowledge). It is the ability to apply valuable and viable knowledge, experience, understanding, and insight while being prudent and sensible. It is focused on our own minds; the synthesis of our experience, insight, understanding, and knowledge. The appropriate use of knowledge to solve human problems. It is knowing when and how to apply knowledge.

Word processing Creating documents using a word processing software package such as Microsoft Word.

Workaround A way invented by users to bypass the system to accomplish a task. Usually indicate a poor fit of the system or technology to the workflow or user. Devised ways to beat a system that does not function appropriately or is not suited to the task it was developed to assist with; for example, one might remove the armband from the patient and attach it to the bed if the bar code reader fails to interpret bar codes when the bracelet curves tightly around a small arm.

World Wide Web (WWW) An international network of computers and servers that offers access to stored documents written in HTML code, and access to graphics, audio, and video files.

Worm A form of malicious code. A self-replicating computer program that uses a network to send multiple copies of itself to other computers, subsequently tying up bandwidth and incapacitating networks.

Yottabyte (YB) A unit of information or computer storage equal to one septillion bytes.

Youth Risk Behavior Surveillance System (YRBSS) An epidemiologic survey conducted by the CDC to identify and track the most common health risk behaviors that lead to illnesses and mortality among youth.

Zettabyte (ZB) A unit of information or computer storage equal to one sextillion bytes.

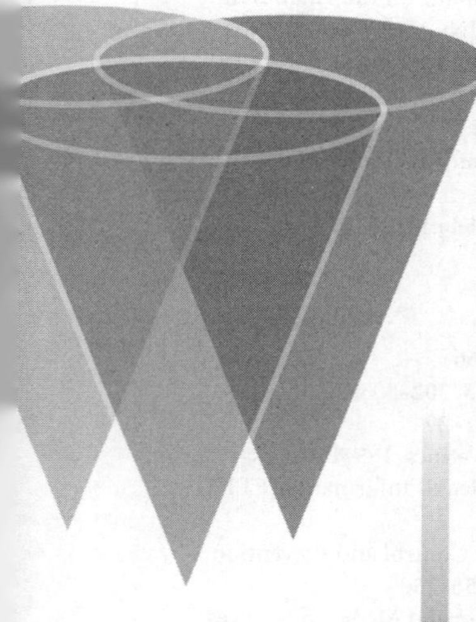

Index

A